Language and HIV/AIDS

CRITICAL LANGUAGE AND LITERACY STUDIES
Series Editors: Vaidehi Ramanathan, *University of California, USA*; Bonny Norton, *University of British Columbia, Canada* and Alastair Pennycook, *University of Technology, Sydney, Australia*

Critical Language and Literacy Studies is an international series that encourages monographs directly addressing issues of power (its flows, inequities, distributions and trajectories) in a variety of language- and literacy-related realms. The aim with this series is twofold: (1) to cultivate scholarship that openly engages with social, political and historical dimensions in language and literacy studies, and (2) to widen disciplinary horizons by encouraging new work on topics that have received little focus and that use innovative theoretical frameworks.

Full details of all the books in this series and of all our other publications can be found on http://www.multilingual-matters.com, or by writing to Multilingual Matters, St Nicholas House, 31-34 High Street, Bristol, BS1 2AW, UK.

Other books in the series:
Collaborative Research in Multilingual Classrooms
Corey Denos, Kelleen Toohey, Kathy Neilson and Bonnie Waterstone
English as a Local Language: Post-colonial Identities and Multilingual Practices
Christina Higgins
The Idea of English in Japan: Ideology and the Evolution of a Global Language
Philip Seargeant

CRITICAL LANGUAGE AND LITERACY STUDIES
Series Editors: Vaidehi Ramanathan, Bonny Norton and Alastair Pennycook

Language and HIV/AIDS

Edited by
Christina Higgins and Bonny Norton

MULTILINGUAL MATTERS
Bristol • Buffalo • Toronto

Library of Congress Cataloging in Publication Data
A catalog record for this book is available from the Library of Congress.
Language and HIV/Aids/Edited by Christina Higgins and Bonny Norton.
Critical language and literacy studies: 5
Includes bibliographical references and index.
1. AIDS (Disease)--Prevention--Study and teaching. 2. HIV infections--Prevention--Study and teaching.
I. Higgins, Christina. II. Norton, Bonny
RA643.8.L36 2009
614.5'99392–dc22 2009033460

British Library Cataloguing in Publication Data
A catalogue entry for this book is available from the British Library.

ISBN-13: 978-1-84769-220-7 (hbk)
ISBN-13: 978-1-84769-219-1 (pbk)

Multilingual Matters
UK: St Nicholas House, 31-34 High Street, Bristol, BS1 2AW, UK.
USA: UTP, 2250 Military Road, Tonawanda, NY 14150, USA.
Canada: UTP, 5201 Dufferin Street, North York, Ontario, M3H 5T8, Canada.

The policy of Multilingual Matters/Channel View Publications is to use papers that are natural, renewable and recyclable products, made from wood grown in sustainable forests. In the manufacturing process of our books, and to further support our policy, preference is given to printers that have FSC and PEFC Chain of Custody certification.TheFSCand/orPEFClogoswillappearonthosebooks where full certificationhasbeengrantedtotheprinterconcerned.

Typeset by Techset Composition Ltd., Salisbury, UK.

Contents

Contributors

Thabisile Buthelezi is an associate professor and head of School of Education Studies, at the University of KwaZulu-Natal, South Africa. Her teaching and research interests are in the areas of language education, gender and media, HIV/AIDS in education and sexuality education, including sexualities in Africa. Her most recent book chapters are 'Dimensions of Diversity: Educating Urban Township Learners, A Case of Umlazi Township School in Durban, SA', which appeared in the *International Handbook of Urban Education* edited by W. Pink and G. Noblit, and 'Providing Leadership for Managing HIV and AIDS in Schools', which appeared in *Developing Consciously Competent HIV/AIDS Educators in the African Context* by L. Woods. Email: Buthelezit10@nu.ac.za

Ángeles Clemente has been working for more than 20 years at the Facultad de Idiomas at the Universidad Autónoma 'Benito Juárez' de Oaxaca in the city of Oaxaca, Mexico. Her areas of research and teaching are in applied linguistics and second language acquisition. Her research focus has moved from a socio-cognitive approach in learning towards a socio-cultural focus on activities of learning English as an additional language. This shift in her research interests can be noted in her current book (co-authored by M. Higgins) *Performing English with a Post-Colonial Accent: Ethnographic Narratives from Mexico* (2008). Email: angelesclemente@gmail.com

Naydene de Lange is professor and holds the newly established HIV/AIDS Research Chair in the Faculty of Education at Nelson Mandela University Port Elizabeth, South Africa. Her research focuses on HIV/AIDS using visual participatory methodologies. She has headed the editing of a book, *Putting People in the Picture: Visual Methodologies for Social Change*, as well as co-authored a book, *Picturing Hope*. She publishes in international and national journals, and heads up and collaborates in various funded research projects. She is also co-director of the Centre for

Visual Methodologies for Social Change at UKZN and an NRF-rated researcher. Email: Delangen@nu.ac.za

Martina Drescher is a full professor of General Linguistics and Linguistics of Romance Languages at the University of Bayreuth (Germany). She has also taught at the Université Laval (Québec/Canada) and at the University of Ouagadougou (Burkina Faso). Her recently published books concern health communication in sub-Saharan Africa (*Kommunikation über HIV/ AIDS. Interdisziplinäre Beiträge zur Prävention im subsaharischen Afrika* co-edited with Sabine Klaeger, 2006), discourse markers (*Les marqueurs discursifs dans les langues romanes* co-edited with Barbara Frank-Job, 2006), language and emotions (*Sprachliche Affektivität*, 2003) and genres (*Textsorten im romanischen Sprachvergleich*, 2002). Her research interests include interactional linguistics, discourse analysis and sociolinguistics, with a particular emphasis on Canadian and African varieties of French. Email: martina. drescher@uni-bayreuth.de

Mark Finn is a senior lecturer in psychology at the University of East London. Since completing his PhD at the Centre for Critical Psychology (University of Western Sydney), he has held two research posts at Cardiff University in the Health Communication Research Centre (with Srikant Sarangi) and the School of Social Sciences. With a predominant research interest in the discursive productions and regulations of non/normative intimate relationships, he has also conducted published research into fatherhood and masculinity, health-related quality of life and transgenderism. Mark's current research is to do with the therapeutic engagement with practices of open non-monogamy. Email: m.finn@uel.ac.uk

Sarah Flicker is engaged in an exciting and innovative program of research that focuses on teen HIV prevention and support. More broadly, she is interested in community-based participatory methodologies and is active on a variety of research teams that focus on adolescent sexual health with youth in Canada and most recently in South Africa. Dr Flicker works across methodologies (qualitative, quantitative and arts-based) and seeks to partner with youth, students and allied practitioners on action research agendas. Currently, she is an assistant professor in the Faculty of Environmental Studies at York University and an Ontario HIV Treatment Network Scholar. Email: flicker@yorku.ca

Christina Higgins is an assistant professor in the Department of Second Language Studies at the University of Hawai'i at Manoa, where she teaches courses in sociolinguistics, discourse analysis and intercultural communication. Her recent research has focused on communication in

NGO-sponsored HIV/AIDS prevention and awareness education in Tanzania, where she has investigated the discursive construction of local and global worldviews. In her book *English As a Local Language: Post-Colonial Identities and Multilingual Practices* (Multilingual Matters), she has also explored the role of language and popular culture in awareness efforts in hip-hop lyrics about HIV/AIDS and in public health advertisements. Email: cmhiggin@hawaii.edu

Michael James Higgins is an anthropologist from the United States who has been conducting urban ethnographic research in the city of Oaxaca for more than 40 years. He is a professor emeritus of anthropology from the University of Northern Colorado in Greeley, Colorado. His research has focused on issues of gender, sexuality, ethnicity and social class dynamics among the urban poor and working class of the city of Oaxaca. Currently he is involved in collaborative ethnographic research with Ángeles Clemente on language, culture and identity in Oaxaca. He has co-authored a book with Clemente, *Performing English with Post-Colonial Accent: Ethnographic Narratives from Mexico* (2008). Email address: mjhiggi55@hotmail.com

Rodney Jones is associate head of the Department of English at City University of Hong Kong. His research interests include youth cultures, computer-mediated communication, multimodal discourse analysis, discourse and sexuality, and health communication. He has published numerous academic articles, book chapters and short stories and is co-editor of *Discourse in Action: Introducing Mediated Discourse Analysis* (Routledge, 2005) and *Advances in Discourse Studies* (Routledge, 2008). Email: enrodney@cityu.edu.hk

Shelley Jones is an assistant professor in the Department of Curriculum and Instruction at the State University of New York, Potsdam. She teaches courses in literacy, social studies education, and educational research in the Master of Science in Teaching program based in Ottawa, Ontario. Her research and pedagogical interests include gender, education and international development, global education, global citizenship and multimodality. Her recent research has focused on educational challenges and opportunities for girls and women in rural Uganda. Email: jonessk@potsdam.edu

Maureen Kendrick is an associate professor in the Department of Language and Literacy Education at the University of British Columbia. Her research focuses on literacy and multimodality as social practice, literacy and international development, and digital literacies. She is author of *Converging Worlds: Play, Literacy, and Culture in Early Childhood* and co-editor of *Portraits* *of Literacy Across Home, School, and Community.* She has also written numerous journal articles and book chapters on literacy and multimodality in local and global contexts. Currently, she is researching digital literacy practices in secondary English language classrooms involving Canadian immigrant and refugee students and Ugandan students. Email: maureen. kendrick@ubc.ca

Noushin Khushrushahi received her Master of Arts in Asia-Pacific Policy Studies from the University of British Columbia, Canada, where she focused on gender and human rights policy. Her research and policy interests include HIV/AIDS prevention and management policy, anti-human trafficking policy and human rights. Email: noushink@gmail.com

Henrike Körner is a senior research fellow in the National Centre in HIV Social Research at the University of New South Wales in Sydney, Australia. She has worked in English language and literacy education and has a background in systemic functional linguistics. Her research focuses on gay men's discourses of 'risk' in the context of HIV infection, doctor/patient interactions, HIV/AIDS as it affects people from culturally and linguistically diverse backgrounds, representation of HIV and hepatitis C-related issues in the medical and popular media. Her most recent work is concerned with general practitioners diagnosing depression in gay men, and discourses of depression. Email: h.korner@unsw.edu.au

June Larkin is vice principal, New College and teaches in the Women and Gender Studies and Equity Studies Programs at the University of Toronto. She is a co-coordinator of the Gendering Adolescent AIDS Prevention (GAAP) Project that brings together youth, community workers, policy makers, students and researchers in Canada and South Africa on projects that use participatory approaches to working with young people in relation to sexuality, HIV prevention and AIDS awareness. Her research is in the areas of gender, youth and HIV; adolescent sexuality; and arts-based approaches to HIV education with youth. Email: june@utgaap.org

Claudia Mitchell is a James McGill professor in the Faculty of Education, McGill University, and an honorary professor, University of KwaZulu-Natal. Her research focuses on the use of visual and other participatory methodologies such as photo-voice, community video, particularly in addressing gender and HIV and AIDS, teacher identity and the culture of girlhood within broader studies of children and popular culture and media studies. She is the co-author/co-editor of a number of books, including *Teaching and HIV&AIDS in the South African Classroom* (with K. Pithouse)

Contributors xi

and *Putting People in the Picture: Visual Methodologies for Social Change* (with N. DeLange and J. Stuart). She is a co-founding editor of *Girlhood Studies: An Interdisciplinary Journal* (with J. Reid-Walsh and J. Kirk). Email: claudia.mitchell@mcgill.ca

Relebohile Moletsane is director of the Gender and Development Unit at the Human Sciences Research Council (HSRC), South Africa. She has extensive experience in teaching and research in the areas of curriculum studies and gender and education, including gender-based violence and its links to HIV and AIDS and AIDS-related stigma, body politics, as well as on girlhood in the era of AIDS in Southern African contexts. She is co-author (with Claudia Mitchell, Ann Smith and Linda Chisholm) of the book *Methodologies for Mapping a Southern African Girlhood in the Age of Aids* (Rotterdam/New York/Taipei: Sense Publishers). She holds an honorary Associate Professorship in the Faculty of Education at the University of KwaZulu-Natal, Durban South Africa. Email: rmoletsane@hsrc.ac.za

Annabelle Mooney is a senior lecturer in sociolinguistics at Roehampton University. She works in the fields of language and religion, globalization, law and gender. She is currently working on the language of human rights, considering legal, linguistic and semiotic approaches. Recent publications include 'Boys will be boys: men's magazines and the normalisation of pornography' (*Feminist Media Studies*) and 'Death Alive and Kicking: Dianne Pretty, legal violence and the sacred' (*Social Semiotics*), which addresses the issue of voluntary euthanasia in relation to the implicitly religious foundations of contemporary legal human rights. Email: a.mooney@roehampton.ac.uk

Harriet Mutonyi is a lecturer in the Faculty of Education, and coordinator of the Teaching and Learning in Higher Education program at Uganda Martyrs University. Her recent research work has focused on issues of health literacy, HIV/AIDS, gender and the role of Ugandan youth in dealing with these issues. Some of her works have been published in *Alberta Journal of Educational Research, Compare Journal of Comparative Education* and *Diasporic, Indigenous, and Minority Education* (DIME). Email: mutonyi@umu.ac.ug or hmutonyi@yahoo.com

Bonny Norton is a professor and distinguished university scholar in the Department of Language and Literacy Education, University of British Columbia, Canada. Her award-winning research addresses identity and language learning, education and international development, and critical literacy. Her current research investigates the use of innovative technology in east Africa. Recent publications include *Identity and Language Learning* (Longman/Pearson, 2000), *Critical Pedagogies and Language Learning* (Cambridge University Press, 2004, with K. Toohey) and *Gender and English Language Learners* (TESOL, 2004, with A. Pavlenko). Her website can be found at http://lerc.educ.ubc.ca/fac/norton/

Srikant Sarangi is a professor of language and communication and Director of the Health Communication Research Centre at Cardiff University. He is also a professor in language and communication at Norwegian University of Science and Technology, Trondheim (2009–2011). His research interests are in applied linguistics and institutional/professional discourse studies (e.g. health care, social welfare, bureaucracy, education, etc.). He is author and editor of ten books, guest editor of five journal special issues and has published over 150 journal articles and book chapters. He is the editor of *Text & Talk* as well as the founding editor of *Communication & Medicine* and (with C.N. Candlin) of *Journal of Applied Linguistics* and three book series. Email: sarangi@cardiff.ac.uk

William Savage works globally as an organizational and community development facilitator with international and local non-governmental, inter-governmental, international and government agencies. His recent areas of experience are HIV and AIDS, maternal health and child rights. William is the co-editor of Longman's 1997 *Language and Development: Teachers in a Changing World*. Having lived most of his life in the Marshall Islands, Hawai'i, Saudi Arabia, Thailand and Cambodia, in 2008 he moved home to Louisiana. William is a practitioner and certified teacher of Kundalini Yoga and has taught in Southeast Asia, California and the southern USA. Email: williamsava@gmail.com

Jean Stuart is a lecturer in media, and director of the Centre for Visual Methodologies for Social Change, in the Faculty of Education at the University of KwaZulu-Natal, South Africa. She has recently completed a PhD that explores, with preservice teachers, ways of working with visual arts-based approaches for addressing HIV and AIDS. Her research interests include using participatory and arts-based approaches that position participants as cultural producers to address socio-cultural aspects of health issues. Email: Stuartd@ukzn.ac.za

Abbreviations

ABC   Abstain, Be faithful, use Condoms
AIDS   Acquired Immunodeficiency Syndrome
AMREF African Medical and Research Foundation
ARV/ART Antiretroviral Therapy
COESIDA *Consejo Estatal para la Prevención y Control del SIDA* (Mexico)
CONASIDA *Consejo Nacional para la Prevención y Control del SIDA* (Mexico)
CSW   Commercial Sex Workers
GAD   Gender and Development
HIV   Human Immunodeficiency Virus
LSE   Life Skills Education
MSM   Men who have Sex with Men
NACO National AIDS Control Organization (India)
NARI   National AIDS Research Institute (India)
NGO   Non-governmental Organization
PEPFAR President's Emergency Plan For AIDS Relief (USA)
PIASCY Presidential Initiative on AIDS Strategy for Communicating to Young People (Uganda)
TASO   The AIDS Support Organization (Uganda)
UNICEF United Nations Children's Fund
USAID United States Agency for International Development
VCT   Voluntary Counseling and Testing
WHO   World Health Organization
WID   Women in Development

Preface

Devoted to exploring a host of issues around HIV/AIDS in various geographic and virtual domains (Uganda, Tanzania, India, Australia, Andaman Islands, online contexts and visual arts) and through different analytic modes (discourse analysis, first-person accounts and ethnographic data), this volume probes questions around sex, sexuality and their fraught articulations. It does so primarily to call our attention to how experiences of HIV embodiment impact subjectivities, including the formation of and resistance to cultural norms. While medically oriented scholarship in applied sociolinguistics has called our attention to complex language-related concerns in medical and social work domains (Hall *et al.*, 2006; Hamilton, 1994; Makoni & de Bot, 2006; Manderson & Stirling, 2007; Sarangi & Roberts, 1998), this volume with its exclusive focus on HIV/AIDS ushers in a focus that is as yet unprecedented. A key point here is not just how death and grief loom large around this condition, but how issues of discrimination and suffering are coded in local cultural norms around patriarchy, and how AIDS patients and their caregivers move both themselves and discourses about their condition to more uplifting domains. It is this cluster of issues that this volume so evocatively probes.

As Higgins and Norton point out in their introduction, at the heart of their book is 'local knowledge'. Foregrounding the political nature and uses of local knowledge to contest prevailing views about HIV/AIDS, the various readings do not assume that the local is naturally formed, waiting for the researcher to interpret it. Instead, the focus is on how local knowledges are produced by local subjects navigating societal and cultural strictures around AIDS: condom use (Jones and Norton), keeping *rakhels* (Kushrushahi), cartoons and classes contesting biomedical explanations (Drescher, Mutonyi and Kendrick), learning about AIDS online (Jones) or switching languages to speak of sex (Clemente and Higgins). In each instance, the aim of such knowledge production is to transform our conceptualizations about 'normal', 'functioning' bodies. As the various pieces in the volume evocatively point out, the stability of notions such as 'normal bodies' is, of course, predicated on the silencing of voices that threaten the status quo or are not given a chance to be heard (Mitchell *et al.*, Finn and Sarangi, Mooney, this volume). The need, then, for such locally grounded views to emerge is all the more imperative.

This focus on local knowledges permits us to not only address the very contextually bound nature of 'knowing' – of searching for ways to address a life-threatening condition – but of how our ways of knowing are partially shaped by what is/is not viewed as 'knowledge' by domains of social study. Speaking openly about one's sexuality (Savage) or finding ways to address it online (Jones) or through the visual arts (Mitchell *et al.*) pushes at the borders of the 'impermissible'; by openly articulating the consequences of how people with AIDS negotiate human relations, institutional mandates, neo-liberal ideologies and changing conditions of their bodies, this volume presents HIV-related realities in their complexities while also underscoring how our knowledge-making emerges from our modes of inquiry.

What this brings us to, then, is unpacking the 'local' in knowledge-making. Given the volume's focus on uncovering the myriad intersecting forces around sex, sexuality and HIV, the readings prod us into thinking about the local as relational, temporally bound and contextual (rather than as scalar or spatial). One way in which it accomplishes this alternate orientation to 'local knowledge-making' is by highlighting the issue of power in cultures. By consistently moving the discussion to probing the tensions around which open articulations of HIV-related concerns are constrained, the volume makes us see how various kinds of suppressions lead to a proliferation of very local social discourses (of abstinence, patriarchy, condom use and health-related visual images) in different geographic contexts. Such a move is by no means ordinary. First, it helps us realize how the localness of AIDS (including knowledge-making regarding it) emerges only in relation to an understanding of the same in another context. In other words, the power of local knowledge-making emerges from its connections to other grounded articulations in other geographic domains. Second, it calls into question ways in which social discourses suppress rights: the right to speak openly about the condition and/or one's sexuality, to be accorded societal respect, to seek medical aid and to contest prevailing forces of marginalization. As Michelman (1996) points out, the having of rights depends on a receipt of a special sort of recognition and acceptance of one's status in a particular social community. We are not born equal; we become equal as members of a group on the strength of or decision to guarantee ourselves and each other mutually equal rights.

Certainly, each of the essays in this volume underscores both the politics of local knowledge-making about HIV/AIDS and guaranteeing patients and their caregivers rights that are often denied them (cf. Savage, Körner, Higgins, this volume). The volume successfully deracializes HIV/AIDS – a condition about which most would agree we need global awareness – while respecting very divergent geographic articulations. It jolts us not only into recognizing the social urgency of the condition and the need to speak openly of these concerns, but also into making substantive connections between conceptualizations of locality and the realities around AIDS. This book is a significant contribution to our understanding of how knowledge in HIV/AIDS education has to be considered through a focus on language, discourse and semiotics. While there may be global, medical solutions to alleviate the threat of HIV/ AIDS, the way it is understood, the way we talk about it and teach it and the way it is lived and experienced are deeply local.

Vaidehi Ramanathan, Alastair Pennycook, Bonny Norton

References

Hall, C. Slembrouck, S. and Sarangi, S. (2006) *Language Practices in Social Work: Categorization and Accountability in Child Welfare*. New York: Routledge.

Hamilton, H. (1994) *Conversations with an Alzheimer's Patient: An Interactional Sociolinguistic Study*. Cambridge: Cambridge University Press.

Makoni, S. and de Bot, K. (2006) *Language and Aging in Multilingual Settings*. Clevedon: Multilingual Matters.

Manderson, L. and Stirling, L. (2007) The absent breast: Speaking of the mastectomied body. *Feminism and Psychology* 17 (1), 75–92.

Michelman, F. (1996) Parsing "A right to have rights." *Constellations: An International Journal of Critical and Democratic Theory* 3 (2), 200–209.

Sarangi, S. and Roberts, C. (1998) *Talk, Work and Institutional Order: Discourse in Medical, Mediation, and Management Settings*. New York: Mouton de Gruyter.

Tanner, L. (2006) *Lost Bodies: Inhabiting the Borders of Life and Death*. Cornell: Cornell University Press.

Introduction

Applied Linguistics, Local Knowledge and HIV/AIDS

CHRISTINA HIGGINS and BONNY NORTON

This volume focuses on the role of language, discourse and semiotics in the construction of knowledge in HIV/AIDS education in different regions of the world, within the broader framework of applied linguistics and public health. The contributions examine the production, location and utilization of local knowledge in educational settings vis-à-vis discourses that are transmitted through official channels such as medical and health professionals, non-governmental organizations (NGOs) and international agencies. Defining HIV/AIDS education broadly, the volume examines the construction of HIV/AIDS education as a discourse within educational contexts that shapes knowledge about the disease, and the emergence of competing and cross-cultural ideologies that are co-constructed in educational settings. The central goal of the volume is to provide a collection of studies that yields helpful insights into the discursive construction of knowledge about HIV/AIDS, while demonstrating how the tools of applied linguistics can be exercised to reveal a deeper understanding of the production and dissemination of this knowledge. Our goal is to democratize the construction of knowledge about HIV/AIDS through sensitive, emic analyses that give priority to the voices of people, including youth, who are not typically sanctioned as producers of such knowledge.

The chapters use a range of qualitative methodologies to critically explore the role of language and discourse in educational contexts in which various and sometimes competing forms of knowledge about HIV/AIDS are constructed. The authors draw on discourse analysis, ethnography and social semiotics to interpret meaning-making practices in HIV/AIDS education around the world, analyzing formal and informal educational practices in Australia, Burkina Faso, Cambodia, Hong Kong, India,

South Africa, Tanzania, Thailand and Uganda. The contributors examine both the forms of knowledge that are present among communities affected by HIV/AIDS and the forms of knowledge conveyed by health experts that are meant to help prevent the spread of HIV. By exploring both sets of knowledge, the chapters explore how 'professional' discourses of sexual health and prevention interact with 'lay' discourses, and they highlight important practical concerns that result from the gaps between these two sets of knowledge. Many of the chapters demonstrate that target audiences do have an awareness of official knowledge about HIV/AIDS, but they also reveal the salience of local knowledge for these populations. The analyses offered seek to make sense of the challenges that educators, health practitioners and target populations face as a result of these co-present forms of knowledge, and to make recommendations for change.

In this Introduction, we begin by locating the volume within a broad literature on language and public health, and then turn to a consideration of research on HIV/AIDS and applied linguistics, more specifically. Next, given our interest in the intersection between local and global discourses on HIV/AIDS, we turn to a consideration of the ways in which applied linguists have addressed local knowledge across diverse research sites, and the implications this research has for investigations of HIV/AIDS. We conclude the chapter with a discussion on the organizing principle of the volume and its overall structure, with chapter summaries.

Language and Public Health

A comprehensive review of literature indicates that the relationship between language and public health is of great interest to a wide range of scholars, many of whom would not necessarily define themselves as applied linguists. Although the focus of our review is on the research that falls broadly within the applied linguistics community, it is useful to consider the research of other scholarly communities with an interest in language and public health, as a reminder that applied linguists are not working in isolation, as we attempt to grapple with a highly complex and important topic. To this end, we have made a tripartite distinction between three bodies of literature and have characterized each with reference to its proximity to the field of applied linguistics. At the most distant from applied linguistics is a body of research on language and public health that targets specific professionals such as doctors, nurses and health practitioners, and is found in journals such as *Advances in Nursing Science*, the *British Medical Journal* and the *Journal of General Internal Medicine*.

The second body of research, associated with the social sciences, has greater affinity with applied linguistics, and includes the disciplines of education, psychology, sociology and anthropology. It is published in journals such as *Adult Learning, American Psychologist, Annual Review of Sociology* and *Health Communication*, many of which are familiar to applied linguists. The third body of research falls within the broad field of applied linguistics, and is published in a wide variety of journals, including *Applied Linguistics*, the *Journal of Sociolinguistics*, the *Journal of Language and Social Psychology* and *Research on Language & Social Interaction*. Extensive research on language and public health is published in each of these three scholarly communities, and helps locate the HIV/AIDS chapters in this book within a larger framework.

In research that targets the health profession, there are a number of lines of inquiry that address the relationship between language and public health. Going back to the 1980s, health researchers such as Mishler (1984) have been intrigued by doctor–patient interaction, and have made detailed investigations of the ways in which the medical interview seeks to resolve differences between the technical–scientific standpoint of the physician, on the one hand, and the patients' location in the concerns of everyday life, on the other. To investigate this relationship, Mishler draws on extensive analysis of tape-recorded medical interviews to better understand how clinical work is undertaken. More recently, related research includes a focus on doctor–patient communication in aboriginal communities (Towle, 2006) and the needs of patients who have limited English language skills (Ngo-Metzger *et al.*, 2003; Partida, 2007; Saha & Fernandez, 2007). Whereas Partida (2007) makes the case that overcoming language barriers is essential to quality health care, Ngo-Metzger *et al.*'s (2003) research, and that of Saha and Fernandez (2007), addresses the role of interpreters in overcoming language barriers. The language practices of adolescents, as another focal group, have also attracted the attention of health researchers. Harvey *et al.* (2008) found, for example, that the use of email may be an important resource for adolescents who struggle to articulate their health challenges. A corpus linguistic analysis of a million-word adolescent health email database in the United Kingdom, drawn from a UK-hosted and doctor-led website, found that email has much potential for supplementing face-to-face encounters between adolescents and health professionals. The underlying assumption of much of this research is that a critical language and discourse study can advance medical inquiry in that it provides a framework in which the relationship between health, discourse, power and society can be examined (Boutain, 1999).

In social science research, which is more directly related to the field of applied linguistics, we learn that there is extensive research on health communication and its impact on people's health (Vahabi, 2007), with physician–patient interaction being a key theme in the literature. In their review of 30 years of research in the area of physician–patient interaction, Heritage *et al.* (2006) describe the changes in orientation to research on this topic, documenting the transition from a doctor-centered emphasis to a more contemporary focus on the social, moral and technical dilemmas that doctors and patients need to face together. The work of West (1984) has been particularly influential in this transition. With respect to the literature on HIV/AIDS, the narrative productions of HIV/AIDS patients are insightfully researched, and scholars such as Leonard and Ellen (2008) analyze the ways in which the narratives of HIV-positive patients are shaped by social and institutional practices. Eggly (2002), in fact, makes the case for an expanded definition of 'narrative' in physician–patient communication. In her view, narratives can be redefined with respect to the narrative forms that emerge through the co-construction of key events, the repetition and elaboration of key events and the co-constructed interpretation of key events.

The challenges of second language speakers who seek access to medical services are also of much interest to social science researchers. Based on a sample of 1747 patients, Kung (2004), for example, found that language, among a number of other factors, was an important consideration in mental health service use by Chinese Americans. Likewise, Evans' (2001) research found that immigrant/refugee parents in the USA who had limited English skills, had difficulty communicating with health care providers. Our review of the social science literature suggests, however, that such challenges are not restricted to migration contexts. In the African context, in which ex-colonial languages are often official languages, the development of health literacy is seen to be a particular challenge (Underwood *et al.*, 2007), particularly with reference to sexual health literacy (Jones & Norton, 2007). Drawing on their longitudinal research with Ugandan schoolgirls, Jones and Norton (2007) make the case that poverty and sexual abuse severely constrain sexual health options for many young African women, notwithstanding their knowledge of the health risks associated with unsafe sex. With regard to other health challenges in Africa, such as malaria, Kendrick and Mutonyi (2007) have argued that local modes of communication can be an important resource in promoting improved health care practices.

Although much of social science research investigates the interaction between health care providers and patients, there is also great interest in the ways in which medical practitioners consult one another in an attempt to reach a consensus on the diagnosis and treatment of patients. An important study by Atkinson (1995), for example, draws attention to the nature of the medical talk that takes place between hematologists, that is, medical practitioners who specialize in problems of the blood system, with a view to better understanding the way in which medical knowledge is produced and reproduced. As Atkinson argues, a great deal of modern medical work takes place away from the patient and the consultation, and it is important to understand the way in which talk constructs medical knowledge in a variety of clinical and laboratory settings.

Within the broad field of applied linguistics, interest in language and public health has been gaining momentum, and there are four areas of research that have received particular attention in this body of research. First, as in other disciplines, there is much applied linguistic research that is focused on the study of discourse in medical settings. Scholars such as C. Candlin and S. Candlin (2002, 2003), for example, have been particularly active in framing applied linguistics debates on health communication. Their 2002 special issue of the *Journal of Language & Social Interaction* on 'Expert talk and risk in health care' examines the expertise with which practitioners and their clients manage risk situations in genetic counseling, nursing and medical practice (Candlin, 2002; Linell *et al.*, 2002; Peräkylä, 2002; Sarangi & Clarke, 2002). Their 2003 article in the *Annual Review of Applied Linguistics* is a state-of-the-art overview of research methodologies and analytical procedures in healthcare communication. Taking nursing as a central example, the article highlights the importance of and inherent challenges in interdisciplinary collaboration among applied linguists, professional practitioners, and researchers from other fields. In a similar vein, J. Coupland *et al.* (1994) and Sarangi and Roberts (1999) draw on a range of analytic tools, including conversation analysis, to investigate the nature of discourse in medical settings, and are particularly interested in the role of talk in creating workplace practice and relationships.

Second, like most research by scholars in other disciplines, as discussed above, there is considerable research within applied linguistics on the challenges of non-native speakers in health care settings. The research by Cameron and Williams (1997) on non-native speaker–native speaker interaction in medical settings is particularly important in this regard, in that it has found that while there is great potential for cross-cultural miscommunication, communicative success can be achieved through inferencing, creative communication strategies and professional knowledge. Related to health care communication between non-native and native speakers are the challenges of interpretation and translation, an area of research taken up by scholars such as Davidson (2000). In his research on the role of interpreters in Spanish–English medical discourse, Davidson makes the case that interpreters are not 'neutral' linguistic translators, but active participants in the process of diagnosis.

Third, applied linguistics research on public health has also turned its attention to challenges associated with particular medical conditions such as Alzheimer's disease, diabetes and epilepsy. In this regard, Hamilton's (1994/2005) sociolinguistic research on Alzheimer's disease was ground-breaking for drawing on open-ended, naturally occurring conversations between the researcher and an Alzheimer's patient, over four-and-a-half years, to offer an alternative approach to psycholinguistic studies of groups of patients in clinical settings. Ramanathan's (1997, 2008) research on Alzheimer patient discourse has also been innovative, in that it investigates the ways in which memories, personal life histories and narratives inform identity constructions. Her joint research with Makoni (Ramanathan & Makoni, 2008), which addresses the biomedical experiences of people suffering from diabetes and epilepsy, argues persuasively that applied linguistics research should 'bring the body back' in more humanistic ways. Her forthcoming book *Bodies and Language* promises to be seminal in this regard (Ramanathan, 2010).

Fourth, the analysis of media and health is also receiving increasing attention. Koteyko *et al.* (2008), for example, draw on discourse analysis and corpus linguistics to examine the ways in which debates on the MRSA 'superbug' are represented in the media in the United Kingdom, and the significance of the different storylines through which discourses of blame, responsibility and urgency have been depicted. Similarly, researchers in New Zealand (Lawrence *et al.*, 2008), who have examined the way in which tuberculosis (TB) is represented in the media, make the case that media coverage often serves larger political goals and that the case-by-case analysis in the media obscures more challenging discourses, such as the relationship between TB and poverty. Such findings resonate with many themes in the research on HIV/AIDS in applied linguistics.

HIV/AIDS in Applied Linguistics

HIV/AIDS has been an object of study for sociolinguists and discourse analysts for approximately two decades. Most of this research has examined contexts relevant to gay men in resource-rich nations, and the bulk of this research has focused on stigma, risk and sexual identification in face-to-face interactions. Maynard (2003), Peräkylä (1995) and Silverman (1990, 1997) use conversation analysis to examine how the process of counseling is interactionally constructed in ways that embody assumptions about the purpose and practice of HIV tests among counselors and their clients. Leap (1995) also studies HIV counseling sessions, focusing on features of grammar and discourse that reveal clients' understandings about the pandemic and its effects on their lives. Beyond counseling contexts, Jones *et al.* (2000) study the narratives of HIV/AIDS patients in Hong Kong to explore the role of culture in disclosure in the Chinese context. Their study demonstrates the importance of methodology in the analysis of HIV/AIDS, and the larger project demonstrates how such research can be used to develop associated training materials for caseworkers to highlight the cultural facets of talking about the disease. Other discourse-based studies that analyze the sensitive areas of disclosure, stigma, and risk are Jones (2002), which examines how speakers frame their activities when handing out informative pamphlets to men they identify as gay in Hong Kong's city parks, and Jones and Candlin (2003), which explores the situatedness of risk by analyzing the stories that gay men tell of their sexual experiences.

Surprisingly, applied linguistics research on HIV/AIDS in resource-poor contexts is a much more recent development. In a review of sociolinguistic research in public health domains in sub-Saharan Africa, Djite concludes that there is a 'relative dearth of sociolinguistic studies in the area of health' (Djite, 2008: 94) despite the millions of people who are infected across this continent. While studies are indeed still relatively few in number, applied linguists have begun to turn their attention to HIV/AIDS in non-western contexts, focusing specifically on the creation of knowledge as it is constructed in language and multimodal semiotic systems (e.g. Drescher, 2007; Kendrick & Hissani, 2007; Kendrick *et al.*, 2006; Mitchell, 2006; Mitchell & Smith, 2003; Mooney & Sarangi, 2005; Norton & Mutonyi, 2007). These studies reveal the presence of differing worldviews and perspectives at the levels of institutional structures and in the form of cultural practices. Attention to these competing discourses marks an important re-focusing in research on HIV/AIDS since the international agencies that fund the majority of prevention and education programs have increasingly acknowledged the need to address the particularities of local contexts and cultures in order to achieve progress in appropriate ways (Craddock, 2004; Farmer, 1994).

Although the shift in research on HIV/AIDS to non-western contexts seems to be an obvious reason to underscore the role of culturally sensitive discourses and differing worldviews, the scope of geographic contexts addressed in this book makes it clear that research in any geographic setting must take into account the role of context in the production of knowledge. For resource-poor contexts, this may often mean considering how education efforts intersect with the availability of resources, gender relations and cultural belief systems that differ from west-based, biomedical perspectives. However, as several chapters in this volume clearly illustrate (e.g. those of Jones, Körner), the production of knowledge in resource-rich contexts is not necessarily in line with official discourses about HIV/AIDS prevention either. Consequently, it is crucial that applied linguists consider how lay knowledge of all kinds interacts with authorized discourses about HIV/AIDS.

Local Knowledge

Cultural anthropologist Clifford Geertz is well known for his description of culture as highly contextual acts of interpreting symbols. Consequently, for ethnographers, 'sorting through the machinery of distant ideas, the shapes of knowledge are always ineluctably local, indivisible from their instruments and their encasements' (Geertz, 1983: 4). His description of local knowledge highlights the impossibility of separating knowledge from context and expresses the need for analysts to interpret acts of meaning-making *in situ*, in relation to the networks of social, economic and political factors that shape social practices. Local knowledge has circulated in anthropology for several decades, and it has influenced numerous fields including post-colonial studies, public policy and human geography, and recently, applied linguistics. Across these domains, local knowledge refers to *ways of knowing* that people negotiate in their own terms that are typically outside the boundaries of 'accepted' or 'authoritative' paradigms. Rather than gaining knowledge from published accounts or legitimized experts, all forms of local knowledge are grounded in personal familiarity and derived from lived experience.

Canagarajah (2002) offers the most comprehensive discussion of local knowledge in applied linguistics. Here, he summarizes the growth of this concept in the social sciences and humanities, noting how it has moved beyond Geertz's anthropological use of the term to refer to the social practices of particular communities to its circulation in analyses of social life in a range of social, academic and professional spheres, including science and medicine. He argues that enlightenment-inspired empiricism led to a crisis for local knowledge, explaining that 'as modernism establishes geopolitical networks and a world economy that foster its vision of life, all communities are pressed into a uniform march to attain progress' (Canagarajah, 2002: 245). Although he draws attention to the imbalances in political and economic power that allowed certain forms of knowledge emanating from the west to become synonymous with global knowledge, Canagarajah is just as quick to point out the danger of drawing clear boundaries between the local and the global. While local knowledge has been relegated to a secondary position, it has changed as a result of its interaction with the global through processes of hybridity and adaptation. In other words, the search for local knowledge must be tempered with an understanding that both the local and the global are discursive processes.

Although the term was not necessarily used, local knowledge has been an area of interest in educational linguistics and educational anthropology in the form of 'home' and 'school' literacies. Early research in this area focused mostly on oral literacies in school and home contexts and the consequences for academic success (e.g. Gee, 1990; Heath, 1983; Michaels, 1981). More recent work situated in the New Literacy Studies framework (e.g. Lankshear & Knobel, 2003; Street, 1995) has shifted the focus of attention to literacies that young people employ in their cyberworlds, where they participate in massively multiple online player games, interact with others in online forums and craft fan fiction (e.g. Black, 2005; Brass, 2008; Gee, 2003; Lam, 2000; Thorne, 2008). Relatedly, Pennycook's (2007) work on hip hop as a global, transcultural resource advocates the inclusion of local knowledge in the form of 'hiphopography' as a way for educators to engage with important literacy practices in students' communities beyond school walls.

Another area in applied linguistics in which questions about local knowledge have become increasingly relevant is English language teaching (ELT), as the exportation of west-based methods and materials from the center to the periphery has been identified as a continued act of imperialism by the west (cf. Canagarajah, 2005; Edge, 2006; Holliday, 2005; Kumaravadivelu, 2005; Lin & Luke, 2006; Phan Le Ha, 2008; Ramanathan, 2005). In this research, scholars have questioned the ideological supremacy of the 'native speaker' teacher, the appropriacy and feasibility of communicative language teaching and the teaching of western culture as a goal of ELT. They have also challenged the view that local practices such as grammar translation, choral recitation, and a focus on reading and writing over oral skills is somehow 'backward' or in need of modernization, and they have convincingly argued for the need to appreciate local methods and materials in light of local values.

The present volume builds on these emerging lines of research that find value in incorporating local knowledge into theories of language and in educational theory and practice. All of the contributions here seek to broaden the ways in which knowledge about HIV/AIDS is understood through studies of how knowledge is authorized, disseminated, contested and, ultimately, transformed. Since HIV/AIDS emerged as a crisis in the 1980s, most prevention efforts have worked to achieve biomedical understandings among high-risk populations through community-based education and voluntary counseling and testing services. In these educational settings, health educators typically give epidemiological explanations about the disease and provide information about what measures can be taken to prevent its spread. Biomedical approaches have been dominant due to the paradigm in which HIV/AIDS is centrally located in the western world, that is, the paradigm of natural science (Kalipeni *et al.*, 2004). As Thomas Kuhn (1962) explained many years ago, knowledge about diseases is typically thought of as science based, construed in medical discourses, or in ways of talking that refer to agreed-upon boundaries that classify and categorize physical and biological phenomena. In a Kuhnian sense, then, the biomedical paradigm for HIV/AIDS reinforces borders of official knowledge and actively devalues other ways of knowing. Research in medical anthropology and related fields offers many examples of the under-appreciation of local knowledge in prevention campaigns sponsored by NGOs, and many researchers argue that the exclusion of local knowledge seems due in large part to the fact that NGO funding relies on donors such as UNICEF and the World Bank, the very agencies that produce the most official discourses about HIV/AIDS prevention (Green, 2003; Pfeiffer, 2004; Setel, 1999).

HIV/AIDS education remains the single-most important tool in the battle against the spread of the virus. Yet, while large sums of money are used year after year to fund educational campaigns that seek to get messages of prevention and behavior change across to high-risk populations, little is known about how these messages are communicated or what discourses emerge in response. This volume aims to provide a better understanding of these issues across a wide range of settings, by exploring HIV/AIDS education in both resource-rich and resource-poor nations, among homosexual and, heterosexual populations, and in formal and informal educational contexts.

Organization of the Volume

The volume is organized into four sections and 12 chapters that examine different perspectives on the place of local knowledge in HIV/AIDS education.

Section 1: Constructions of knowledge about HIV/AIDS

The first section of the book explores the kinds of local/lay and global/professional knowledge that are produced among high-risk populations, and the degree to which local populations align with global and local discourses of sexual health and cultural practices.

In Chapter 1, William Savage opens the volume with his own reflective narrative as an HIV-positive gay man who has spent many years working as a community development facilitator and educator in Southeast Asia. His chapter eloquently shows how autobiographical narratives are a form of knowledge construction about the disease, and how narratives such as his can form the basis of educational outreach efforts from a highly personalized perspective. Framing his contribution around location, self and journey, he explores how he and others living with HIV/AIDS get located, and how this influences how people learn about, understand and perceive them. His chapter is a moving portrayal of his own personal transformation from someone living in fear to a place where he can reach out to people, and his story demonstrates the power of narrative as a source of knowledge, compassion and site for potential healing.

The chapters that follow in this section provide more traditional research-based accounts of the construction of local knowledge in educational practices. In Chapter 2, Harriet Mutonyi and Maureen Kendrick draw on social semiotics (Kress & Jewitt, 2003) and visual anthropology to examine the use of drawing as a tool for interpreting Ugandan students' conceptualizations of HIV/AIDS. While some global discourses of HIV/AIDS prevention are present in the drawings, Mutonyi and Kendrick's analysis shows that many of the drawings highlight the transactional nature of sexuality among Ugandan youth, an aspect of sexual relationships that is part of Uganda's social landscape, and hence part of Ugandan youth's local knowledge about the disease.

In Chapter 3, Ángeles Clemente and Michael Higgins explore the gap between how HIV/AIDS is defined and acted upon by the official health agencies of Oaxaca, Mexico, and how these discourses are processed by a group of young students at the state university who are studying to become English language teachers. Using interviews, Clemente and Higgins investigate how university students respond to the national AIDS council's messages of prevention alongside local discourses that treat men's unabated sexual desires as the source of HIV transmission. The authors treat the interviews as performances (Butler, 1999; Pennycook, 2004) in which students imagine their future interactions with sexual partners, and they investigate how students respond to these discourses in both Spanish and English. They explain that the students are able to perform different identities in each language, thus making sex 'safer' or 'less safe' to talk about.

In Chapter 4, Henrike Körner analyzes the discursive construction of risk in a corpus of gay men's accounts of sexual exposure to HIV in a study carried out in Sydney, Australia that was based on semi-structured, in-depth interviews. Drawing on Bakhtin's notions of *heteroglossia* and *dialogism*, and appraisal theory from systemic functional linguistics, she describes the heteroglossic backdrop against which gay men's accounts of sexual exposure to HIV and their perceptions of 'risk' are constructed. She discusses the intertextuality in gay men's accounts of sexual exposure to HIV by describing how they resonate with the safe sex discourse of health promotion in the gay community, risk reduction strategies such as negotiated safety, and the discourse of epidemiology and biomedicine in the form of viral load tests and advances in antiretroviral treatments. However, she also finds that these discourses are enmeshed with individuals' experiences of the HIV epidemic as well as individuals' own sexual histories.

Section 2: Gendered practices in the spread of HIV/AIDS

In the second section of the book, three chapters investigate discourses of gender and HIV/AIDS in India, Tanzania and Uganda, respectively. The authors argue that the position of women in HIV/AIDS discourses and practices is highly troubling, and that it reflects wider patriarchal relations at both local and global levels. In Chapter 5, Noushin Khushrushahi examines the public discourses that point fingers at infected female individuals for their 'un-Indian' morals and behavior. Taking a Foucaultian perspective, she examines the discursive context that shapes the manner in which some sex workers in India conceive of and respond to HIV/AIDS intervention messages by exploring how these women engage, decode and respond to the information given in three government-sponsored pamphlets.

Next, in Chapter 6, Christina Higgins examines how a large NGO in Tanzania has responded to initiatives to focus on gender relations rather than gender-sensitive education by investigating how the discourses of sexual responsibility are discursively constructed and re-entextualized with discourses of gender at HIV/AIDS education sessions. Employing an ethnographically informed approach to critical discourse analysis (Blommaert, 2005), she analyzes educational sessions at a *madrassa* (Islamic school), in plays performed at community bonanzas and during life skills classes that are meant to alter risky behaviors through raising awareness. Higgins argues that each of these contexts provides evidence that women and girls are discursively constructed as the target of NGO-sponsored educational efforts, and yet these efforts do little to distribute the discourses of gender and responsibility more fairly among male and female Tanzanians.

In Chapter 7, Shelley Jones and Bonny Norton call into question many of the assumptions upon which sexual health policies are developed internationally by discussing their research on health literacy involving 15 schoolgirls in rural Uganda. Although these students were well informed about the risks and responsibilities of sexual activity and HIV/AIDS, Jones and Norton explain that these young women's options were severely constrained by poverty, sexual abuse and systemic gender inequities. Taking a post-structuralist perspective, Jones and Norton assert that ownership of discourses of health literacy is determined not only by who speaks and who listens, but also by who is included and who is excluded in discourses of power. Accordingly, they critique health education's concern with the dissemination of information and the teaching of various life skills by reporting aspects of their longitudinal research, which reveals that many Ugandan girls cannot actively apply their knowledge to practice, and hence remain excluded from discourses of empowerment.

Section 3: The place of local knowledge in HIV/AIDS educational practices

The third section of the book investigates ways in which knowledge about HIV/AIDS and its prevention is disseminated in formal and informal educational settings. Exploring the relationship between global/professional and local forms of knowledge, the authors in this section show how target populations make sense of the messages of prevention that surround them, and they compare how local knowledge and professional forms of education are taken up among communities.

In Chapter 8, Rodney Jones uses *mediated discourse analysis* (Norris & Jones 2005; Scollon, 2001) to examine how gay men in Hong Kong talk about HIV/AIDS in online chat rooms and internet forums. Jones argues that much of what people learn about HIV/AIDS does not come from formal educational channels, but rather from private or semi-public interactions with peers in settings such as internet chat rooms. He concludes that if HIV/AIDS educators wish to understand how to implement community-based prevention efforts, they must understand how people talk about and teach one another about HIV/AIDS in their everyday lives, and how community constructions of HIV/AIDS and the risks associated with it appropriate, adapt and contest more official constructions from media and public health discourses.

Next, in Chapter 9, Martina Drescher analyzes a corpus of French data from classroom interactions in Burkina Faso between a trainer and future communicative agents in HIV/AIDS prevention campaigns. She focuses on the different types of reformulations and their contribution to the emergence of two competing knowledge systems in the context of a series of asymmetrical interactions characterized by a transfer of knowledge in the medical domain. Her analysis shows that reformulations operate as *contextualization cues* (Gumperz, 1982) that help to construct an opposition of two potentially competing knowledge systems in these training sessions, that is, biomedical or global knowledge on the one hand, and traditional or local knowledge on the other.

In Chapter 10, Claudia Mitchell, Jean Stuart, Naydene DeLange, Relebohile Moletsane, Thabisile Buthelezi, June Larkin and Sarah Flicker describe aspects of several projects their research team has undertaken over the past three years that seek to provide opportunities to develop new literacies with young people and their teachers in South Africa. They discuss a variety of visual methods that have at the center the idea of engagement through participation, including photo-voice and participatory video. The authors describe how such literacies are critical in relation to seeing how young people themselves frame issues around stigma, voluntary counseling and testing, gender violence and safe sex practices, but also in relation to ways of 'getting the message out' in culturally relevant ways to peer audiences. Their chapter describes how the projects create the opportunity for community literacy practices that speak to the concept of voice and to the role of participation within a context that acknowledges the particularities of the pandemic.

Section 4: Institutional responses to HIV/AIDS

In the final section of the book, two chapters consider how NGOs and governmental institutions in India have responded to the HIV/AIDS epidemic. In Chapter 11, Mark Finn and Srikant Sarangi explore discourses of empowerment and neoliberalism circulating in Indian NGOs that rely on western constructions of the rational individual to empower HIV-positive persons. They explore the operations of 'knowledge' and 'empowerment' as key modalities of a global knowledge of acceptable HIV-positive health. They argue, more specifically, that the knowledge-based decision strategy of empowerment functions to inculcate a specific way of knowing and being in the decision-making individual, who is subjectified in and by the responsible assimilation of particular truths about health, identity and quality of life. They assert that the very idea of living an empowered life and of being able to make healthy decisions is for many HIV-positive people in India an unrealistic fantasy, and they suggest alternatives that would challenge discourses of neoliberalism in discourses of HIV/AIDS.

Finn and Sarangi's critique of institutional discourses provides an interesting prelude to the final chapter, Chapter 12, by Annabelle Mooney, who describes the success of government-sponsored education in the Port Blair region of the Andaman Islands, a region with low HIV prevalence compared to mainland India. Mooney argues that education as discoursed by the government has provided benefits to residents of the Andaman Islands. In her chapter, she carries out a semantic–pragmatic analysis of several prevention signs, and she explains that these signs explain the conditions that need to be in place for their messages to be understood and taken up. Corroborating her reading of these signs with interviews and fieldwork data, she argues that the signs can be understood as indexing the resilient and robust social environment present in and around Port Blair. Mooney's chapter provides a compelling contrast with Finn and Sarangi's analysis of discourses in mainland India, and the two very different perspectives reveal how significantly context matters in interpreting messages about HIV/AIDS prevention.

These 12 chapters reveal that local knowledge is always present, sometimes even in the form of authorized discourses about HIV/AIDS. However, most of the chapters show that local knowledge remains in competition with official discourses about HIV/AIDS in formal and informal domains of education, and most of the chapters reveal that local knowledge is largely eclipsed in favor of official discourses about HIV/AIDS. While a volume of this nature does not strive to make grand generalizations about the place of local knowledge in the prevention of HIV/AIDS, we believe that understanding how knowledge is constructed among various populations can helpfully inform any and all efforts to prevent the spread of HIV. What the findings presented here do seem to have in common is that greater inclusion of unauthorized voices can lead to deeper understandings about why some educational practices have greater success than others. It is our hope that this volume will inspire those working in the field of HIV/AIDS prevention to listen carefully to these voices.

References

Atkinson, P. (1995) *Medical Talk and Medical Work: The Liturgy of the Clinic*. London: Sage.

Black, R.W. (2005) Access and affiliation: The literacy and composition practices of English language learners in an online fanfiction community. *Journal of Adolescent & Adult Literacy* 49, 118–128.

Blommaert, J. (2005) *Discourse*. Cambridge: Cambridge University Press.

Boutain, D. (1999) Critical language and discourse study: Their transformative relevance for critical nursing inquiry. *Advances in Nursing Science* 21 (3), 1–8.

Brass, J.J. (2008) Local knowledge and digital movie composing in an after-school literacy program. *Journal of Adolescent & Adult Literacy* 51, 464–473.

Butler, J. (1999) Performativity's social magic. In R. Shusterman (ed.) *Bourdieu: A Critical Reader* (pp. 113–129). London: Blackwell Publishers.

Cameron, R. and Williams, J. (1997) Sentence to ten cents: A case study of relevance and communicative success in non-native speaker interactions in a medical setting. *Applied Linguistics* 18, 415–455.

Canagarajah, S. (2002) Reconstructing local knowledge. *Journal of Language, Identity, and Education* 1, 243–259.

Canagarajah, S. (ed.) (2005) *Reclaiming the Local in Language Policy and Practice.* Mahwah, NJ: Erlbaum.

Candlin, C. and Candlin, S. (2002) Expert talk and risk in health care. (Special issue.) *Research on Language & Social Interaction* 35 (2), 115–219.

Candlin, C.N. and Candlin, S. (2003) Healthcare communication as a problematic site for applied linguistic research. *Annual Review of Applied Linguistics* 23, 134–154.

Candlin, S. (2002) Taking risks: An indicator of expertise? *Research on Language & Social Interaction* 35 (2), 173–193.

Coupland, J., Robinson, J.D. and Coupland, N. (1994) Frame negotiation in elderly patient consultations. *Discourse & Society* 5, 89–124.

Craddock, S. (2004) Beyond epidemiology: Locating AIDS in Africa. In E. Kalipeni, S. Craddock and J. Ghosh (eds) *HIV & AIDS in Africa: Beyond Epidemiology* (pp. 1–10). Malden, MA: Blackwell.

Davidson, B. (2000) The interpreter as institutional gatekeeper: The social-linguistics role of interpreters in Spanish-English medical discourse. *Journal of Sociolinguistics* 4 (3), 379–405.

Djite, P.G. (2008) *The Sociolinguistics of Development in Africa.* Clevedon: Multilingual Matters.

Drescher, M. (2007) Global and local alignments in HIV/AIDS prevention trainings: A case study from Burkina Faso. *Communication and Medicine* 4, 3–14.

Edge, J. (ed.) (2006) *(Re)locating TESOL in an Age of Empire.* London: Palgrave.

Eggly, S. (2002) Physician-patient co-construction of illness narratives in the medical interview. *Health Communication* 14 (3), 339–360.

Evans, S. (2001) How do ESL students in two Pittsburgh neighborhoods talk about the situations they face as limited English proficiency (LEP) parents? *PAACE* (Pennsylvania Association for Adult Continuing Education). *Journal of Lifelong Learning* 10, 55–63.

Farmer, P. (1994) Aids-talk and the constitution of cultural models. *Social Science and Medicine* 38, 801–809.

Gee, J. (1990) *Social Linguistics and Literacies: Ideology in Discourses.* New York: Routledge.

Gee, J. (2003) *What Video Games have to Teach us about Learning and Literacy.* New York: Palgrave.

Geertz, C. (1983) *Local Knowledge: Further Essays in Interpretive Anthropology.* New York: Basic Books.

Green, E.C. (2003) *Rethinking AIDS Prevention: Learning from Success in Developing Countries.* Westport, CT: Praeger.

Gumperz, J.J. (1982) *Discourse Strategies.* Cambridge: Cambridge University Press.

Hamilton, H. (1994/2005). *Conversations with an Alzheimer's Patient: An Interactional Sociolinguistic Study.* Cambridge: Cambridge University Press.

Harvey, K., Churchill, D., Crawford, P., Brown, B., Mullany, L., Macfarlane, A. and McPherson, A. (2008) Health communication and adolescents: What do their emails tell us? *Family Practice* 25 (4), 304–311.

Heath, S.B. (1983) *Ways with Words: Language, Life and Work in Communities and Classrooms*. Cambridge: Cambridge University Press.

Heritage, J., Maynard, D., Cook, K. and Massey, D. (2006) Problems and prospects in the study of physician–patient interaction: 30 years of research. *Annual Review of Sociology* 32 (1), 351–374.

Holliday, A. (2005) *The Struggle to Teach English as an International Language*. Oxford: Oxford University Press.

Jones, R. (2002) A walk in the park: Frames and positions in AIDS prevention outreach among gay men in China. *Journal of Sociolinguistics* 6, 575–588.

Jones, R. and Candlin, C. (2003) Constructing risk across timescales and trajectories: Gay men's stories of sexual encounters. *Health, Risk & Society* 5, 199–213.

Jones, R.H., Candlin, C.N. and Yu, K.K. (2000) *Culture, Communication and Quality of Life of People Living with HIV/AIDS in Hong Kong*. Hong Kong: The AIDS Trust Fund of Hong Kong and the Centre for English Language Education and Communication Research, City University of Hong Kong.

Jones, S. and Norton, B. (2007) On the limits of sexual health literacy: Insights from Ugandan schoolgirls. *Journal of Diaspora, Indigenous, and Minority Education* 1 (4), 285–305.

Kalipeni, E., Craddock, S., Oppong, J. and Ghosh, J. (eds) (2004) *HIV and AIDS in Africa: Beyond Epidemiology*. Malden, MA: Blackwell.

Kendrick, M. and Hissani, H. (2007a) Letters, imagined communities, and literate identities. *Journal of Literacy Research* 39, 195–216.

Kendrick, M., Jones, S., Mutonyi, H. and Norton, B. (2006) Multimodality and English education in Ugandan schools. *English Studies in Africa* 49, 95–114.

Kendrick, M. and Mutonyi, H. (2007b) Meeting the challenge of health literacy in rural Uganda: The critical role of women and local modes of communication. *Journal of Diaspora, Indigenous, and Minority Education* 1 (4), 265–283.

Koteyko, N., Nerlich, B., Crawford, P. and Wright, N. (2008) 'Not rocket science' or 'no silver bullet'? Media and government discourses about MRSA and cleanliness. *Applied Linguistics* 29 (2), 223–243.

Kress, G. and Jewitt, C. (2003) Introduction. In C. Jewitt and G. Kress (eds) *Multimodal Literacy* (pp. 1–18). New York: Peter Lang.

Kuhn, T. (1962) *The Structure of Scientific Revolutions*. Chicago: University of Chicago Press.

Kumaravadivelu, B. (2005) *Understanding Language Teaching: From Method to Post-Method*. Mahwah, NJ: Erlbaum.

Kung, W. (2004) Cultural and practical barriers to seeking mental health treatment for Chinese Americans. *Journal of Community Psychology* 32 (1), 27–43.

Lam, W.S.E. (2000) Second language literacy and the design of the self: A case study of a teenager writing on the Internet. *TESOL Quarterly* 34, 457–483.

Lankshear, C. and Knobel, M. (2003) *New Literacies: Changing Knowledge and Classroom Learning*. Buckingham, England & Philadelphia: Open University Press.

Lawrence, J., Kearns, R., Park, J., Bryder, L. and Worth, H. (2008) Discourses of disease: Representations of tuberculosis within New Zealand newspapers 2002–2004. *Social Science and Medicine* 66 (3), 727–739.

Leap, W. (1995) Talking about AIDS: Linguistic perspectives on non-neutral discourse. In H. ten Brummelhuis and G. Herdt (eds) *Culture and Sexual Risk: Anthropological Perspectives of AIDS* (pp. 227–238). Sydney: Gordon and Breach.

Leonard, L. and Ellen, J. (2008) 'The story of my life': AIDS and 'Autobiographical occasions'. *Qualitative Sociology* 31 (1), 37–56.

Lin, A. and Luke, A. (eds) (2006) Postcolonial approaches to TESOL. (Special volume.) *Critical Inquiry in Language Studies* 3, 65–200.

Linell, P., Adelsward, V., Sachs, L., Bredmar, M. and Lindstedt, U. (2002) Expert talk in medical contexts: Explicit and implicit orientation to risks. *Research on Language & Social Interaction* 35 (2), 195–218.

Maynard, D. (2003) *Bad News, Good News: Conversational Order in Everyday Talk and Clinical Settings.* Chicago: University of Chicago Press.

Michaels, S. (1981) 'Sharing time': Children's narrative styles and differential access to literacy. *Language in Society* 10, 423–442.

Mishler, E. (1984) *The Discourse of Medicine: The Dialectics of Medical Interviews.* Norwood, NJ: Ablex.

Mitchell, C. (2006) In my life: Youth stories and poems on HIV/AIDS: Towards a new literacy in the age of AIDS. *Changing English* 13, 355–368.

Mitchell, C. and Smith, A. (2003) Sick of AIDS: Literacy and the meaning of life for South African youth. *Culture, Health & Sexuality* 5, 513–522.

Mooney, A. and Sarangi, S. (2005) An ecological framing of HIV preventive intervention: A case study of non-government organisational work in the developing world. *Health* 9, 275–296.

Ngo-Metzger, Q., Massagli, M., Clarridge, B., Manocchia, M., Davis, R., Iezzoni, L. and Phillips, R. (2003) Linguistic and cultural barriers to care. *Journal of General Internal Medicine* 18 (1), 44–52.

Norris, S. and Jones, R. (eds) (2005) *Discourse in Action: Introducing Mediated Discourse Analysis.* London: Routledge.

Norton, B. and Mutonyi, H. (2007) 'Talk what others think you can't talk': HIV/ AIDS clubs as peer education in Ugandan schools. *Compare* 37, 479–492.

Partida, Y. (2007) Addressing language barriers: Building response capacity for a changing nation. *Journal of General Internal Medicine* 22, 347–349.

Pennycook, A. (2004) Performativity and language studies. *Critical Inquiry in Language Studies: An International Journal* 1, 1–19.

Pennycook, A. (2007) *Global Englishes and Transcultural Flows.* London and New York: Routledge.

Peräkylä, A. (1995) *Aids Counselling: Institutional Interaction and Clinical Practice.* Cambridge: Cambridge University Press.

Peräkylä, A. (2002) Agency and authority: Extended responses to diagnostic statements in primary care encounters. *Research on Language & Social Interaction* 35 (2), 219–247.

Pfeiffer, J. (2004) Condom social marketing, Pentecostalism, and structural adjustment in Mozambique: A clash of AIDS prevention messages. *Medical Anthropology Quarterly* 18, 77–103.

Phan Le Ha (2008) *Teaching English as an International Language: Identity, Resistance and Negotiation.* Clevedon: Multilingual Matters.

Ramanathan, V. (1997) *Alzheimer Discourse: Some Sociolinguistic Dimensions.* Mahwah, NJ: Lawrence Erlbaum.

Ramanathan, V. (2005) *The English-vernacular Divide: Postcolonial Language Politics and Practice*. Clevedon: Multilingual Matters.

Ramanathan, V. (2008) Applied linguistics redux: A Derridean exploration of Alzheimer life histories. *Applied Linguistics* 29 (1), 1–23.

Ramanathan, V. (2010) *Bodies and Language: Health, Ailments and Disabilities*. Bristol: Multilingual Matters.

Ramanathan, V. and Makoni, S. (2008) Bringing the body back in body narratives: The mislanguaging of bodies in biomedical, societal, and poststructuralist discourses on diabetes and epilepsy. *Critical Inquiry in Language Studies* 4 (4), 283–306.

Saha, S. and Fernandez, A. (2007) Language barriers in health care. *Journal of General Internal Medicine* 22, 281–282.

Sarangi, S. and Clarke, A. (2002) Zones of expertise and the management of uncertainty in genetics risk communication. *Research on Language & Social Interaction* 35 (2), 139–171.

Sarangi, S. and Roberts, C. (eds) (1999) *Talk, Work and Institutional Orders: Discourse in Medical, Mediation and Management Settings*. Berlin: Mouton.

Scollon, R. (2001) *Mediated Discourse: The Nexus of Practice*. London: Routledge.

Setel, P.W. (1999) *A Plague of Paradoxes: AIDS, Culture, and Demography in Northern Tanzania*. Chicago: University of Chicago Press.

Silverman, D. (1990) The social organization of HIV counselling. In P. Aggleton, G. Hart and P. Davies (eds) *AIDS: Individual, Cultural and Policy Perspectives* (pp. 191–211). Lewes: Falmer.

Silverman, D. (1997) *Discourses of Counselling*. London: Sage.

Street, B. (1995) *Social Literacies: Critical Approaches to Literacy in Development, Ethnography and Education*. London & New York: Longman.

Thorne, S.L. (2008) Transcultural communication in open internet environments and massively multiplayer online games. In S. Magnan (ed.) *Mediating Discourse Online* (pp. 305–327). Amsterdam: John Benjamins.

Towle, A. (2006) Doctor–patient communications in the aboriginal communities: Towards the development of educational programs. *Patient Education and Counseling* 63 (3), 340–346.

Underwood, C., Serlemitsos, E. and Macwangi, M. (2007) Health communication in multilingual contexts: A study of reading preferences, practices, and proficiencies among literate adults in Zambia. *Journal of Health Communication* 12 (4), 317–337.

Vahabi, M. (2007) The impact of health communication on health-related decision-making: A review of evidence. *Health Education* 107 (1), 27–41.

West, C. (1984) *Routine Complications: Troubles in Talk between Doctors and Patients*. Bloomington: Indiana University Press.

Chapter 1

Lengths of Life: Stories of Being with HIV

WILLIAM SAVAGE

Introduction

The premise of this chapter is that an effective way for people to understand about HIV and AIDS is for them to learn to listen to and tell stories of what it is like to be infected with the virus and/or affected by the epidemic. Framed around life, location, self and journey, I narrate parts of my story of learning to live and be well as an HIV-positive gay man. While this is a reflective essay on my experiences, I also reference additional perspectives in the other 11 chapters about living and working with HIV and AIDS around the world. In many ways, all of the chapters in this collection are also stories; in some the faces of the people are easily seen, and in others we need to look carefully at and through the numbers and descriptions for the faces to emerge. As Rodney Jones (this volume) points out, 'If AIDS educators wish to understand how to implement truly "community based" prevention efforts, they must understand how people talk about and teach one another about HIV in their everyday lives, and how community constructions of HIV and the risks associated with it appropriate, adapt and contest more official constructions from media and public health discourses'.

Although colleagues in our various fields continue to debate the place of autobiography and narrative inquiry in research, it is not my intention here to review that dialogue. Rather I want to celebrate some of what listening to and telling stories offer us as people who work at or are intrigued by the intersection of education and applied linguistics and HIV and AIDS, what Pavlenko (2007: 166–167) refers to as 'attention to ways in which storytellers use language to interpret experiences and position themselves as particular kinds of people'. It is among my purposes to be part of what Bell (2002: 209, referencing Canagarajah, 1996) highlights as an 'opportunity for marginalized groups to participate in knowledge construction in the academy'.

Lengths of Life

'My name is Bill Savage and I tested positive for HIV in December 1995.' I had gone to Sydney, Australia, from where I lived and worked in Bangkok, uncertain at that time as to what might happen if I tested positive as a foreign resident of Thailand. For years I had lived with the fear of getting tested, and somehow knew that I was positive. I was in Sydney for six months of residence at the university where I started a PhD program. It was toward the end of that stay and just before I was to return to Bangkok and to my Thai partner of over five years, that I made an appointment to get tested.

Clearly busy with his daily appointments, my diagnosing doctor took just enough time for me during that first session, talking with me as a counselor might, asking about my family's medical history and any difficult circumstances in our lives. Feeling at ease with him, I spoke about my mother having Huntington's disease and having been in a nursing home for seven years (she would die less than a year later). I talked about my own fears of having Huntington's, ever since finding out that Mom had it, back in 1975 when I was 15, and living with that dread for the 20 years since, then at 35, the age around which my mother and grandmother had started showing the symptoms. I told him about Laura, the second of my three younger sisters, murdered two-and-a-half years before, shot in the back of the head in a restaurant robbery, and how she and I had been so close, at the time the only person in my family I had told that I was gay.

The doctor no doubt said more than what I remember, but this is what stays with me: 'With all that you've been through, and with what I feel from you today', he said, 'I sense that you are a self-healer and that will be useful, whether you test positive or negative'. We moved from our chairs around his desk to an examining table, upon which I sat as he prepared the syringe. Watching as he inserted the needle in the vein of my arm, and seeing my blood flow into the vial, a wave of relief washed over me. The fear of getting tested disappeared instantly; no longer was I its prisoner, and soon there would be no uncertainty about my HIV status. That was my first lesson in what to do with fear, one I had to keep learning again and again as each of the next fears came into and left my life one after another.

A week later I returned to the doctor's office for the results. I was sitting in the reception area waiting for my appointment when the doctor came in to speak with the receptionist, saw me and from the look on his face and the way he greeted me, I knew that I was HIV-positive. When he actually told me a few minutes later, I am not sure today whether I was thinking about death, but I do remember a deeply subconscious refrain of 'you go to Sydney, you test positive, you die'. The remaining time with the doctor was spent discussing clinical details, numbers, a few further tests for any opportunistic infections, and how I might follow up these life-changing results once I got back to Thailand. I called my partner and told him and also a close friend at the international university where I worked, thinking that at least one person at my workplace should know.

When I got back to Bangkok, through another close friend, I found a doctor who treated HIV-positive people at his clinic and began a seven-year relationship with him in which I would go in every six months for CD4 and viral load testing. (CD4, or T-cells, are the white blood cells responsible for the body's immune system response, while the viral load measures the amount of virus in the blood.) Over that time, the CD4 counts remained in the normal range and the viral loads fluctuated from low to higher and back again, although for those years, neither number ever reached a point where going onto the antiretroviral (ARV) drugs was recommended. I was made much more unwell by fear and by the slow dawning realization of dark sides of my psyche that were at play. In retrospect, I understand that I was mentally unwell.

In those early years, I told few people that I was HIV-positive, only the closest of friends. It felt much the same as when I first came out and began to accept myself as gay – when I tested positive for homosexuality – with the consuming fear of what people's reactions would be. I now see that this was all also part of my own coming to terms with deeper parts of myself, and that I had a lot to work on that I was not yet even acknowledging. I was certainly not taking care of myself, continuing what I now consider to be destructive behaviors, and not seeking ways of being mentally, emotionally and spiritually grounded. One of the strongest fears was telling my father about my HIV status. Laura had been killed in 1993; the oldest of my three younger sisters Sandy started showing the symptoms of Huntington's around the time I got tested and my mother died with that disease in October 1996. How could I possibly add to my father's sadness?

In December 2003, eight years after my diagnosis, I got the first disappointing test results from my doctor in Thailand, the CD4s showing a decreasing trend over that year and the viral load increasing. It occurred to me that I was 'not going to get away with it after all', *it* being not taking care of myself. In short, the results scared life back into me. On a single day, I stopped smoking, decided not to drink alcohol anymore, got off caffeine, went back to my swimming, yoga and meditation practices, and got my diet back on track by returning to my vegetarian ways. What was important was that these were the very things I had been struggling with for decades, all the things I wanted to continue doing or not doing, the characteristics of the sort of person I wanted to be and now was closer than ever to being.

The doctor asked me to come back in three, rather than six, months for the next tests, in March 2004. Those results were 378 for the CD4s, a further large drop, the first time below the normal range, and nearing the treatment-indicative 350 mark. The viral load was 32,000, a big drop from what it had reached three months earlier. My first thoughts upon hearing that news could have been 'well, that didn't work', *that* being the lifestyle changes of three months. But my reaction was, rather, how happy I was that I had finally been able to overcome those struggles, how much more mentally well I was, to be able to hear those results and deal with the realities of the situation.

My doctor asked me to come back in a month for another round of tests and suggested that I start thinking about going onto the ARV treatment, which has always been an inevitable next phase for me. In the meantime, I went on holiday to Australia to meet my father and stepmother from Louisiana, which allowed me to visit my diagnosing doctor again. He confirmed that 350 was the current CD4 number below which doctors were advising people to go on the drugs. He also talked about my being a 'long-term slow progressor', as my Thai doctor had done, and that people were no longer referred to as 'non-progressors' since everyone with HIV is progressing to some degree. The Sydney doctor also said how he thought that it was significant that I had been able to overcome my substance addictions and work on (what I have come to think of as) my mental (in)capacity to engage in healthy behaviors, and that this would have a long-term impact on my well-being.

Back in Bangkok for the next tests in April 2004, the CD4 number was 38, and the viral load went down a bit to 27,000. Again, I was able to get these results with a measure of acceptance I was happy to experience, and I went shortly after that to buy pill boxes to start the ARVs. My doctor referred me to another doctor at the HIV center at one of the best hospitals in Thailand. He wanted me to see the new doctor right away, as if there was no time to lose. An HIV-positive friend who has been doing well on the drugs for years and with whom I had been in e-mail contact throughout all of this, implored me in a message to 'stop reading this message and get yourself to the hospital and onto the drugs'. But I just did not feel the urgency. In fact, to this day, I have never been sick in a way obviously related to being HIV-positive, and I felt good.

When I met the new doctor for the first time, he looked at the current numbers and the past trend, and said, 'Yes, it is time for you to go onto the drugs – what are you doing next week?' I was leaving for a short work trip to Nairobi the next day. He advised against starting the drugs while traveling since we would not know whether there would be any side effects, and he suggested that we take another round of tests so that he would have a baseline for his work with me.

When he called the numbers up on the screen when I next saw him in May 2004, he asked, 'This is amazing, what have you been doing?' The CD4s were up to 820 and the viral load was down to 7000! I responded that it was either amazing or the 38 was a mistake, which does happen with these tests. Still, the trend over the past year had been a decreasing CD4 count. The appointment ended with the doctor saying that there was no way I should start the ARV treatment with numbers like those. So it seemed to be just me, the power of positive and wholesome living, and the love and respect of and for a lot of people in my world.

In July 2004, I took a first big step by coming out to myself and others as an HIV-positive person at the 15th International AIDS Conference that was held in Bangkok. I went along to sessions for HIV-positive people, spent time in the lounge set up for positive people and played a role in the conference as writer, director and emcee of the opening program of the AIDS Film Festival. In the script, I even allowed a tacit acknowledgment of my own HIV status by saying, 'As we will hear in a moment, this week's film screenings show us faces, names, lives and identities; they tell us other people's stories, and they will remind us, once again, of who we are and what we should be doing, as people living with, affected by and concerned with HIV and AIDS'.

In August 2004, a second important step was to tell my father and step-mother about being HIV-positive. I went to Louisiana for a three-week visit and decided to tell them on the second night I was there. I just said it: 'I want you to know that I am HIV-positive; I have known for nine years; and I am healthy'. The way they responded lifted the burden and block-age to telling other people, to being open and out about my status. They were caring, loving, supportive and curious. In fact, I wondered whether they had understood what I had told them. Did they even know what HIV was? They had and they did. My father said that he was sorry that I had HIV, that he had much to learn about it, but mostly he was sad to know that I had carried this alone for that many years before I felt I could tell him. I sensed again what 'freedom from fear' is; our relationship changed fundamentally, and the new level of authenticity brought strength and togetherness a little over a year later when my sister Sandy died unexpectedly prematurely with Huntington's disease.

For the next three years, the CD4 counts remained within the normal range and the viral loads continued to fluctuate as they always had. I stayed with my changed lifestyle and in November 2005 started doing Kundalini Yoga, which was to become the practice through which I continued to transform myself and my life. In August of 2007, the viral load leapt from an already-high 165,000 to over 400,000, which seemed like an awful lot of virus! Because the CD4s were still above the range of concern, my doctor suggested that I come back in a couple of months for another test. At that time, in October 2007, while the viral load had dropped to 159,000, the CD4s had come down to 475. Knowing that I was about to make the move to live in New Orleans in December, the doctor suggested that I consider going onto the ARVs that day, so that he could monitor me over the next two months in Thailand. I immediately got started on a Kundalini Yoga set of a vigorous exercise sequence called 'immune fitness' and a powerful meditation called 'immune system booster: the inner sun', and the test results were almost identical to the time before. The changes I made in my lifestyle the first time were easy in comparison with the more subtle ones that would be necessary this time, taking all of my practices to their next levels, as I continue to seek that still, quiet place that has come to be my intended destination and destiny.

I realized at that time that I had created a story for myself that going onto the ARVs was a failure. Having been healthy for 12 years without them meant that I had failed if and when I needed to start the drugs. In reality, it is a blessing that they are available to me. More deeply, I have come to realize that I have been making choices to change and to heal, to continue a difficult journey of discovery: Who is this self? Can I break free of what is holding me back from a path to well-being? This has little to do with being HIV-positive or not. And so the next step into the unknown was my arrival at my new home in New Orleans, uncertain as to what awaited me. Through providential circumstances I met the young man who would become my doctor, discovered that I was eligible as an HIV-positive uninsured resident of Louisiana for affordable care and treatment, and had another round of tests that affirmed that it was time to start the ARVs, which began in February 2008. With the gift of the advances in HIV science over the years, I began on Atripla, a single daily pill with the combination of efavirenz, emtricitabine and tenofovir. The only side effect

I have experienced so far on the medication is the feeling of having increased energy levels, which my late sister Sandy's sister-in-law, a physical therapist, articulated for me as: Now I am taking these drugs to fight the virus, so I do not have to do that myself any more and can use my own energy for my health and my life. After two months, my viral load had come down to 266 from over 200,000 and the CD4 count had increased from 370 to 440, and so I embarked on the next leg of this journey.

There are two among the many dimensions of this experience that I want to conclude my story-thus-far with: fear and a notion of 'lengths of life'. I have come to believe that how people live their lives, and how they experience other people's, is determined in part by how they deal with fear: their own and their responses to other people's. As I mentioned early in my narrative, actually having the HIV test done enabled me finally to face a long-standing fear, and to learn what that feels like, as I applied and continue to apply that learning to each fear as it has arisen. These have mostly centered around the knowledge that there was something about me that if other people knew, there would be uncertain reactions and consequences: colleagues, superiors and administrators at my place of employment; acquaintances and government officials in the country where I lived as a foreigner; long-time and newer friends in various places around the world; my immediate and extended family in the United States and even people I had not yet met. There was something about me that I and a few other people knew and I had the nearly-debilitating experience over the years of feeling like I was not being my authentic self. Along with the fear of hiding this piece of information was a deeper fear of becoming ill, of dying and of death.

The idea of 'lengths of life' dawned on me when I was swimming one day. A lifelong distance swimmer, I feel most myself physically when I am in the water, typically putting in 1 to over 2 km at a time. During the last few laps of freestyle, stroking with all the strength I can muster, I repeat as a mantra, 'These are the lengths of life, as long I am HIV-positive and can swim like this, I will be alright'. As I have learned and changed and grown over these years of living with HIV, I have come to think of my existence in terms of how it measures across time, and how it plays out in phases of changing identity and purpose. Lengths of life: between regular CD4 and viral load tests, each time in awe of the power of 'the numbers' to color my perception of well-being; between the beginnings and ends of yoga sets and 40-day yoga practices; between the inevitable start of taking the ARVs and the current thinking on them about life expectancy; between seeing loved ones this time and the next and between being uncertain about what comes next and reaching out to embrace what is possible. What gifts these lengths of life are! Who was it that said that, besides death, the things all of us share are the breath of air, the taste of water and time?

Transforming Locations

The first sentence of my story – 'My name is Bill Savage and I tested positive for HIV in December 1995'. – is a tribute to people I met at the 2004 AIDS Conference in Bangkok. They are from Uganda and were representing The AIDS Support Organization (TASO). At each conference event they appeared at, they first stood in a line and introduced themselves by saying their names, when they tested HIV-positive and when they joined TASO. The audiences did not learn anything else that was personal about these 10 or so people, but they witnessed their energy as they watched them dance and sing with exuberance. It is now a cliché to talk about how for so long being HIV-positive was like a death sentence. Yet this persists even as advances are made in the prevention and treatment of HIV infection. This misconception lingers strongly even as we are able to see and document how people are living healthy full lives with HIV. As recently as December 1, 2007, World AIDS Day, the United Nations Secretary General called for an end to the stigma and discrimination surrounding HIV and AIDS, for to many of us, this, and not the virus, is what is killing people.

It must have been at the AIDS Conference, and blessed with the gift of meeting people like the TASO friends, that I began to realize how different my story of being HIV-positive was from many other people's, coming as I do from a world of relatively more privilege, less vulnerability and no experience of stigmatization or discrimination. What HIV-positive people do share in their stories are fear and pain, and what many of us are doing with that has given our lives new purposes. I knew that I could play a small part – in ways that I could not even imagine then – by telling my own story along with those of others. The world needs to hear HIV-positive people themselves narrating their own experiences so that others can understand. So a question is: How do people living with HIV and AIDS locate themselves and get located by others? The assumptions here are that people cannot possibly understand about HIV and AIDS without hearing people's stories, and that people infected with the virus and affected by the epidemic cannot realize their healing and transformative potential without being able to tell their stories. It is about putting a human face on HIV and AIDS. There are many sources of people's stories in a variety of media, and I will highlight a few here that have had a powerful impact on me, as examples of the sorts of narratives that educators and researchers could use to broaden perceptions of the world of HIV and AIDS.

The Asia Pacific Leadership Forum of UNAIDS published a two-volume set called *Portraits of Commitment*, one from South Asia (UNAIDS, 2004b) and the other from Southeast Asia (UNAIDS, 2004a). They contain stories and photographs of young people, religious and spiritual leaders, entertainment and sports figures, community activists, public servants, educators, business people and health workers. These pioneers 'are leading a response to the HIV/AIDS epidemic in their communities and countries [and] reflect about why they speak out and are committed to action. A few of them have HIV in their blood. All have it some way in their lives' (UNAIDS, 2004a: 1). They 'tell how AIDS has made them a better doctor, researcher, legislator, citizen or person' (UNAIDS, 2004b: 9), how AIDS has helped them see who they want to be, such as Sapana Pradham-Malla, a 42-year-old woman lawyer from Nepal, who writes: 'When I hear their voices, their stories, then I'm inspired to take up a fight for their rights' (UNAIDS, 2004b: 47).

Similar in appearance and format – although closer to the lived reality of HIV – is a publication called *Unheard Voices, Hidden Lives* (International HIV/AIDS Alliance, 2006). Through the Alliance's Frontiers Prevention Project, representatives of organizations of men who have sex with men, sex workers and HIV-positive people participated in workshops in Cambodia, Ecuador and India. They were given cameras and training and asked to use photography to tell the stories of their lives and their communities. The intention of the collection of striking images and words was that 'the experiences of people living at the frontiers of the global HIV epidemic are all too often unheard and unseen. The individuals in this book ... invite us to share, in their own images and words, their experiences, hopes, and fears of living in a world irreversibly touched by HIV' (International HIV/AIDS Alliance, 2006: 3). Fear and hope, two commonly juxtaposed experiences of HIV, are reflected in this excerpt from Chet Thol, a 45-year-old HIV-positive man from Cambodia: 'I remember when I first became aware that I was infected with HIV. I was very afraid that people in my community would come to know about my status. Later on, when I dared to show my face to the community, then my life got better' (International HIV/AIDS Alliance, 2006: 19).

A contrasting medium is a DVD called *Living Art: HIV/AIDS at Center Stage* (Smith, 2005), produced as a documentary of the cultural program of the 2004 AIDS Conference in Bangkok, with this written on the disk: 'a dynamic view of the innovative use of culture and the arts in the global response to the AIDS epidemic'. It is rich in its presentation of the diversity of the arts that permeated every corner of the international conference: music, theater, painting, electronic media, performance, design, dance (our friends from TASO inspire on-screen as they do in person) and even aerial acrobatics with the Ribbon of Hope, a gigantic red AIDS ribbon on which breathtaking feats were performed by an HIV-positive artist. Each person featured and interviewed in the DVD's stories shared the sentiment that people need to be touched in as many ways as possible, and the arts can reach into our humanity in ways that the sciences cannot. The research reported in this book also presents a range of artistic expression including cartoon drawings (cf. Harriet Mutonyi & Maureen Kendrick, this volume); drama and role plays (cf. Christina Higgins, this volume); and photo-voice and video (cf. Claudia Mitchell *et al.*, this volume).

The most powerful storytelling medium is meeting people affected by HIV in person. In November 2007, I went with workshop participants to visit Baan Gerda, a purpose-built village about four hours' drive north of Bangkok. Its residents include 75 children and 18 adult 'parents', all HIV-positive, who live together in a community that was started by a German former businessman and his Thai wife. Well integrated into the neighboring villages and schools, it is an example of how stigma and discrimination can be lessened when HIV-negative people have a chance to meet and know positive people. The children are all AIDS orphans or abandoned and the parents are either AIDS widows or HIV-positive couples, and they are all on ARVs. Our workshop was part of the planning process of an international child NGO (non-governmental organization) I regularly work with, as they outlined an HIV strategy for their programs across Asia. In dialogue with the staff of Baan Gerda, the participants were struck by how their questions were responded to with such honesty. When asked how long the children were expected to live, the reply was, 'We don't know, but then none of us know that'. Questioned about the other children's reactions when one of their friends died with AIDS, the answer was, 'It seems our children handle death better than the adults'. The lasting impression of Baan Gerda was that it is a place of life, joy and hope. In the communal dining hall are a series of before-and-after photographs of children when they first arrived, ill with AIDS, and after a short time on ARVs. There was a boy named Oy, next to whose photos were numbers indicating an increase in CD4 count from 23 to 958. We later met Oy on his way from school to lunch, a healthy-looking, smiling child, walking, chatting and laughing with his friends.

New Life Friends Memories (Phongphit, 1999) is a book-length translated collection of life stories of poor HIV-positive people in Thailand, all of whom found themselves eventually as members of New Life Friends, a community-based organization for HIV and AIDS support. In the book's foreword, Thai social critic Prawes Wasi engages and inspires us with these words:

> While reading the book you are now holding, try, if you can, to involve your mind, spirit, and wisdom ... People who have encountered death, but do not die, have undergone a spiritual transformation that makes them seem like new persons ... HIV-positive people who have come so close to death that they have risen beyond the fear of dying are simply enlightened. They possess energy to give life, and energy to contribute to the betterment of society (p ii) ... Do not be surprised if, in the future, we hear news of HIV-positive people attaining enlightenment ... Freedom has become their immunity, warding off even negative societal attitudes, which are comparable to diseases (p iii).

Among the many enlightened words from *New Life Friends*, listen to these from a woman named Sonthaya (Phongphit, 1999: 53–54):

> I am glad to have written [my story] since it has allowed me to have a chance to recall my life. Sometimes it has been painful, but it has helped me discover myself and string together my forty long years. Writing an autobiography brings pain, but bitterness becomes a healing – the more bitter it is, the more curative it becomes. After finishing my story, I felt relieved. I did not need to forget or pretend to forget the past. This was my own life.

A powerful argument for telling and listening to stories of experiences of HIV is because this is healing, not only for HIV-positive storytellers, but also for those who can be healed of misconceptions, misunderstandings, prejudices, stigmatization and fear, and ultimately, idealistically and optimistically, for the world. Margaret Wheatley writes:

> I believe we can change the world if we start listening to one another again. Simple, honest, human conversation. Not mediation, negotiation, problem-solving, debate, or public meetings. Simple, truthful conversation where we each have a chance to speak, we each feel heard, and we each listen well (Wheatley, 2002: 3). "You can't hate someone whose story you know." You don't have to like the story, or even the person telling you their story. But listening creates a relationship. We move closer to one another (Wheatley, 2002: 91) ... If we can speak our story and know that others hear it, we are somehow healed by that. (Wheatley, 2005: 218)

From these deeply personal interpretations of the healing capacity of storytelling, we reach out to the curative power of stories to change others' perceptions about us and to join us together. 'Imagining a person's life as a collage of stories challenges the notion that there are some specifications somewhere about what a person is supposed to be like', writes Ann Jauregui (2007: 108). And Adam Kahane (2004: 102) writes: 'When people choose to tell a personal story . . ., they are revealing something of themselves. They are sharing what matters to them . . . Furthermore, because (in Carl Rogers' paradoxical phrase) "what is most personal is most universal", these stories also illuminate the source of . . . shared commitment.' As Pavlenko (2007: 180) summarizes:

> Several characteristics make autobiographic narratives into unique and appealing foci of applied linguistics inquiry. They are interesting and thus have aesthetic value and can engage the readers. They are accessible and thus can appeal to larger audiences. They are also textual and thus have reflective value for their authors and for the readers who are encouraged to imagine alternative ways of being in the world. Most importantly, they are transformative as they shift the power relationship between researchers and participants, and between teachers and learners, making the object of the inquiry into the subject and granting the subject both agency and voice.

A powerful example of what is possible at an interface of education and research, language and stories, people and insight, and HIV and AIDS is Patti Lather's (1997) account of the writing of and reaction to *Troubling the Angels: Women Living with HIV/AIDS*, which she co-wrote with Chris Smithies (1997). The book is a collection of women's narratives about 'the day-to-day realities of living with the disease, relationships, efforts to make sense of the disease in their lives, death and dying issues, and the role of support groups' (Lather, 1997: 286). The book is complex: two prefaces, one about the book, and another about the women; narrative chapters of the interview data; sidebars containing resources, information, demographics and references; 'angel inter texts and illustrations that use the reemergence of angels in popular culture, especially AIDS discourses' (Lather, 1997: 286); subtext commentary, where the authors tell stories of carrying out the research; writing by the women themselves and an 'epilogue that updates the reader on each of the women and the support groups and includes their reactions to the desktop published version of the book' (Lather, 1997: 287). The book is inspirational in numerous ways, for example, the academic risks that it took in 'break[ing] down the usual codes we bring to reading' (Lather, 1997: 287), articulating 'the capacity of AIDS to shock us into a different relation with the future' (Lather, 1997: 291), and 'saying yes to life in the face of disaster, sickness, murder, cruelty and senseless death (Lather, 1997: 293).

A Wholeness of Self

I have become increasingly aware that my wellness has been related to the ever closer unity between my personal and professional selves, to the power of questions that are emerging to guide my growth toward authenticity and wholeness, and to an understanding and acceptance of realities of life in its psychological, emotional and social dimensions. Central to this awareness has been the struggle toward more honesty, trust and risk-taking in all relationships.

After my diagnosis in 1995, a notion began formulating in my mind, stimulated by reading somewhere what the Vietnamese Buddhist monk Thich Nhat Hanh said about people needing to find the one big idea that would drive their lives. Mine was a question: 'What sort of person do I want to be?' I could ask what sort of friend, professional, brother, facilitator, son, colleague, partner, citizen or teacher do I want to be. I suppose it was as these thoughts were coming together that I also realized that becoming infected with HIV was a gift. And if it was a gift, then it had to be shared, which meant that I would need to start telling more people, and bringing it more into my world as a part of my self, and to the outer world by sharing my personal story of HIV. To reach such a place of wholeness, I would need to find ways of not just balancing my personal and professional selves, but of bringing them together as one. Yet I am once again soberingly reminded of places and perceptions of privilege by Mark Finn and Srikant Sarangi (this volume): 'The very idea of living an empowered life and of being able to make healthy decisions is for many HIV-positive people in India an unrealistic fantasy'.

I had a conversation with a dear friend who worked for a health-related international NGO on a project in South Africa, engaging with straight men around issues of violence against women in domestic relationships and how this interfaced with HIV. My friend talked about the typical sorts of factors that determine whether men go for HIV testing, for example awareness, cost, access, location and confidentiality. When he reached a pause in his description, I said, 'My experience of finally taking myself to get tested had little to do with any of that'. It had much more to do with fear and a subconscious recognition I now have that what led me to unsafe sexual behaviors lay deep and dark in my psyche, in a place that we do not often let ourselves dwell and that we certainly do not talk about with others. I can see how I was subconsciously telling myself that I would rather die of AIDS than live with Huntington's disease, and how if my sister could do it (die), then so could I; such was the profound impact of those circumstances on me. I do not think that there was a direct link between these kinds of psychological sentiments and not practicing safe sex: 'I'm not worried about condoms because these two things have happened to me'. Rather, there was a mental unwellness that seemingly disabled me from being protective of myself and others. Just writing that scares me now, and I will certainly spend the rest of my days trying to understand and learning to accept. The point I was trying to make to my friend was that it is not just about practicing safe sex or getting tested or other program interventions. It is also about the complexity of individual people. As other contributors to this volume write: 'For safe sex messages to be successful, promoting condom use alone is not enough' (Henrike Körner), and it is not enough to 'assume that knowledge of unsafe sexual practices will lead to changes in behavior and lifestyle' (Shelley Jones and Bonny Norton). So much of the work done in HIV treats people in their general populations and constructed norms of behavior. Where are the efforts at working with the realities of people's lives and perceptions of their selves?

Journeying from Fear to Healing

I close this chapter by reflecting on the part of life's journey that has taken me professionally from being a language teacher and academic to being a facilitator in the context of organizational and community development, and on a personal transformation from living in fear to wanting to reach out to people, groups and communities with a curiosity about all the potentials for healing that may be possible.

After a few fits and starts in trying to figure out 'what I was going to be', I completed an MA in English as a second language at the University of Hawai'i in the mid-1980s, taught English for almost a year in Saudi Arabia and then in August 1989 took up a faculty position at the Asian Institute of Technology near Bangkok, Thailand. The center I worked in was fertile ground for exploring alternative language learning and teaching approaches, enabling me to have the experience of writing and publishing in the field, including a few efforts that seemed to have stood out in their time, such as Savage and Storer (1992) and Kenny and Savage (1997). What those and other pieces of work had in common, in retrospect, was creating the conditions through which people could find their voices, where divergent viewpoints could be expressed and heard, and different experiences lived and valued. This took me along a path of becoming what might be called an organizational and community development facilitator, working with international and local NGOs, international organizations (various United Nations entities) and government agencies, involving strategic planning, communications strategies and resource mobilization, among other initiatives, and in fields such as agriculture, child rights and fisheries, among others.

In early 2006 I had my first opportunities to work as an HIV-positive facilitator with two HIV-related organizations, one based in Bangkok and the other in Dhaka, Bangladesh. In putting together the back-to-back strategic planning process designs (the first a retreat and the second a workshop), I thought that if the two organizations were going to be able to work through what needed to happen to realize the kind of change in their professional space that they envisioned for themselves, they would have to 'get personal' about it, to rediscover who they all were as individuals, as people and as colleagues. Did they really know, had they ever heard about, what other people's motivations were for working with HIV and AIDS? Had they ever had a chance to tell anyone else why they had chosen this work? It seemed to me that we needed a session in each event where people would tell each other stories of their own experiences of HIV.

Inspired by the work of Adam Kahane, who wrote about taking groups of workshop participants outdoors to shift the spaces of talking and listening, I was happy when retreat participants asked whether we could hold any of the sessions outside, located as we were up in the mountains about two hours from Bangkok. We walked up to a ridge-with-a-view, and three groups of six or seven sat under shade trees several meters apart and told each other their HIV and AIDS stories. I walked among the groups and listened to a few stories from each, emotionally moved with others as I heard the wide range of people's experiences. We all came back together in a circle at the largest shady spot and people from each group talked about how they felt as they listened to the stories, how they had decided to share them and some examples. We ran the storytelling session in a similar way during the second organization's workshop, though occupying rather different spaces inside their staff house in Dhaka.

When the participants in both events had finished reporting back to each other, I suggested that since I had asked them to tell their stories, I wanted to tell my own. I spoke about the learning that I had done over the years since I tested HIV-positive in December 1995, how I had responded to the great fears as they entered and left my life one after the other, how I had come to know what it meant to need and want and begin to change one's life. I wrapped up my story by talking about fear, and how we might face and overcome it through honesty (becoming our authentic selves), trust (in ourselves, in others and others in us) and risk (deciding to do what seems impossible, as long as it is with pure intentions). My story seemed to resonate with people in both groups, many of whom spoke afterwards about appreciating the honesty it implied, the trust it showed I had in them, the risk I must have known I was taking to make my relationship with them more personal, while working together in a professional space. Honesty, trust and risk – all of these came up in discussions time and again during the two events.

At first I thought there had to be something special that an HIV-positive person could bring to a group of people who work in the field of HIV and AIDS. I now understand that it is not the reality of being positive, which is just a fact, a piece of information, but rather what someone has done with that to change themselves. One could imagine a person living with HIV not having a story that would be helpful in any way to another group of people, just as there are HIV-negative people with stories that are. What are the possibilities for bringing people together so that we are 'working with difference', bringing together and working through different perceptions, opinions, knowledge, experiences and ways of working? As Adam Kahane (2004: 127) writes, 'Our job as facilitators and leaders is simply to help create a clean, safe space. Then the healing will occur'. I am curious about all the kinds of healing that may be possible. What follows is one last story, when I authentically felt myself in a place that was both personal and professional, and healing.

On the final afternoon of my visit to Dhaka for the HIV strategy workshop there, I was asked to meet with some members of a self-help group for HIV-positive people that the organization had been supporting. One of their leaders was in our strategy workshop and felt that my story would be helpful to his friends. We gathered in a meeting room, about 20 people altogether, women and men whom I perceived to represent different socioeconomic circumstances and sexualities, including one of the organization's staff who acted as our Bangla–English interpreter.

I began the session by telling my story in much the same way as I had done during the strategic planning workshops. Facilitated by our interpreter, other people told their stories. As I listened to each woman and man in turn, I was once again reminded of how vastly different most people's realities of being HIV-positive are from mine. A man sitting across the table from me spoke last, with a story not unlike those told by others that evening. If we listed all of the worst possible things that could happen to a person who tests positive for HIV in Bangladesh, they had happened to him. His name was published in the newspaper; he was violently ostracized from his village, family, wife and children; he lost his employment, was refused entry into hospital and ended up utterly alone. As part of its HIV work, the organization monitors these sorts of occurrences, finding people whose names are made public, bringing them to a safe place and eventually working with their communities to try to create the conditions under which people can return. This man and his community were such a case.

Once he had finished speaking, our interpreter suggested that we could all ask each other questions about our stories. The first and only one came from this man across the table, who asked me, 'Are you married?' Assuming I had made my homosexuality clear when I told my story, I said, 'No, I'm gay'. The interpreter asked me to phrase my response a different way, as he would not be able to translate 'gay'. 'OK', I thought quickly, 'In 25 words or less, what does it mean to be gay?' 'Tell him I'm not sexually attracted to women', I said. The man looked at me as if he had heard something repugnant about me, and then as quickly his countenance changed from hateful to something between sadness and compassion.

With tears in his eyes, he spoke: 'I have just told you all a story of my experience of being HIV-positive. I ended by saying that the most important thing I have learned is that I never again want to judge or be judged by other people as happened to me. And yet, when I heard what Bill said, I immediately thought badly of him, and then I just as suddenly was aware of what I had done. So what I have learned from this is that, no matter how far we think we've come, we always have a long way to go'. We all sat in that still, quiet place until we got up to thank each other and bid each other farewell.

References

Bell, J.S. (2002) Narrative inquiry: More than just telling stories. *TESOL Quarterly* 36 (2), 207–213.

Canagarajah, A.S. (1996) From critical research practice to critical research reporting. *TESOL Quarterly* 30, 321–331.

International HIV/AIDS Alliance (2006) *Unheard Voices, Hidden Lives*. Brighton: International HIV/AIDS Alliance.

Jauregui, A. (2007) *Epiphanies: Where Science and Miracles Meet*. New York, NY: Atria Books; Hillsboro, OR: Beyond Words Publishing.

Kahane, A. (2004) *Solving Tough Problems: An Open Way of Talking, Listening, and Creating New Realities*. San Francisco: Berrett-Koehler Publishers, Inc.

Kenny, B. and Savage, W. (eds) (1997) *Language and Development: Teachers in a Changing World*. Essex: Addison Wesley Longman.

Lather, P. (1997) Drawing the line at angels: Working the ruins of feminist ethnography. *Qualitative Studies in Education* 10 (3), 285–304.

Lather, P. and Smithies, C. (1997) *Troubling the Angels: Women Living with HIV/AIDS*. Boulder, CO: Westview.

Pavlenko, A. (2007) Autobiographic narratives as data in applied linguistics. *Applied Linguistics* 28 (2), 163–188.

Phongphit, S. (1999) *New Life Friends Memories*. Chiang Mai, Thailand: AidsNet.

Savage, W. and Storer, G. (1992) An emergent language program framework: Actively involving learners in needs analysis. *System* 20 (2), 187–199.

Smith, J. (director/producer) (2005) *Living Art: HIV/AIDS at Center Stage* (DVD). Auckland, New Zealand: Southern Moon Productions.

UNAIDS (2004a) *From Southeast Asia and the Pacific: Portraits of Commitment – Why People Become Leaders in HIV/AIDS Work*. Bangkok: Asia Pacific Leadership Forum on HIV & AIDS, UNAIDS.

UNAIDS (2004b) *South Asia Portraits of Commitment*. Bangkok: Asia Pacific Leadership Forum on HIV & AIDS, UNAIDS.

Wheatley, M.J. (2002) *Turning to One Another: Simple Conversations to Restore Hope to the Future*. San Francisco: Berrett-Koehler Publishers, Inc.

Wheatley, M.J. (2005) *Finding Our Way: Leadership For an Uncertain Time*. San Francisco: Berrett-Koehler Publishers, Inc.

Chapter 2

Ugandan Students' Visual Representations of Health Literacies: A Focus on HIV/AIDS Knowledge

HARRIET MUTONYI and MAUREEN E. KENDRICK

Introduction

In this chapter, we focus on the insightful and multi-layered ways in which Ugandan youth use cartoon drawings to represent the social, cultural, psychological and physiological context of their HIV/AIDS knowledge. Uganda is considered the first African country to success-fully reduce the rates of HIV infection in the larger populace (Stoneburner & Low-Beer, 2004; USAID, 2002). The apparent success for combating the spread of HIV/AIDS in Uganda has been partly due to the use of various media for communicating messages about AIDS that are sensi-tive to the socio-cultural world of Ugandans. The messages are geared towards having an HIV-free generation in Uganda. Therefore the messages are designed to (1) increase individual and community awareness of HIV/AIDS risk and to take appropriate health action; (2) stimulate and support community action to control HIV; and (3) advocate for an enabling environment for the prevention and control of HIV in Uganda (IEC Unit, Ministry of Health, 2002). In 2005, the Presidential Initiative for AIDS Strategy for Communicating to Youth (PIASCY) was launched. The initiative aims at promoting behavioural change among youth through open discussions that address their particular cultural, social and political challenges. Ugandan youth are particularly targeted in public HIV and AIDS messages because they are the most vulnerable population for new infections (Ministry of Education and Sports/PIASCY, 2005).

To have an effective communication strategy that penetrates the whole population strata (rural-urban), and is consistent with cultural ideologies (oral and written), multi-modal forms of representation have been used in public HIV/AIDS messages including visual (e.g. advertising billboards, cartoons and television), oral (e.g. radio presentations) and embodied (e.g. drama presentations). Although students in Uganda have been exposed in the wider society to such multi-modal tools of representation, they are rarely given opportunities to use these available modes within classrooms where language remains the predominant form of representation. Kress (2000) provides some insights into why language is privileged in many cultures. He writes:

> There is a general assumption that language is a communicational and representational medium which is fully adequate to the expression of anything that we might want to express: that anything that we think, feel, sense, can be said (or written) in language. (Kress, 2000: 193)

Given that students bring to the classroom knowledge and meaning-making tools that have been constructed and developed from their everyday lives outside school, our challenge as researchers was to design a study that enabled students to transform their knowledge into modes of representation that fully express their understandings of HIV/AIDS.

Research consistently shows that drawing as a means of investigating what students know has the potential to modify verbal knowledge as the dominant mode of representation (Peterson, 1997). Only a limited number of educational researchers, however, have used visual images such as drawings to investigate students' knowledge and understanding of particular topics and concepts (Peterson, 1997; Prosser, 1998; Weber & Mitchell, 1995; Wetton & McWhirter, 1998). In this study, we examine the use of drawing as a tool for understanding students' conceptualizations of HIV/AIDS by addressing the question: 'How do Ugandan Senior Three Students use cartoons to represent their knowledge of HIV/AIDS?' Students were asked to produce 'cartoons' rather than drawings because they indicated that they associate the word drawing with 'artistic' drawing and they were not 'talented' in this way. Cartooning, on the other hand, allowed them to draw what they call 'stick images' without paying special attention to positioning and spatial relationships from a purely aesthetic perspective. For all of these secondary students, cartooning was a familiar mode of communication used extensively in public education campaigns that target youth. As such, the students did not have preconceived notions of school-sanctioned standards for how cartoons should look or how they should function. We present 11 illustrative examples that exemplify the kinds of visual narratives that this group of students constructed.

Context

In order to reach the youth, HIV/AIDS-related programs were introduced into school curricula and extracurricular activities in Uganda in 1994 (Mirembe, 2002). The government of Uganda also initiated the 'sex education policy' in 2002 as a way of protecting school children from HIV/AIDS and early pregnancies (Nakazinga, 2004). The major objectives of these programs and policies were to help teachers provide information on HIV/AIDS, train girls to avoid sexual advances from men and create awareness about the dangers of early pregnancies. Private individuals have also joined the struggle to provide a forum for the exchange of knowledge. For example, the 'Straight Talk' newspaper and radio talk shows funded by UNICEF and USAID provide such forums. Although the programs are aimed at empowering girls, there are other unaccounted for factors that may hinder the girls from attaining the full benefits of such programs.

In Uganda, designated family members traditionally introduce sex education when young people are preparing for marriage. For this reason, the sex education policy has had only limited community support. Nakazinga (*New Vision*, Oct 2004) reports that there are some people who argue that sex education at early stages works against cultural values. The report quoted one elder of the community Kyazike, saying 'sex and its education is sacred, it should be taught to those preparing for marriage not pupils in primary schools'. Because of the sacred place sex education has traditionally held within communities, talking about sex publicly in many African communities is considered taboo (Fuglesang, 1997). Some studies show that with sex being a taboo topic, some teachers fear to transgress these cultural barriers and provide sex education even though they are mandated to do so (Kinsman *et al.*, 2001; Kiwawulo, 2004).

Theoretical Perspectives

When students are asked about their understandings of particular topics, ideas and concepts, they respond by presenting 'representations' (Bruner, 1964). Gilbert and Boulter (2000) refer to such representations as mental models – personal cognitive representations held by an individual. The only way to understand students' mental models of a particular phenomenon is by eliciting one or more of their expressed models of that phenomenon (Reiss *et al.*, 2007). Although there are multiple ways of collecting information about students' understandings of scientific phenomena, the vast majority of these methods rely on talking or writing. The need to take a completely fresh look at multiple modes of representation in theories of communication and to re-evaluate how we use different symbol systems to represent meaning has been well argued by Kress (2000). He stresses that it is critically important for this new agenda to include the full range of semiotic modes and a full understanding of their potentials and limitations in particular societies.

In this research, we adopt what has been referred to in education as a multi-modal perspective, which assumes that 'meanings are made, distributed, received, interpreted and remade in interpretation through many representational and communicative modes – not just through language' (Kress & Jewitt, 2003: 1). We draw on social semiotics, which, according to Kress and van Leeuwen (1996), is an attempt to explain and understand how signs are used to produce and communicate meanings across social settings from families to institutions. Signs created through drawings simultaneously communicate the here and now of a social context while representing the resources individuals have 'to hand' from the world around them (Kress, 1997; Vygotsky, 1978). The meanings also reflect reality as imagined by sign makers and influenced by their beliefs, values and biases.

Visual anthropology also broadly informs our understanding of multiple modes of representation within specific social and cultural settings. Visual anthropologists contend, 'much that is observable, much that can be learned about a culture can be recorded most effectively and comprehensively through film, photography or by drawing' (Banks & Murphy, 1997: 14). They also argue that neglecting visual data may be a reflection of the Western bias (the privileging of the intellectual over the experiential or phenomenological) or neglecting the importance of visual phenomena across cultures. Their position does not require that visual methods be used in all contexts but used where appropriate, with the caveat that appropriateness may not be obvious from the outset of the study. Traditionally, researchers rather than research participants have used visual modes for recording culture. We view our participants as co-researchers and put the visual tools for drawing in their hands to enhance our understanding of their HIV/AIDS knowledge.

Research Methodology

This is an interpretive qualitative case study (Gallagher & Tobin, 1991; Merriam, 1998; Stake, 1995, 1998; Yin, 2003) involving Senior Three (S.3) or

Grade 11 biology classes from four Eastern Ugandan high schools. The four schools varied in status and represented typical public high schools in Uganda; that is, girls-only boarding, boys-only boarding, mixed-boarding and mixed-day schools. S.3 classes were selected because HIV/AIDS is part of the S.3 biology curriculum and, more importantly, this age group is considered highly at risk of contracting HIV/AIDS (Uganda AIDS Commission, 2002). The participants were those studying biology at the S.3 level who were willing to take part in the study. Biology students were chosen because the aim of the research was to investigate students' understandings of HIV/AIDS, including how their prior knowledge and experience impact student interaction with classroom instruction on HIV/AIDS (see Mutonyi, 2005).

Discussion of HIV/AIDS issues directly related to sexual issues is generally taboo, and adults and young people (adolescents included) do not talk easily about sexual matters in formal settings, particularly in the presence of outsiders (Nyanzi*et al.*, 2001). The research design therefore required a methodology that provided an atmosphere of safety, allowing students to express their knowledge of HIV/AIDS, sexuality and social behavior. One section of a questionnaire was developed to allow students to use both text and drawing to convey their understanding of HIV/AIDS (Anderson, 1990). The question was 'What would be your own slogan for HIV/AIDS? Illustrate in a cartoon form the message your slogan would convey about HIV/AIDS. Explain the message your cartoon is conveying'. In total, 160 students completed the questionnaire; 120 of these students (62/75 boys and 58/85 girls) completed the cartoon portion of the questionnaire. In this chapter, we focus exclusively on the cartoons as visual representations of the students' HIV/AIDS knowledge.

We use an adaptation of Warburton (1998) analytic framework to explore what the cartoons as mediated images might mean. Warburton suggests that the analysis of cartoons from a research perspective centers on two categories of questions: (1) what are we actually looking at? and (2) what can we say about it and how can we make use of it? Using these questions as an overarching guide, the drawings were collaboratively coded and analysed by both researchers through the following levels of interpretation: *initial description* (What visual and textual material is contained within the cartoon? Who and what are represented?), *immediate connotation* (What does the cartoon count for publicly? What does the image/text signify?), *systemic connotation* (What is the place and status of the cartoon with respect to the communication system or systems it is part of? What are the connotations of the image/text?), *establishing narrative threads* (For what/whom was the cartoon intended?

What is the relationship between the cartoon and broader discourses on HIV/AIDS?).

To extend the analysis, we used Jewitt and Oyama's (2001) framework for analysing health-related visual images, focusing particularly on the underlying assumptions of gender representations that can be deduced from the cartoon drawings. In the analysis, we include general concepts of narrative visual analysis in relation to participants (e.g. represented/non-represented and interactive participants) (Jewitt & Oyama, 2001; Kress & van Leeuwen, 1996). The combination of descriptive frameworks used in the analysis allowed us to uncover a visual narrative that was not initially evident. These narratives helped us raise questions about the possible meanings of the cartoons in relation to broader theories and discourses on health literacy and public and cultural constructions of HIV/AIDS.

In the following section, we present our analysis of 11 cartoon drawings (by five boys and six girls), which are used as illustrative examples of the predominant themes portrayed by this group of 120 students in their visual conceptualizations of HIV/AIDS.

Findings

The students' visual depictions of their conceptualizations of HIV/ AIDS were categorized into four groups: *Prostitutes and Sugar Daddies* (transactional sexual relationships), *Learning the ABCs* (HIV/AIDS prevention knowledge), *Fighting Stigmatization in Community Relations with HIV-Positive Persons*, and *The New Reality of HIV/AIDS*. The drawings also had gendered messages especially in relation to *learning the ABCs*. Details of the gendered nature of the drawings are included in the analysis and discussion of the cartoons.

Prostitutes and sugar daddies

Of the 120 students, 30 (17 girls and 13 boys) portrayed men or women (of different age groups) in transactional sexual relationships such as prostitution or relationships between older men and younger women. The various ways such relationships are shaped were represented in these three selected drawings.

Cartoon 1: Abel (male)
Abel's cartoon portrays prostitution as a transactional sexual relationship and how it leads to the spread of HIV/AIDS (Figure 2.1). The picture can be divided into left and right portions. On the left, two people (one

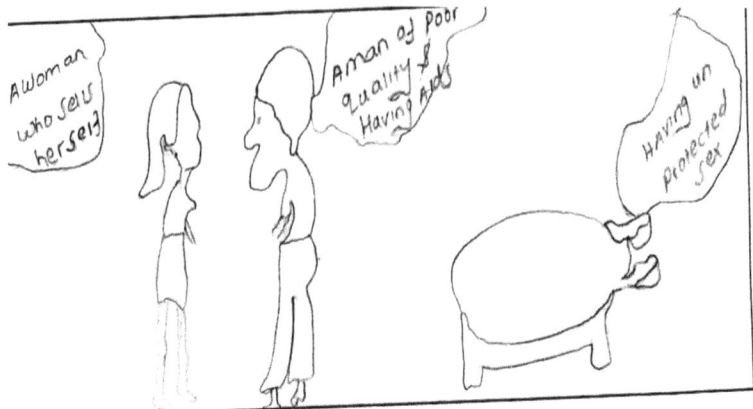

Figure 2.1 Abel

female and one male) are having a conversation and on the right, they are
having sex. The picture proceeds in a time sequence: on the left, the man
and woman are negotiating a sexual relationship and on the right, they are
engaging in sex. The accompanying text reads: 'a woman who sells herself'
and 'a man of poor quality and having AIDS' 'having unprotected sex'.
These represented participants are the subject of the cartoon's main narrative, that is, the role transactional sex plays in the HIV epidemic in Uganda.
The first narrative is that prostitutes expose themselves to HIV infection
because of the type of clients they serve. Abel knows that having protected
sex through condom use with an HIV-infected person prevents HIV transmission. His cartoon, however, indirectly raises the paradoxical question
of what options for protected sex exist for prostitutes if their clients refuse
to use condoms. Put differently, how can they ensure their own protection
but fulfill the wishes of their clients as well? The woman is depicted as a
victim. The salient message is that HIV can be preventable for males if
they choose to use a condom.

Cartoon 2: Tolophina (female)
    Tolophina includes a series of pictures linked to the narrative captions:
'I am worried my friend Susan have HIV/AIDS' and 'Susan on streets
with other men b'se she had arrived at Kampala'. On the left side of the
picture, two people – Susan and a man – are depicted as engaged in a
sexual transaction (Figure 2.2). 'How much are you going to pay me?' is
written in Susan's speech bubble; her extended arm directed towards the
man communicates her active role in soliciting the interaction. The man's

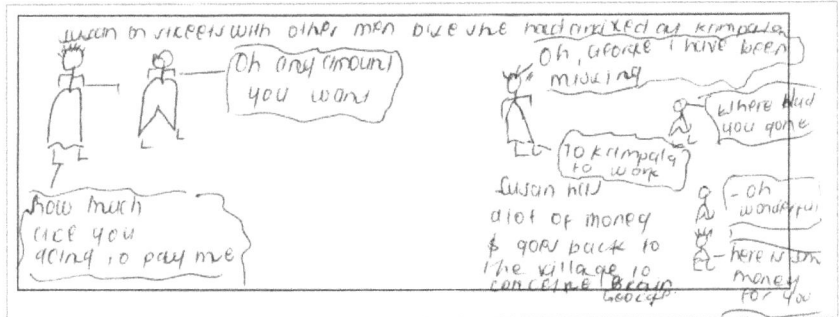

Figure 2.2 Tolophina

body is positioned away from Susan, which indicates a more passive role in the interaction. In the second frame of the cartoon, Susan's body positioning creates a direct line to George, the boy, and again establishes her active role in the interaction. George's body directed away from the girl adds to the narrative the possibility of someone or something that is not represented in the picture. In the final frame of the narrative, Susan is represented in a position of power over George. The representation of Susan in an active role in initiating transactional relationships to earn money and in maintaining romantic relationships with the lure of money emphasizes the vulnerability of all those who have sex with prostitutes rather than the vulnerability of the prostitutes themselves. This notion of vulnerability is further emphasized by the unknown in relation to George's gaze and body positioning in both the second and third sequence of the narrative.

The narrative portrayed in Tolophina's cartoon also represents the link between socio-economic status and HIV/AIDS, and how HIV gets spread among urban and rural people in Uganda. The narrative indicates that George and Susan had been friends in the village, but Susan ends up going to Kampala to work as a prostitute. Often, girls from poor families might resort to prostitution to survive, which may very well be the case with Susan. The cartoonist makes reference to Kampala because of the status it most likely carries in the conversation with George, who may never have been to the city. Prostitution in Uganda is most predominant in Kampala. Because of these circumstances, Tolophina is concerned that Susan has been exposed to possible HIV infection. George, on the other hand, is portrayed as innocent and in love with Susan, who takes advantage of his trust. He happily accepts the money she earns as a prostitute, possibly because he is also poor. Despite the central messages of sexual faithfulness in the Ugandan HIV campaign, this cartoon portrays some of the circumstances under which partners may be unfaithful. Tolophina depicts the girl as the actor rather than the more typical victim. She also portrays the rural male as vulnerable to the city savvy female.

Cartoon 3: Klere (female)

Central to Klere's cartoon are two people: one man and one girl. The written title for the cartoon reads, 'I would say no to sex [abstain from sex]' (Figure 2.3). The man is offering something to the girl, saying, 'Please have this [tea and sugar] I love you. I want to have sex with you'. The action created by his outstretched arms is blocked on his left by the girl's gesture of refusal, who says, 'I don't want free things are dangerous they can make one get HIV/AIDS'. The man's outstretched right arm, however, establishes the possibility of a non-represented participant or a network of participants, which links the viewer into the narrative as a possible recipient of the gifts. This 'sugar daddy' relationship whereby young girls are lured into a sexual relationship with an older man by offers of gifts is a transactional sexual relationship not dissimilar to prostitution. According to the students who participated in this study, the men are often older and the gifts are usually related to what the girls need or want, for example, clothing or jewelry or sometimes school fees. This cartoonist's message advocates for abstinence by saying no to gifts.

The Ugandan HIV/AIDS curriculum is geared towards empowering young women to say no to the pressures to have sex. Refusing a gift gives

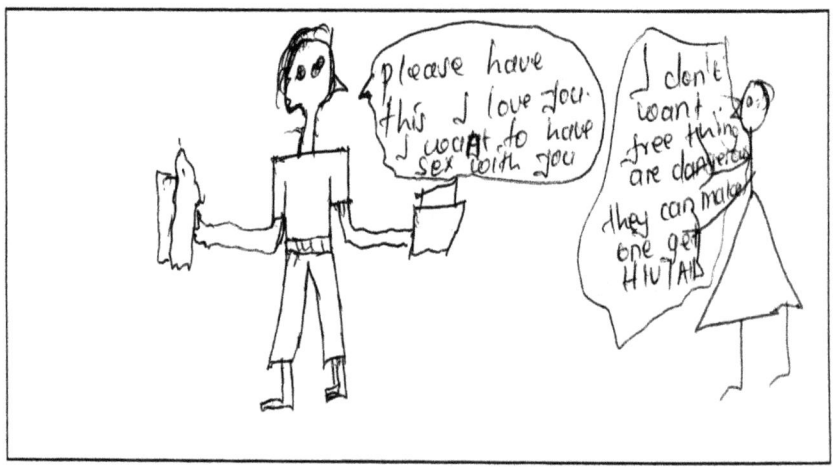

Figure 2.3 Klere

girls the ability to say no without any consequences. The other message embedded in this cartoon is the slogan 'love is not sex', found in the school compounds of the students who participated in this study. The slogan is meant to empower young people not to associate sex with love or love with sex but rather, to instill in them the abstinence slogan 'true love waits', a simplistic way of saying no to sex. The cartoon also empowers a woman to say no to sex if she is not ready. Klere's cartoon communicates that both genders have a role to play in the prevention of HIV/AIDS; by choosing abstinence and insisting that girls can resist the pressure of having sex by refusing gifts from men, she also positions herself as a role model for other girls.

The three cartoon drawings in this section illustrate the pressures young girls face in avoiding HIV/AIDS. According to the new HIV/STD statistics of Uganda, young people aged between 15 and 25 years are 9 times more vulnerable to HIV infection (Ministry of Health [MoH], 2006). The risk is heightened by the cross-generational relationships or 'sugar daddy' relationships that the students have illustrated in their cartoon drawings. The highest prevalence rates of HIV/AIDS are among men who are 45 years and older, and these are reported to be the ones luring young girls into sexual relationships (Mason, 2007). By including non-represented participants, these students vividly depict cross-generational relationships as creating an environment of risk for young girls.

Learning the ABCs

Using condoms

Although some of the students in the questionnaire responses suggested that condom use as a method of HIV prevention is controversial, several of the cartoons focused on condom use as an effective measure against HIV/AIDS. Out of the 120 students, 30 boys created cartoons relating to education programs on condom use for young people. None of the girls represented condom use in their cartoon drawing, which showed a gendered understanding on who needs to know about condom use. Examples include:

Cartoon 4: Opio (male)

Opio's cartoon portrays a learning environment (Figure 2.4). The instructor at the front is male and appears to be ill. His finger, which points to his audience, is raised in an instructional gesture. The audience is sitting on the ground/floor and in close proximity to the instructor who is saying, 'You boys, many people are dying so abstine [abstain]'. The cartoonist's

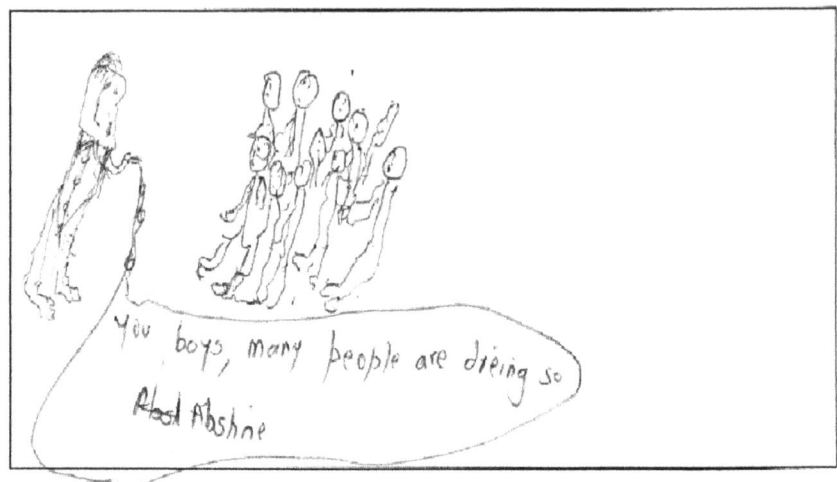

Figure 2.4 Opio

explanatory text states 'Many people in Uganda today are being killed by AIDS because it has no medicine so abstine or have protected sex'. The intended audience, 'you boys', is clearly all male. The group of boys leans rigidly away from the instructor, which raises questions about fear and stigmatization of those with HIV/AIDS.

HIV-infected persons conduct many of the community education programs in Uganda; it is the role of these instructors to caution others not to get infected. They tell their stories and how the disease has affected them both physically and emotionally, and advise the listeners not to follow the same path. The central message portrayed by Opio's cartoon is abstinence, but if one cannot abstain, then use condoms. Clearly, Opio knows that condom use is effective in HIV prevention. His choice of a male audience for his message reflects the reality that it is the men who have the option of using condoms for protected sex, something that women need not learn about.

Cartoon 5: Mugoya (male)

Like Opio, Mugoya's cartoon features a male instructor, in this case, sitting on a stool (Figure 2.5). He is holding a package labeled CD (condom); the gaze of the instructor and audience is directed at the condom. Behind the instructor is a flipchart on a stand upon which is written 'HIV/AIDS/ Use of condoms'. The caption, rather than just mentioning condoms as an HIV/AIDS preventative, emphasizes that people are actually being taught

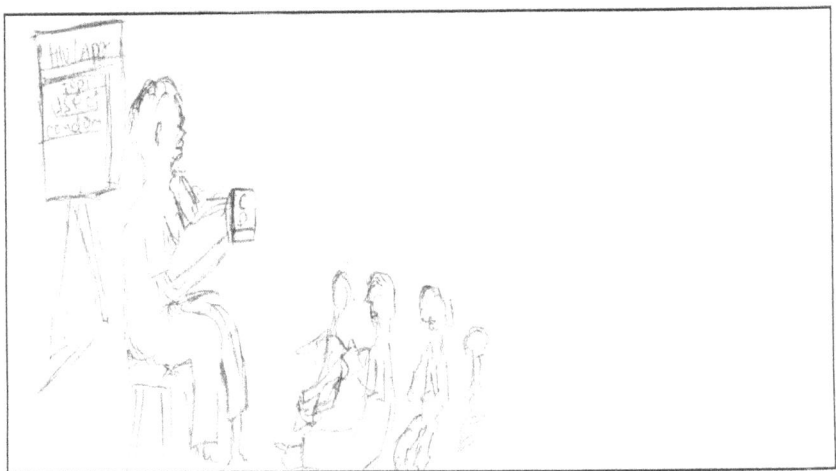

Figure 2.5 Mugoya

how to use a condom. The audience is sitting on the ground near the instructor. Of particular interest is the audience composition, which includes both males and females. The depiction of the instructor in a seated position establishes a sense of trust and equality with the audience.

Mugoya has internalized condom use as an effective measure against HIV infection. In relation to the larger national HIV campaign, he focuses on the C from the ABC formula (Abstinence – Be faithful – Condom use) used in Uganda. Although more recent efforts have emphasized an AB strategy, Mugoya's cartoon recognizes that those who are sexually active need to know about condom use. The inclusion of women in the audience could also mean that the cartoonist advocates for the importance of informing women about condom use as an option for preventing HIV/AIDS.

Cartoon 6: Opondo (male)

Opondo's cartoon is set outdoors amidst a heavy downpour (Figure 2.6). There are three people: one wrapped in a condom, sheltered from the storm; the other two standing side by side in the rain without protection. The cartoonist uses metaphor to convey his message about HIV/AIDS prevention. The rain is labeled 'AIDS/HIV'; the person wrapped in the condom is labeled 'protected sex', whereas the unsheltered people are labeled 'unprotected sex'. The accompanying text reads, 'To stay safe from HIV/AIDS simply abstain from sex or use condoms'.

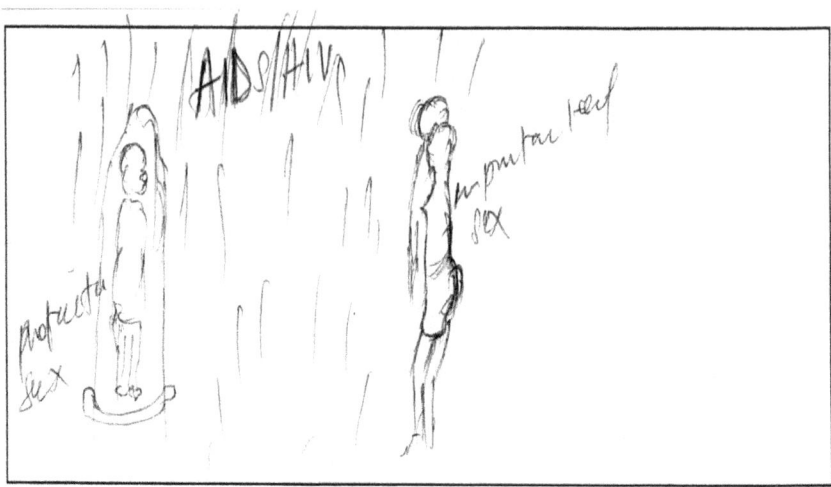

Figure 2.6 Opondo

Similar to several other cartoonists, Opondo demonstrates that he knows that condoms prevent HIV/AIDS and that unprotected sex makes one vulnerable to infection. The person wrapped in the condom does not appear wet while the ones without shelter are soaked, symbolizing their vulnerability to infection. The cartoonist respects the cultural approach to educating people about condom use without being explicit about it. Specifically, he uses rain to represent body fluid and a human life instead of a phallic object (e.g. a banana) to communicate how condoms protect against HIV/AIDS. Literature on African learning states that it is only a wise child who can understand the subtleties of such metaphors (Boateng, 1983; Kanu, 2006; Reagan, 2005); this cartoon shows a high level of creativity and cultural sensitivity in a message that moves beyond more common media messages.

Trying to abstain

Whereas boys tended to create messages that portray condoms as an effective measure against HIV/AIDS, girls more typically focused on abstinence. In total, 40 students, the majority of whom were females (30 girls and 10 boys) pointed out the importance of abstinence for youth. Abstinence messages took the following forms:

Cartoon 7: Wangoye (female)

The caption for this cartoon reads, 'To stay safe, abstain from sex' (Figure 2.7). On the left side of the picture is a young woman, smartly

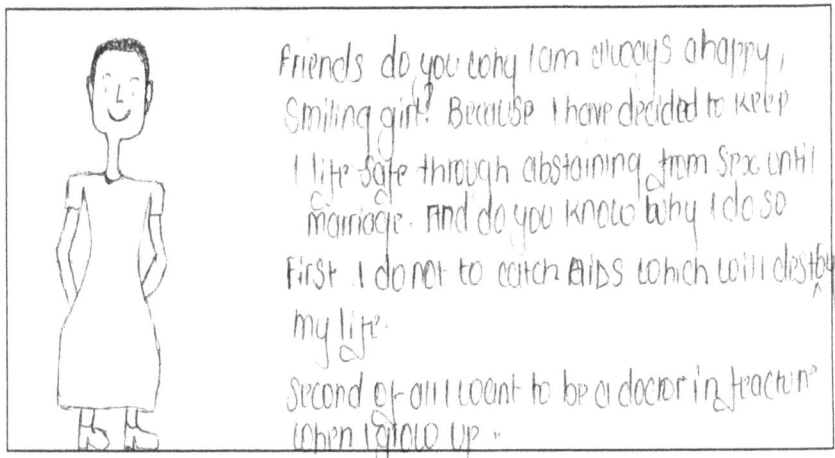

Figure 2.7 Wangoye

dressed in a long short-sleeved dress and high-heeled shoes. Her hair is short. She directs her gaze to the viewer as an interactive participant: 'Friends do you [know] why I am always a happy smiling girl? Because I have decided to keep life safe through abstaining from sex until marriage. And you know why I do so. First I do not catch AIDS which will destroy my life. Second of all I want to be a doctor in future when I grow up'. The text explains why the young woman is smiling and is full of confidence. The cartoonist has internalized the message of abstinence and has made it her option. The message is personalized but includes interactive participants.

To the majority of young females, abstinence is seen as the best preventative option, and cartoons such as this are aligned with public messages about ensuring a bright future by avoiding exposure to HIV/AIDS infection. Numerous billboards tout attractive lifestyles that feature high school and post-secondary graduates who are said to have abstained, attained an education and secured successful careers. Wangoye wants her audience, most likely other young girls, to know that she could be featured on such a billboard. She is abstaining, concentrating on her academics and focusing on her future life as a doctor. Her persuasive message here is that HIV/AIDS can interfere with these goals.

Many of Uganda's HIV-related messages target youth and the national campaign promotes affirmative action for girls and young women through empowerment. Wangoye's cartoon, which emphasizes her ability to make decisions about her sexual health and future, epitomizes this message of empowerment even though the only preventive method over which women have some degree of power is abstinence.

Cartoon 8: Nandudu (female)

Nandudu's cartoon includes three represented participants (Figure 2.8). On the left side of the frame, she has drawn one boy and one girl who are standing together and smiling. 'We are happy coz of abstaining', they say in unison. On the right side, but some distance away, is a pregnant girl. She is frowning, 'Oh my! I wish I had abstained from sex'. The caption for the cartoon is: 'Abstinence is the best way to stay safe'. Nandudu's message emphasizes abstinence and includes pregnancy as one of the additional challenges of early sex faced by young girls.

Again, Nandudu's cartoon demonstrates the limited options young girls have against HIV prevention other than abstinence. In addition, although she draws a girl and a boy making a 'we' statement, there is an absence of a represented male participant linked to the drawing of the pregnant girl infected with HIV/AIDS. There are two possible meanings here: the abstinence message may be more pertinent for young girls than their counterparts who have the option of condom use; and, young girls who become pregnant/contract HIV/AIDS are unlikely to have the support of the baby's father. The inclusion of both males and females in this cartoon emphasizes the need for partnerships in preventing HIV/AIDS infection (and early pregnancy). In this cartoon, Nandudu

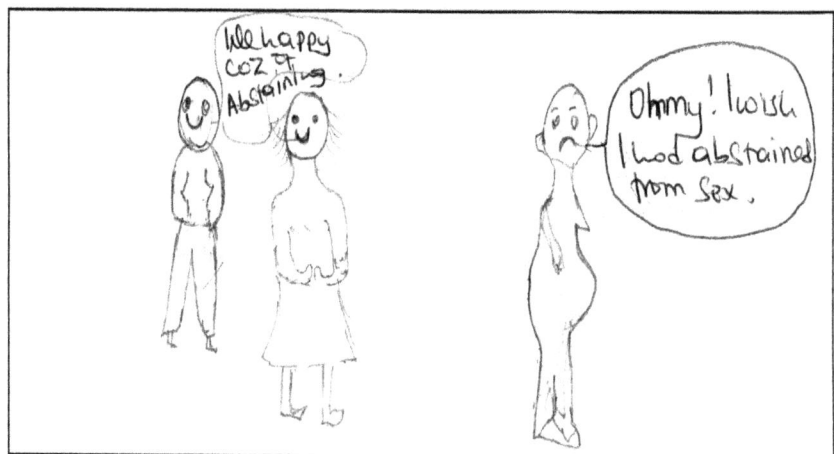

Figure 2.8 Nandudu

positions herself as a role model for other girls. Her inclusion of the happy male youth in this narrative simultaneously challenges boys to choose abstinence. The cartoon highlights Nandudu's in-depth knowledge of the health risks associated with early sexual activity.

Generally, the students have internalized messages about how to avoid HIV infection. The boys demonstrate high awareness of HIV prevention measures that include condom use, which counters the common speculation that abstinence messages are predominant in HIV/AIDS education campaigns for youth. The girls also demonstrate a high awareness of preventive measures although they opt for abstinence. Our conclusion is both the boys and girls concentrate on the preventive measure of which they are in control. In addition, the students' cartoons reveal situations such as prostitution, blind trust in romantic relationships and rape, where knowledge about preventive measures is not applied.

Fighting stigmatization

Also represented in the students' cartoons were messages targeting the larger populace. These messages focused on the attitudes of people towards infected persons and the need to provide home and community care for infected persons. These messages were represented by 10 students, six of whom were girls; the majority of the drawings depicted girls as the primary caregivers of infected persons, as shown in the examples that follow.

Cartoon 9: Musiku (female)
Musiku's cartoon features two represented participants, both female (Figure 2.9). One is drawn larger and closer to the viewer than the other; the action of her outstretched arm initiates an interaction between the women. The title of the cartoon, 'Let's fight stigma we should stop discriminating people with HIV/AIDS because themselves did not want to have it' is the ideal, whereas the kind of stigmatization represented in the cartoon is the current reality for many people with HIV/AIDS in Uganda: 'You look at you, am I the one who told you to have it. It's upon you'. A further explanation is offered by the following: 'The cartoon is simply talking about discrimination of people with HIV/AIDS. The fat woman was saying that she was tired of washing the sister's clothes of feaces and she is not the one who told her to acquire it. So she should suffer with it like she wanted it'.

The attitude of blame is one of the key issues now being addressed in national campaigns in Uganda. It is reported that many communities treat infected persons negatively because it is believed that they did not heed

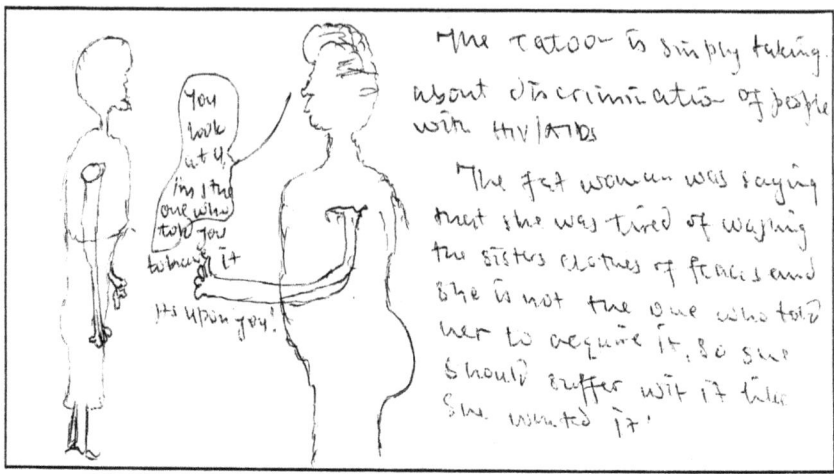

Figure 2.9 Musiku

the information on prevention (Cohen, 2003). Musiku's cartoon message provides a rare glimpse at the frustration and stress primary caregivers face each day in looking after infected persons. The stress patients face while dealing with the attitudes of their caregivers and other members of the community is also represented here.

Stigmatization remains one of the major challenges in Uganda's HIV/AIDS campaigns. In particular, the question of who provides counseling for those who are looking after infected relatives needs to be addressed. Members of the community often isolate families because they have an infected patient in the home. In some communities, families themselves place blame on the infected persons for bringing shame to the family and the resultant isolation. Stigmatization within families may also prevent proper care for patients because family members will not want to share anything with the infected person for the fear that they may become infected.

How do caregivers deal with isolation? In this cartoon, the strategy is to blame the patient for the misery. Musiku's message is one of sympathy for the infected person; hence she focuses on the anti-stigma campaign. The cartoon is intended to appeal to the compassionate nature of those responsible for caring for HIV-infected persons. The cartoonist's intimate knowledge of how infected persons are sometimes treated by relatives suggests that this scenario may be very familiar to her. She depicts both caregiver and patient as female; their relationship may be indicative of female rivalry within a family. When the patient is male, there is often some differential treatment between males and females in relation to how girls respond to the role of caregiver.

Cartoon 10: Namuwaya (female)

In Namuwaya's cartoon, there are two represented participants; the one standing is dressed like a nurse, the other, labeled AIDS, is kneeling on the ground (Figure 2.10). The viewer's attention is immediately drawn to the hand-holding gesture between the two women, emphasizing their physical and emotional connection. The gaze of both women is directed at the viewer, inviting engagement and possibly empathy. The nurse explains, 'I help the patient with food, medicine let me say caring for the patient. I advise the patient'. The cartoon title reads: 'Helping people suffering from HIV/AIDS'. This cartoon, like the previous one, deals with stigmatization, but with a positive demonstration of how to relate to infected persons. In addition, the cartoon informs us of the quality of health care that needs to be provided for infected persons, as outlined in the national communication strategies (IEC, 2004). Of particular interest is that Namuwaya represents herself in the cartoon through the use of 'I' statements. Her personalization of messages about how to treat infected persons may be indicative of her awareness that quality of patient care can boost immunity, or possibly even her desire to undertake a career as a nurse.

Unlike Musiku's cartoon, Namuwaya focuses on nurses as primary care providers, demonstrating a professional, rather than family, approach

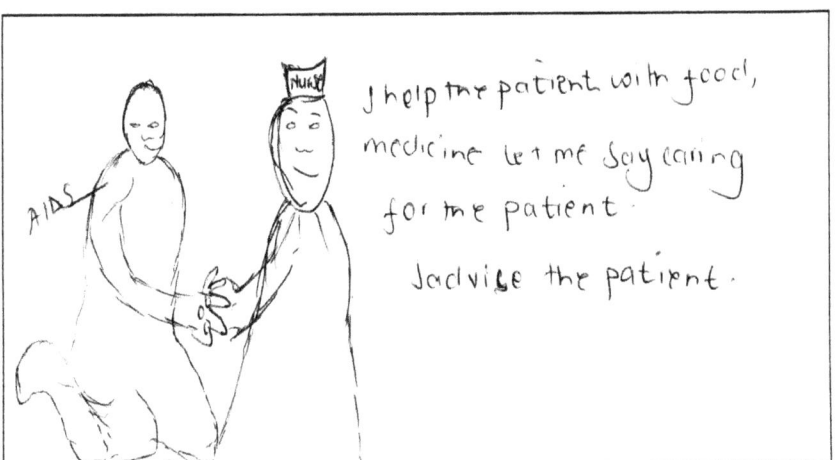

Figure 2.10 Namuwaya

to relating to HIV/AIDS-infected persons. The role of a nurse in this capacity is highlighted in the accompanying caption. The choice to portray a female patient may signify that Namuwaya, as a nurse, is comfortable providing care to a female patient. Her choice may also reflect current statistics, which indicate that more females are seeking medical care and counseling in Uganda than their male counterparts. Statistics also show that more women are infected than men. Perhaps it is because of these various factors that the cartoonist imagines becoming a nurse and championing the cause of helping people living with HIV/AIDS.

Generally both Musiku and Namuwaya's cartoons position women as primary care providers for infected persons. This is a common phenomenon in many communities, particularly in Uganda and other African countries. While both cartoons focus on fighting stigmatization, Musiku's cartoon reveals the harsh realities of the communities' attitudes towards infected persons whereas Namuwaya calls upon professionals to provide more compassionate care for infected persons. The absence of represented males in both cartoons may be revelatory not only in terms of primary care provision but also in terms of gender construction where females are viewed as more compassionate or nurturing.

New reality of HIV/AIDS

Ten of the students' drawings (5 boys and 5 girls) concentrated on the realities of HIV/AIDS in Uganda ranging from issues of increased poverty and the vulnerability of girls to increased numbers of orphans in Uganda. The last cartoon from those selected pictures provides an example.

Cartoon 11: Awiya (female)

Awiya's cartoon is comprised of six sequential images that create a narrative (Figure 2.11). The first image shows a person standing, and the caption reads 'AIDS patient'. In the second, the patient is lying down: 'AIDS has put me down' is written under the image. In the third image, two people are carrying a garbage can, 'picking dirty things of the street'. The fourth image shows two coffins: 'Parents dead' is written underneath. In the fifth image, there are two young children, '... also infected thru breast feeding'. In the final image showing two coffins, we are told, 'Children later on die'. These images represent the story of a family; it begins with infected parents and ends with children left as orphans. The title caption states 'AIDS, AIDS, AIDS! What a killer disease killing young and old, leaving us to suffer'. In verbally explaining the cartoon, Awiya used the words 'me' and 'us', suggesting that the cartoon message is of personal significance.

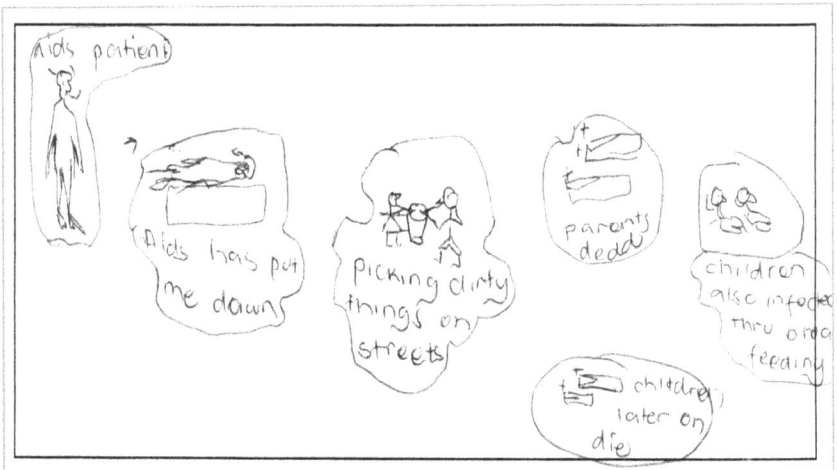

Figure 2.11 Awiya

This narrative raises awareness about the new realities of HIV/AIDS in Uganda: mother-to-child transmission, child-headed households, infected children dying of AIDS and increased numbers of street children who have been orphaned by AIDS. National campaigns must now try to address these issues.

Discussion

This study was designed to investigate students' HIV/AIDS knowledge as represented through their visual representations. The central findings are illustrated by the following sub-themes: general knowledge of HIV/AIDS, including sexual health knowledge, representations of self and gender and the vulnerability of HIV/AIDS.

General knowledge of HIV/AIDS

The students overall demonstrated extensive knowledge about the cause, transmission and prevention of HIV/AIDS. Their cartoons narrated messages that dealt with the viral nature of the disease, indicating that public education has indeed penetrated the target population, particularly youth who are in school and perhaps have access to various media used for communication. These findings are consistent with Stoneburner and Low-Beer's (2004) study, which found that HIV/AIDS knowledge levels among the larger Ugandan populace is generally very high due to massive campaigns.

Nature of sexual health knowledge

Some researchers like Burns (2002) have argued that although many Ugandan students have high levels of HIV/AIDS knowledge, they have limited sexual health knowledge in terms of contraceptive use. This is attributed to the fact that matters relating to sexuality are considered taboo topics; as a result, the public is much more comfortable with abstinence messages. From the cartoons represented here, however, it is evident that the students have accessed critical sexual health knowledge such as the use of condoms. Clearly, the media is beginning to break down the barriers of what is considered taboo by publicly discussing sexual health information; indeed, there was open discussion among the students about condom use alongside abstinence. In their cartoons, the students focused on the preventative measure over which they had most control; that is, boys emphasized condom use over abstinence and girls emphasized abstinence exclusively. In contrast, in contexts where students are expected to represent their HIV/AIDS knowledge through spoken or written language alone, they are less open about discussing taboo topics such as sexual activity and condom use.

Representations of self and gender

Many students represented themselves in their cartoons through the use of 'I' or 'me' statements in the accompanying explanations. These cartoons simultaneously carry both a private and public message. For instance, the girls often portrayed themselves as moralistic in cartoons dealing with abstinence. Their messages serve not only as a reminder to themselves that abstinence is their best option for protecting themselves against HIV/AIDS, but also that girls in general should serve as 'good girl' role models. Part of the 'good girl' identity also involves being nurturing and caring, as represented in cartoons focusing on how to support HIV-positive family members. The message in these cartoons, which included representations of self and other, is that caretaking is the responsibility of girls. Boys also represented girls as primary caregivers for people with HIV/AIDS. In cartoons involving transactional sexual relationships, girls were portrayed as both victim and victimizer. Boys, on the other hand, were primarily represented in positions of power and control, although Tolophina differs by representing George as a victim of

Susan's cunning nature. All of the cartoons represent heteronormative relationships most likely because public messages have focused exclusively on male–female sexual relationships. Indeed, in Uganda, representations of homosexual relationships in public HIV/AIDS education are non-existent. Students have so internalized this sense of normality that they uncritically reproduce it in their images. There is a complete absence of any reference to same gender sex in any of the cartoons.

Vulnerability of HIV/AIDS

Although the students demonstrate a high level of HIV/AIDS knowledge, many of the cartoons represent acute vulnerabilities that prevent application of this knowledge. The most common situation represented was transactional sexual relationships that did not permit girls the right to insist on condom use. Many students represented girls being lured into sexual relationships through prostitution or by men offering them gifts. In these situations, people were most typically portrayed having unprotected sex. In other cartoons, vulnerability to HIV infection was represented in the form of romantic relationships where an unfaithful partner is exposed to HIV/AIDS. The partners do not have protected sex because one of them trusts that the relationship is exclusive. Lastly, some of the cartoons depicted scenarios where girls were exposed to HIV/AIDS through forced – and obviously unprotected – sex. Although most students utilized the opportunity of drawing to represent their understanding of HIV/AIDS, others vented their anger on HIV/AIDS through metaphorical images of HIV/AIDS as a monster they were hunting down with spears or fighting in a boxing ring. Other students portrayed orphaned and homeless children as the new face of HIV/AIDS in Uganda. The urgent need to combat stigmatization was an integral component of many of these HIV/AIDS messages.

Implications for Teachers and Community Leaders

Cartoons as cultural artefacts have considerable potential for HIV/AIDS education in schools and beyond.

(1) They provide an alternative method of accessing students' conceptualizations of health literacies such as HIV/AIDS by making visible the kinds of 'invisible' knowledge, experience and emotion that for personal, social and cultural reasons students may have difficulty in expressing through language alone.

(2) They illuminate the acute vulnerabilities that prevent students from applying their knowledge of HIV/AIDS. By responding to these vulnerabilities, educators and community leaders can take further steps towards helping students prevent HIV/AIDS.

(3) They represent the interface between students' identities and social histories and more public narratives about HIV/AIDS. The diversity of ways in which students portray this interface provides insight into how to validate students' literacies, experiences, cultures and preferred modes of representation in classroom and community contexts.

(4) Use of cartoons can also help teachers transcend cultural barriers in teaching health literacies, including HIV/AIDS. Metaphorical images (e.g. Opondo's) can be used to teach about sex and HIV/AIDS in culturally sensitive ways.

(5) Eliciting students' conceptualizations of emotionally laden topics like HIV/AIDS provides an example on how educators can approach sensitive topics across different cultures. In this study, it was important to consider the sensitivity of the HIV/AIDS as it relates to young people's sexual behavior as well as their experiences with the disease. It was evident that some of the participants had lost their loved ones to HIV/AIDS and were venting their anger in their drawings.

Conclusion

Cartoons are unique cultural artefacts that 'rely on the communication of stereotypes. These synthesize and amplify cultural [and personal] narratives' (Warburton & Saunders, 1996: 307). The students' visual representations of HIV/AIDS knowledge are an intermingling of cultural and personal narratives told to both public and private audiences that allow for the expression of a much fuller range of human emotion and experience than spoken or written communication alone (Kress & van Leeuwen, 1996). Of particular importance is how the cartoons serve to acknowledge the limits of language by simultaneously integrating and transcending taboo cultural practices around discussions of sexuality and condom use. Our findings raise important questions regarding the potentials and limitations of visual and other modes of representation for HIV/AIDS curriculum design and implementation in schools, and in particular, for understanding the relationship between students' own social histories and identities and their interpretation of HIV/AIDS messages. The diversity of ways in which these students 'see' HIV/AIDS demonstrates that cartoons have considerable potential as an untapped pedagogical resource for HIV/AIDS education.

References

Anderson, G. (1990) *Fundamentals of Educational Research*. Basingstoke: Falmer Press.

Banks, M. and Murphy, H. (eds) (1997) *Rethinking Visual Anthropology*. New Haven: Yale University Press.

Boateng, F. (1983) African traditional education: A method of disseminating cultural values. *Journal of Black Studies* 13 (3), 321–336.

Bruner, J. (1964) The course of cognitive growth. *American Psychologist* 29, 1–15.

Burns, K. (2002) Sexuality education in a girls' school in Eastern Uganda. *Agenda* 53, 81–88.

Cohen, S. (2003) Beyond slogans: Lessons from Uganda's experience with ABC and HIV/AIDS. *Reproductive Health Matters* 12 (23), 132–135.

Fuglesang, M. (1997) Lessons for life – past and present modes of sexuality education in Tanzanian society. *Social Science and Medicine* 44 (8), 1245–1254.

Gallagher, J.J. and Tobin, K.G. (1991) Reporting interpretive research. In J. Gallagher (ed.) *Interpretive Research in Science Education* (National Association of Research in Science Teaching Monograph No. 4, pp. 85–95). Manhattan, KS: NARST.

Gilbert, J.K. and Boulter, C. (2000) *Developing Models in Science Education*. Dordrecht: Kluwer.

IEC Unit (2002) *Communication Strategy for IEC – STD/AIDS Control Program*. Kampala: Ministry of Health.

IEC Unit (2004) *The Revised National Strategic Framework for HIV/AIDS Activities in Uganda, 2003/04–2005/06*. Kampala: Ministry of Health.

Jewitt, C. and Oyama, R. (2001) Visual meaning: A social semiotic approach. In T. van Leeuwen and C. Jewitt (eds) *Handbook of Visual Analysis* (pp. 134–156). London: Sage.

Kanu, Y. (2006) Reappropriating traditions in the postcolonial curricular imagination. In Y. Kanu (ed.) *Curriculum as a Cultural Practice. Postcolonial Imaginations* (pp. 203–222). London, Toronto: University of Toronto Press.

Kinsman, J., Nakiyingi, J., Kamali, A., Carpenter, L., Quigley, M., Pool, R. and Whitworth, J. (2001) Evaluation of a comprehensive school-based AIDS education program in rural Masaka, Uganda. *Health and Education Research* 16 (1), 85–100.

Kiwawulo, C. (2004, August 10) Talk to kids about sex [electronic version]. *The New Vision*. Retrieved on 10 September 2005, from http://www.newvision.co.ug/D/9/35/377976

Kress, G. (1997) *Before Writing: Rethinking the Paths to Literacy*. London: Routledge.

Kress, G. (2000) Multimodality. In B. Cope and M. Kalantzis (eds) *Multiliteracies: Literacy Learning and the Design of Social Futures* (pp. 182–202). London: Routledge.

Kress, G. and Jewitt, C. (2003) Introduction. In C. Jewitt and G. Kress (eds) *Multimodal Literacy* (pp. 1–18). New York: Peter Lang.

Kress, G. and van Leeuwen, T. (1996) *Reading Images: The Grammar of Visual Design*. London: Routledge.

Mason, C. (2007) *Fighting Cross-generational Sex*. In *The Monitor* newspaper (November 10) Retrieved from http://www.monitor.co.ug/socpol/socpol10202.php.

Merriam, S.B. (1998) Case *Study Research in Education*. San Francisco: Jersey Boss.

Ministry of Education and Sports/PIASCY (2005) *Lower Post Primary: Student Handbook on HIV/AIDS*. Kampala, Uganda: MoES.

Ministry of Health (2006) *2004–2005 Uganda HIV/AIDS Sero-Behavioural Survey. Prevalence of HIV and Other Sexually Transmitted Infections*. Kampala: Author.

Mirembe, R. (2002) AIDS and democratic education in Uganda. *Comparative Education Volume* 38 (2), 291–302.

Mutonyi, H. (2005) The influence of pre-conceptual and perceptual understandings of HIV/AIDS: A case study of selected Ugandan biology classrooms. Unpublished Master's thesis, University of British Columbia, Canada.

Nakazinga, B. (2004, October 10) Sex education policy threatens to be still birth. *New Vision Newspaper*, pull-out pages on education issues.

Nyanzi, S., Pool, R. and Kinsman, J. (2001) The negotiation of sexual relationships among school pupils in south-western Uganda. *AIDS Care* 13 (1), 83–98.

Peterson, R.W. (1997) Visual memory and language: A study of children's use of art and language to communicate their knowledge of science. Paper presented at the annual meeting of the National Association for Research in Science Teaching, Oak Brooks, IL.

Prosser, J. (1998) *Image-Based Research*. London: Falmer Press.

Reagan, T. (ed.) (2005) *Non-Western Educational Traditions. Indigenous Approaches to Educational Thought and Practice* (3rd edn). Mahwah, NJ: Lawrence Erlbaum.

Reiss, M., Boulter, C. and Tunicliffe, S.D. (2007) See the natural world: A tension between pupils' diverse conceptions as revealed by their visual representations and monolithic science lessons. *Visual Communication* 6 (1), 99–114.

Stake, R. (1995) *The Art of Case Study Research*. Thousand Oaks: Sage.

Stake, R. (1998) Case studies. In N.K. Denzin and Y.L. Lincoln (eds) *Strategies of Qualitative Inquiry* (pp. 86–109). Thousand Oaks: Sage.

Stoneburner, R. and Low-Beer, D. (2004) Population-level HIV declines and the behavioural risk avoidance in Uganda. *Science Magazine* 304, 704–718.

Uganda AIDS Commission (2002) *Combating HIV/AIDS in Uganda Report*. Retrieved on 23 November 2003, from http//www.aidsuganda.org/aids/html.

USAID (United States Agency for International Development) (2002) *What Happened in Uganda?* Retrieved on 24 January 2004, from www.usaids/gov/ourwork/globalhealth/aids/countries/uganda.

Vygotsky, L. (1978) *Mind in Society: The Development of Higher Psychological Processes*. Cambridge, MA: Harvard University Press.

Warburton, T. (1998) Cartoons and teachers: Mediated visual images as data. In J. Prosser (ed.) *Image-Based Research: A Sourcebook for Qualitative Researchers* (pp. 252–262). London: Routledge.

Warburton, T. and Saunders, M. (1996) Representing teachers' professional culture through cartoons. *British Journal of Educational Studies* 44 (3), 307–325.

Weber, S. and Mitchell, C. (1995) *That's Funny, You Don't Look Like a Teacher*. London: Falmer Press.

Wetton, N. and McWhirter, J. (1998) Images and curriculum development in health education. In J. Prosser (ed.) *Image-Based Research* (pp. 263–283). London: Falmer Press.

Yin, R.K. (2003) *Case Study Research: Design and Methods*. Thousand Oaks: Sage.

Chapter 3
Is it Safer to Talk about Sex in Spanish or English? Performing Young Adulthood in Oaxaca, Mexico

ÁNGELES CLEMENTE and MICHAEL J. HIGGINS

Introduction

The overriding theme of this volume is to explore the role of language in the construction of 'local knowledge' about the social realities of HIV/AIDS in various cultural contexts throughout the contemporary world. The construction of these local knowledges often involves a dramatic gap between the AIDS-related discourses performed by health officials and those performed by 'lay' persons dealing with their everyday lives. In this chapter, we discuss the issues of AIDS in the social fields of the post-colonial world of Oaxaca, Mexico. Instead of dealing directly with people afflicted with AIDS, we explore the gap between how AIDS is defined and acted upon by the official health agencies of Oaxaca and how that discourse is processed by a group of young students at the state university who are studying to become English language teachers. What we want to know is how these young university students understand and deal with these realities in the performance of their everyday lives. To understand how the reality of AIDS was factored into their everyday lives, we needed to know their feelings, emotions and perceptions about safe sex. As such, we conducted a series of dialogues in order to explore how their particular views on gender and sexual politics framed their feelings on intimacy and sexuality, and how they do or would discuss issues of safe sex (Cameron, 2007; Nelson, 2006; Pavlenko, 2005; Piller & Takahashi, 2006).[1] Since these are multilingual students with a primary command of Spanish and English, it was relevant to explore which language they would use when discussing these concerns with possible bilingual partners. This, in turn, required a look at the role of their English language education in understanding safe sex. In other words, is talking about sex safer in Spanish or English? Further, did the way these students talk about safe sex reflect or ignore official health discourse on AIDS in Oaxaca?

Setting

For the last several years, we have been working with young students at the *Facultad de Idiomas* in order to explore how they perform English in the multicultural and multilingual context of Oaxaca (Clemente & Higgins, 2008). The *Facultad de Idiomas* is the language teacher training centre for the *Universidad Autónoma Benito Juárez de Oaxaca* (UABJO), the state university of Oaxaca. The BA program in TEFL at the *Facultad* hosts around 600 undergraduate students, most of whom are female. The students come mainly from the city and region of the valley of Oaxaca and they are mostly from a middle or working class context, often being the first in their family to study at the university level. Although some students come from indigenous communities, the majority are from *mestizo* backgrounds (a mixture of European and Indigenous heritages).

The state of Oaxaca is located in the southwest region of Mexico and has a population of over 3.2 million people. It is well known for its ethnic diversity, ecological variety and extreme poverty. The university is located in the city of Oaxaca, which has a population of close to half a million. It is the political, commercial and communication centre of the state. The city is famous for its colonial architecture, ethnic and social diversity and culinary excellence. This city also has many of the characteristics associated with urbanization in Mexico: shortage of housing, limited employment possibilities for 'popular' classes, traffic congestion and political protests (Hernández Díaz, 2007: 35–86).

Shaping of 'Local Knowledge' on AIDS in Oaxaca

The first recognized case of AIDS in Mexico was reported in 1983. Three years later, in 1986, the federal government created CONASIDA (*Consejo Nacional para la Prevencion y Control del SIDA*), a national AIDS council, whose purpose was to coordinate state-level programs dealing with AIDS (Smallman, 2007: 119). During this time, a national program of AIDS education was established throughout the country, which included the distribution of free condoms, attempts at providing free health care and the introduction of new drug treatments (Smallman, 2007: 119). In his book on the AIDS pandemic in Latin America, Smallman argues that the Mexican government and its corresponding health agencies (both federal and state) have responded fairly well to the complexities of this health issue. In 2004, Mexico had a low rate of HIV-positive people, relative to the United States and other Central American countries. Today, Mexico reports 115,651 HIV-positive cases (Cruz-Martínez, 2007: 38). Smallman feels that the overall positive direction of Mexico's response was due to the strong organization of state health programs and support for NGO programs.[2] To illustrate this, he looks at how AIDS was confronted in the state of Oaxaca, where in 2004 there were 2298 reported cases with an approximate 60% death rate (1379 cases). That fell along gender lines at 1866 men and 432 women. Of these cases, close to 40% were in the valley of Oaxaca, 23% were in the Isthmus region and the remaining were found throughout the state (Smallman, 2007: 124–125).

As in other parts of Mexico, in Oaxaca the first occurrences of AIDS were attributed to transmission by gay tourists, and later the spread of AIDS was thought to be a combination of 'culture' of male sexuality and migration. Particularly in Latin America, as in other parts of the world, patterns of male sexuality allow for same sex activity between males so long as there is a clear role distinction between the active partner (the one who penetrates) and the passive one (the penetrated). In these sexual performances, only the passive actor is coded as gay; the active actor claims that his virility is so strong that he can have sex with both men and women (Higgins & Coen, 2008: 130–134). It was assumed that these men were having unprotected sex with other men and then having sex with women, thereby transmitting AIDS. Further, it was found that many of the returning migrants from the United States were HIV positive and that they were infecting their partners in Oaxaca, thus introducing AIDS into the female population (Gutmann, 2007; Smallman, 2007).

At the local level, COESIDA (*Consejo Estatal para la Prevención y Control del SIDA*), the state AIDS agency, defines the AIDS discourse in Oaxaca, and this discourse works to select who can get treatment. The public discourse on AIDS can be seen in the literature offered to the public. In a range of pamphlets addressing AIDS and other sexually transmitted diseases, the common themes are that AIDS can affect anyone; that people's various lifestyles need to be respected; that those at the highest risk are those who do not use condoms, have sex with an infected person or have sex with multiple partners; that the way to avoid or prevent AIDS is absti-nence, fidelity, secure sex (the use of condoms), safe sex (sex with no pene-tration) and honest discussions with one's partner; that AIDS is a sexually transmitted disease which can also be spread through blood and in the process of birthing; and, that all people should get tested.[3]

Smallman feels that the health sector in Oaxaca, working within these assumptions, has responded well. First, all sex workers were required to undergo a monthly check for HIV and could not get a formal work card without such a test. This test was provided by COESIDA. COESIDA also provided testing for the general population, offered counseling and treatment for those who were HIV positive and ran state-wide educational programs on AIDS prevention. Smallman found this program to do the best possible job, considering both its level of funding and the increasing demand of clients.

However, Gutmann (2007) suggests that there is a gap between COESIDA's public discourse and the gritty daily realities of dealing with the crisis of AIDS in Oaxaca. He argues that the COESIDA counseling and medical staffs adhere literally to the cultural discourse of male sexuality mentioned above. That is, they believe that AIDS is transmitted only by sex between men and then spread to women through sex with those same infected men, often their husbands or partners. This belief system sees men as having unabated sexual drives that, if not met by sex with women, will be directed towards sex with other men. This belief is also tied to assumptions about what happens among male migrants in the United States, who through sexual anxiety seek sex with other men or have group sex with prostitutes without using condoms. It is these infected men who, in turn, infect women in Oaxaca. It is assumed that women cannot be the source of infection and that if there were to be infection from contaminated blood or needles, it would be linked back to infected men. This further produces a profile of males whose behavior is seen as 'much riskier' than that of others, and whose behavior would be the cause to eliminate them as candidates for advanced treatment.

Only patients who exhibit compliance are to be given treatments. There are to be no drug users, no alcoholics, no men who have sex with men and no unfaithful men. To receive the treatment, one has to be a good patient, always arrive on time for appointments and demonstrate the willingness to take the medicine in the required time frames. The COESIDA staff often hopes that people will not seek their help, for the reality is that they cannot offer much help to the infected population.

This indicates, in the context of Oaxaca, that AIDS produces a reality of 'death without weeping' (Scheper-Hughes, 1992). Gutmann (2007) states that this cultural analysis utilized by medical personnel acts as a 'cultural condom', in order to contain the disease and to help prevent it from spreading to other populations with presumably less susceptible cultures.

If culture were to be blamed, and if culture could not be changed through institutional remedies, then the best that medical personnel at COESIDA could hope to accomplish for most AIDS patients is to give comfort. This 'cultural condom' also prevents any analysis of the political economy of AIDS in Oaxaca or Mexico. Thus, these deaths are not to be wept for, but rather should be seen as unfortunate outcomes of factors beyond the control of the medical or professional staffs in Oaxaca (Gutmann, 2007). It is within these discursive boundaries that the young students at the *Facultad de Idiomas* compose their own understandings, feelings and actions in terms of AIDS and safe sex.

Our Theoretical Tapestry

In order to interpret the performances of the university students within the discursive boundaries presented above, we have weaved together the following theoretical threads: (1) language performances in everyday life (Pennycook, 2004); (2) the awareness that these multilingual performances are emotionally charged activities (Pavlenko, 2005); and (3) the way such performances engender new imagined communities of linguistic praxis (Kanno & Norton, 2003).

To define what we mean by everyday language performances, we start with Austin's idea that a performative speech act is one 'in which to say something is to do something; or which by saying or in saying something we are doing something' (Austin, 1962: 12). For Pennycook, Austin's comment suggests ways to bring back issues of performance in applied linguistics that can deal with the process of linguistic actions and identity locations and agency (Pennycook, 2004: 7). Drawing upon Butler's work (1999) on identity and gender, Pennycook states that performativity can be seen as a way in which we compose identities as a series of social and cultural performances rather than as an expression of pre-existing identities (2004: 8). The contexts for such performances are local contingencies that frame these identity activities. For the students in this study, how they talk about sexuality is both virtual and real, in Austin's (1962) sense of 'doing something'. Their comments are not per se about actual events, but about how they wish to perform in terms of their desires and wishes.

Insomuch as these everyday language performances are taking place, in a multilingual and multicultural context, we need then to think beyond the hegemony of monolingualism. Pavlenko (2005) is concerned with shifting the focus in language learning studies towards the recognition that all language performances are multilingual, especially in terms of attempting to understand how speakers express the agency of their identities through feelings and emotions. Of interest to our work is Pavlenko's discussion of assumed divided language performance of bilingual speakers, where it is claimed that one's L1 would be the language of emotional expressions and one's additional languages would be used for more concrete or technical expressions. Pavlenko argues that a more textured look at the lived experiences of multilingual performers offers portraits that are complex, varied and framed by the overall context of speech activities (Pavlenko, 2005: 220–243). In her re-reading of various accounts of language and desire among multilingual couples, she found that the choice of language used in terms of emotional performances is scripted in terms of diversity of desires and longings that the various couples bring to their lived experiences, with no expression of simplistic division of languages according to emotion and non-emotional concerns (Pavlenko, 2005: 220–226). These are the kinds of language performances that we encounter in our ethnographic dialogues with these students. Departing from Pavlenko, we are not focusing on how the participants actually use English or Spanish in their dialogues. Rather, we analyze the way the participants perform their projected identities differently with regard to how they discuss their language options.

However, in these performances, the students envision the construction of imagined communities between themselves, their future English students and the world of people with AIDS. Kanno and Norton state that 'imagined communities refer to groups of people, not immediately tangible and accessible, with whom we connect through the power of the imagination' (Kanno & Norton, 2003: 241). In re-working Anderson's (1991) original use of the idea, Kanno and Norton (2003) view the concept of imagined communities as a way to elucidate issues concerning language, identity and education. For them, 'imagined communities are no less real than the ones in which learners have daily engagement and might even have a stronger impact on their current actions and investment' (Kanno & Norton, 2003: 242).

How Students Perform Their 'Local Knowledge' About AIDS

The social realities of the eight students expressed diverse contexts: urban middle class (Dario, Gemma and Claudia), working class (Fernando), rural middle class (Carlos) and rural working class families with developing residential ties to the city of Oaxaca (Carmen, Martha and Rosa). During the time of our study, six of the students were in the last year of the BA program in TEFL and all had a 550 TOEFL in English. Most imagined that they would teach English in the future. We carried out several individual and group conversations with the participants on topics ranging from the overall politics of sexuality in their school community to their personal views about AIDS and how to deal with the information about it. The participants were very eager to talk about these topics; so, in order to select our data, we decided to only analyze and report excerpts that dealt with the issue of language choice in connection to the social realities of HIV/AIDS, giving special importance to their role as future educators. We also decided to include the information that would help to contextualize their local knowledge about this topic.

Dario and Gemma are a heterosexual couple who met at the school and have been together for four years. They are not considering marriage in the near future. They are very committed to their studies, but also enjoy a good sense of humor. Claudia is Martha's best friend and Rosa is Martha's younger sister. All three have decided not to have a partner at school. Likewise, Carmen does not want to mix her personal life with her academic role at the university, and so her partner is from outside the university. The five young women of this study are heterosexual and openly express their view that marriage is not necessarily part of their project of life. In different ways, they have opposed the hopes of their parents, who want to see their daughters marrying soon. Carlos is a heterosexual man who is enjoying his youth, mixing his university studies with his job as a gym trainer. He believes that the combination of these two activities has made him more attractive to girls. Fernando, a homosexual young student, finds the school a safe place, where he feels free to be open; yet he continues to question his sexual orientation because of his perception that women are more stable and honest than men.

The *Facultad de Idiomas* is perceived as one of the more cosmopolitan communities of the university. Most of the students at the *Facultad* seem to accept this observation, expressing pride in this perceived openness and diversity of their social lives. The *Facultad* is considered both by the students within the institution as well as by those in the university at large as a gay-friendly context where sexual libertarianism is expressed freely. Thus, the *Facultad de Idiomas* constitutes a social space where these young students perform their gender and sexuality in a context that contrasts with other social domains within the university and in Oaxaca.

Performing their Gender and Sexuality

Within the diversity of these feelings among these students, there is an emerging discourse that frames their young adulthood in terms of cosmopolitanism, openness and social tolerance, and sentiments about intimacy. Through this discourse, they compose their feelings on fidelity, gayness, virginity, safe sex and the imagined connections between English teaching and the realities of AIDS. Regarding the language for the conversations, we decided to use Spanish, their mother tongue; however, the participants often code-mixed and code-switched. For the sake of consistency, we have translated the data into English (in italics), though we have included some of the original data in Spanish to offer a richer account of the students' perspectives.

Fidelity and commitment

These students approach the question of how to perform fidelity in fairly traditional manners. Carmen also offers a somewhat traditional position in terms of female obligation:

> I like to be monogamous not because of AIDS but because of my principles. I have always thought that way. Fidelity ... I do not know if this is still in or is passé, but I want to be faithful and have a faithful partner. And even if he is not faithful I am going to be faithful. It is one of the main requirements that I ask in a relationship. It is also good because we can prevent a lot of diseases, but for me, it is a matter of my principles.

Fernando also offers a somewhat traditional view, but from the perspective of his changing feelings about his gayness:

> What I look for in a relationship is understanding and acceptance. I want people to accept me the way I am, not to tell me: 'I want you to be this way'. I would like to find someone that makes me feel safe and that wouldn't manipulate me. I think that these features are difficult to find in a Mexican, maybe even in a foreigner. I think that Mexicans still have the idea, even in the gay community, that you are only useful if you are attractive and/or have money. People change and I have changed. Two years ago, I was a 100% sure that I was homosexual. Right now I think that I am bisexual because being gay has not given me much satisfaction.

Gayness and virginity

Where these students start to move away from their somewhat traditional feelings is in the area of sexuality, particularly regarding gayness and virginity. As stated above, the *Facultad* is viewed by many students as a gay-friendly space. Dario says:

> I think that the school is famous for its male homosexuality. Here, there is more freedom of expression and more relations between homos and heteros. At the beginning it felt strange but then you get used to it. I have also noticed that heterosexual guys are very respectful towards gays (both, men and women), there is no discrimination and there are a lot of friendship bonds among everybody.

This gay tolerance is 'gender-marked' in that it clearly accepts male gayness, but with a limited knowledge about female gayness. Gemma says:

> Here at the Facultad, most of the students are women, there are only few men and many of them are gay. Thus, we are in a unique context here. Among the students here, homosexuality is no big deal. I think that the fame of the school is more for its male homosexuality than the female one. Although we are in a very open-minded school we are still more surprised to know that there is a lesbian couple than if there is a male gay couple.

This tolerance is also framed in terms of how open and accepting the straight students are towards the gay students. This can be seen in Fernando's 'gay read' of this openness:

> Here at the Facultad, there are more straight couples than homosexual couples, and the latter are not so open. We all know who's who; it is a 'secreto a voces' [unspoken secrets]. Gay couples are seen as friends, best friends. There are also lesbian couples. In spite of the fact that the school is regarded as a gay school, it is still very uncomfortable to be surrounded by straights. We are not totally open. Straights can be kissing inside the classroom, in the cinema, outside the church and nobody says anything, but gay couples can't. It is still taboo.

Another area where their performances move away from traditional assumptions is in terms of sexual sophistication. This is expressed in Claudia's view on the openness of students at the *Facultad*:

> Some guys in our class say that faithfulness is passé. Unfaithfulness is to be modern, to hang around with several partners. Within the couples there are agreements of non-exclusivity. I guess it is part of the open-mindedness, accepting everything. But they do not criticize me because I think differently. We are open and accept people's ways

of thinking, their ideologies and sexual preferences. People here do not criticize. It is great!

Both the male and female students assume that their classmates are sexually active; they do not place any importance on virginity. Carmen says:

> For young women here at the Facultad, one's virginity is not important. That's an important factor, to talk about sex without inhibitions. Everybody understands you and they give you their opinion, and they help you to understand, to learn. You have more perspectives about sex. You do not get trapped in the circle of "I want to keep myself virgin for my husband."

Even Carlos, who advocated his right to infidelity, is aware that he cannot be concerned about female virginity:

> I do not care about virginity. If I get married I won't care if she is virgin or not. I cannot demand what I do not offer. I have to be realistic. I cannot ask somebody to be a virgin if my life has been full of women, virgin and non-virgin. I don't care. I only care that I love her and she loves me. That's it.

Emotions and the performance of safe sex

The most complex script being composed by these students addresses the issues of sexual responsibility in terms of communication, honesty and safety. They assume that intimate couples should be open and honest with each other and talk about AIDS and their means for protection. Since these students are multilingual (with social experiences with international students), they are aware that they have different sets of languages to use in talking about these issues. Most students suggest that, in the context of bilingual relationships, they would use Spanish to explain their feelings and use English to make sure that what they were attempting to communicate was understandable to their partners. At first their comments seem to express the dichotomy of L1 being used for emotional concerns and L2 for more direct or accurate information (Pavlenko, 2005). However, we suggest a way to read these stories across the grain that offers another perspective.

To begin with, Carlos's views seem to offer the basic dichotomy:

> For prevention, we can say it in Spanish or English, but if I was with a foreigner, I would say it in English. I would say, 'Look, this and that, and we have to take some precautions, we have to be protected'. Everything would be in English. Also it is easier to say that stuff in English than to talk about your feelings.

Fernando also suggests this dichotomy, but stresses that one must be sensitive to the feelings of one's partner:

I do not know if I would have used English or Spanish in an intimate relationship with him. I think that I would have expressed myself in Spanish because it is something so personal, and in my mother tongue these feelings would come out more natural. He would have expressed himself in English, for the same reason. For prevention, I would have used English. I would use English in order not to take risks and to be cautious, but I would not do it briskly.

Rosa stresses that choice of language can be a matter of life or death:

For intimacy I would choose Spanish because I am more confident in it. English is also more direct, Spanish is more emotive, like 'Me gustas'[I like you]. 'Te quiero'[I love you]. 'Eres simpatico'[You're very nice]. For sentimental reasons there are more options in Spanish. For prevention I would use English because he knows English. And it is not just my life which is at risk but both our lives. And it is not only my feelings. In terms prevention, if I fail to communicate I am playing with my life and his life, and you cannot play with that.

The comments of these students do seem to stress that Spanish is their language for expressing feelings and English for conveying information. However, their choice also seems to be based on the fact that their English education has not provided them with the necessary skills to perform their feelings and emotions. Thus, they are not per se expressing this dichotomy between L1 and L2, but are located within it. Spanish is being used to express the accuracy of their emotions and English to ensure that feelings are understood. Further, since they are pondering questions that, as Rosa states, deal with life and death, both languages are being used as they fit the situation being confronted. This makes either language choice emotionally charged enough to demonstrate both concern and accuracy. They are not reproducing a dichotomy but trying to communicate successfully (Clemente & Higgins, 2008). This can be seen in how they attempt to understand the reality of AIDS.

The Shape of Their 'Local Knowledge' on AIDS

These students all seem to have general knowledge about AIDS, but it is something that they feel distant from, as Carmen conveys:

I don't know a lot about AIDS. I have heard about some cases, but not in terms of anyone I know personally. What I have heard has been on

TV or the newspapers. That's why for me it is something very distant; it has not affected me directly. It seems to me to be a societal problem.

Further, few have any personal and social contact with people with AIDS, nor any particular knowledge of groups in Oaxaca who are working on AIDS-related issues. According to Dario:

> Here we do not see that AIDS is a big problem. Dengue is closer to us. It really affects us. You think that AIDS is something that won't happen to us. On the other hand, I think that we do not know much about the latest discoveries in medicine, how to prevent it or how to reduce its growth. That could be a new aspect to talk about and to discuss it more in depth.

Although the official discourses on AIDS in Oaxaca stress that AIDS can affect anyone, it seems that awareness is still closeted by socio-economic class experiences. This is seen in that very few of the students at the *Facultad* have a clear idea of the realities of AIDS, even though the majority of students are from the working class. Interestingly, Martha and Rosa, who come from more humble social conditions than the other students, are the ones who had the most personal contact with AIDS. Martha gives the history of her mother's *compadre* (the godparent to one of her children) who lived with them when Martha was a teenager:

> It was weird when he lived with us at home and he had AIDS. He worked and my mother fed him and at night we used to chat with him. Then my mother realized about the symptoms of his sickness and also some people from our pueblo told her about him, that they saw him in such place doing such and such things that were not proper for a man. My mother got worried about us getting infected. She started to put aside the dishes that he used to eat. I didn't understand why. When I came to understand what was going on, in spite of me being just a teenager, I told her that she was exaggerating. It was something unbelievable for me to be living with someone with AIDS. At that age I thought that AIDS should be very distant, away from home, because at home we were healthy and we knew how to protect ourselves. I tell my little sister to be prepared, to live with the idea that some day she may have a friend, a relative, someone close to her that may have that problem. To be prepared to face that in a more mature way, without prejudices. This experience helped us, because if in the future I meet somebody with that problem I will act in a different way. Now I have more experience and more knowledge of the topic and now I will act differently.

Being Educated and Imagining How to Educate About AIDS

As these youngsters are preparing themselves to be English teachers, they are in a position to be listened to. Besides gaining knowledge about language teaching and the dynamics of the language, classroom knowledge on the subject of HIV/AIDS offers the English teacher a concrete link to real issues of the everyday lives of the students, an important factor for significant language learning.

The participants of this study referred to education on AIDS at two different levels: how they have been educated and how they imagine they would educate their students about AIDS. Talking about their own education, they express that in the context of Oaxaca they officially got to know about AIDS in secondary school. Dario states:

> As I see it, the reason that everybody knows about this topic is because the lectures and talks in secondary and high school and it seems that there is nothing new to know about this problem, that is, one has heard the same about prevention and infection.

Then, Dario illustrates how this information melts with his own realities in Oaxaca:

> AIDS in Oaxaca spreads because of USA migration. Ignorance is the main cause for me. Go to the States, be unfaithful to your wife with a prostitute, come back and infect your family.

At home, according to Claudia's experience, there were no conditions for education on AIDS to take place:

> Here in Mexico it is bad to talk about homosexuality, and you are a whore if you talk about sex. Sexuality is stigmatized; it is like the worst thing in the world. And it is a social problem because, when you are young, they do not teach you how to deal with it, how to take care of yourself. They tell you about colds and about coughs but not about AIDS, not about its causes and effects.

However, as we have seen from Martha and Rosa's story, to have someone near you who is fighting AIDS gives you the opportunity to face that reality. But that does not guarantee that your parents will take it as an educational opportunity. As Rosa states:

> When I turned 18, my mother did not say anything about this disease, although she knew, she was afraid to talk about that. The only thing she said was that I had to be careful, not to get pregnant for the

consequences that that brings: people talk about you, think bad of you. This is the way she was brought up.

At the *Facultad de Idiomas*, as Fernando explains, these youngsters have faced a different situation:

> The school is more open about sexuality. It is a topic that nobody is ashamed of. But there are a lot of problems still. We all have different ideas on sexuality and regard sexuality in a different ways.

Carmen feels that many of them have developed the right attitudes to be more tolerant and not have prejudices about sexual orientations:

> Here, men that are homosexual feel the freedom to say it, and they don't care and they are not judged. We are different from other schools. We are better because of the system, because a lot of our teachers studied here and went to study abroad and came back and they changed, they are different, the way they talk and the way they behave, when they are teaching you can see the difference. In the medicine school or in the law school they are very traditional. When you talk to people here you immediately know that they have a different vision.

However, many like Claudia feel trapped between two different positions:

> I do not know where I would place myself. It is a difficult question; I don't consider myself very open-minded but not very conservative. I am sort of in the middlev. ... These issues are difficult for me, because my family is very macho-oriented and not very tolerant. In my family if somebody admitted that s/he were homosexual, s/he would be literally expelled from the familial group.

As future teachers, these young adults are aware that in the context of teaching English, one could find profound ways to confront and deal with these issues, and by doing so, the teaching of English could be more than empty content; it could be an arena for dealing with real issues of everyday life. First of all, according to Fernando, education of AIDS has to start with facing prejudices:

> As a teacher, I would talk to my students about these issues. First, I want them to understand that they have to respect everybody. That everybody has to make decisions about their personal lives. And that you cannot pressure people to make decisions against their desires, there has to be free will. Sexual diversity is part of the multiculturalism of Mexico and Oaxaca. Everybody is in danger, all

human beings, doesn't matter your sexual orientation. It is not a guarantee to be straight. I would have to make them understand that we are in the same situation and that they shouldn't discriminate, blaming homosexual people for AIDS. I think that fear plus ignorance equals danger.

For Dario, the question is to find a way for students to be open and to be willing to deal with these topics. For him, as he explains, the language classroom provides an excellent opportunity:

Once I planned a lesson on physical functions: go to the toilet, sweat, burp, have sex, things like that. It is necessary vocabulary that it is never taught. So I taught basic words and phrases of an intimate context that help a lot when you live with someone and it helps you to create a lively atmosphere, an interesting lesson. And those are words that stay in your head, if you make a joke it stays in your memory. It's a teaching strategy and creates a friendly atmosphere. They forgot their nervousness. It is part of the language and should not be kept hidden as it did not exist. If you use them in your everyday life, why don't they teach them in the other language? When a teacher teaches them she breaks a barrier. She is no more a strict teacher and they start trusting her. In that context I would explain AIDS, when given the opportunity, naturally, out of a conversation in class.

However, the classroom could provide factual information:

We do not know much about the latest discoveries in medicine, how to prevent AIDS or how to reduce its growth. That could be a new aspect to talk about and to discuss it more in depth.

Dario thinks that teaching a different language provides good opportunities to talk about AIDS:

The teacher has to create the right context to talk about certain topic like AIDS: telling stories, experiences, referring to well-known people. Sometimes it helps to refer to the other culture and ask them to understand it. You can talk about it because there is more openness and also because your students are speaking in English and they think that Americans or Europeans are more open. You could frame it as a health problem, not to be seen as a taboo topic. And you are giving factual information for them to form their own opinion.

But above all, Dario thinks that the teacher has to connect this information with his/her students. Here, he suggests talking about the students' plans to go to the United States, another topic they do not usually discuss:

> I would like to talk about migration with my students. I do not want them to think that they cannot talk about their plans to go to the States, because their classmates would judge them. I want them to discuss the situation of Chicanos. I want to talk about their culture and their art. Bring a Chicano to my class and talk about his/her identity. We could talk about AIDS then. There are statistical studies we can bring to the class. Otherwise you cannot just enter the classroom and say: "Today we'll take about AIDS!"

Finally, Martha critically reflects about English teaching and states that by dealing with these issues, teaching becomes significant as it involves a 'real content' to learn and discuss.

> As a teacher, I feel that I should talk about AIDS, because we are educating, so we have to educate in all areas, for them to be prepared. Supposedly, school is for that, to face the world, and the world we live in has AIDS, a sickness. So we have to talk about that with students, to know how to face life. We should talk about the themes that will really help them. This is what we need here. English is taught through empty content, like 'buying things in a mall'. We have to get real. We have to be realistic, to make the curriculum focus on the reality we are living.

In these various comments we hear how these students are moving from talking about themselves, their feelings and concerns, towards reflecting upon their own education and their future practices as educators by addressing the gaps in people's understandings about AIDS. There are suggestions that what they imagined about the realities of AIDS was not enough, and that they can imagine connecting the various communities of Oaxaca through English teaching in order to express tolerance and compassion for all.

Discussion

We have presented a brief narrative account on the reality of AIDS in Oaxaca and on several multilingual students at the state university who relate to and understand that reality. Drawing from previous ethnography work on how these students perform their gender, sexuality, ethnicity and social class within the multicultural and multilingual context of the

Facultad de Idiomas of the UABJO (Clemente & Higgins, 2008), we have attempted to represent how these performances articulate the students' feelings and emotions regarding the reality of AIDS in their everyday lives, including their use of English (Pavlenko, 2005). Thus, we posed the provocative title of whether it was safer to talk about sex in Spanish or English. For the purpose of discussion, we offer some tentative insights that we have been able to draw from our narrative.

For one, there seems to be a discursive 'gap' between the official and public discourse on AIDS and the manner in which the students in their language performances express their views and sentiments. It would seem that there is no strong link between the two. Even though the various agencies and organizations have been working with the reality of AIDS for more than two decades, these university students were not per se well informed, nor were their realities affected. Although COESIDA felt that it had programs and materials relevant to university students, it was having a minimum impact on these students. One factor is that students felt that over the course of their high school and university education, they had received numerous lectures and warnings on AIDS and hence assumed that they did not need more information. Also, with the exception of Martha and Rosa, the students had no personal or social context with people with AIDS, nor with the organizations dealing with AIDS-related concerns. Ironically, their mother's *compadre* would have been the type of patient denied treatment by COESIDA. Also, reflecting on Guttmann's work, we can conclude that if the official discourse on AIDS had a more critical tone and focused on current political and social factors of AIDS in Oaxaca, then the discourse perhaps might be more attractive to these students.

However, given that these students felt that the reality of AIDS was distanced from them, they had very forthright and innovative ideas on how to use the teaching of English to address the reality of AIDS in the lives of their students. They were able to imagine how, through English teaching, they could connect themselves and their students to the reality of people with AIDS. They used their linguistic agency to imagine a community of tolerance and respect in Oaxaca. Their ideas dealt with socioeconomic issues that ranged from the process of becoming a migrant to the USA, respect for sexual diversity, to a dignified and respectful treatment of people with AIDS. Ironically, without the help of, or connection to, the official discourse on AIDS, they were able to compose their own discourses. We see this 'doing something', in Austin's (1962: 12) sense of the phrase, as an expression of these students' linguistic praxis.

Conclusion: Doing Something!

This 'doing something' leads back to our question of whether sex is safer in Spanish or English. The students were uniquely located in order to ponder this question. All had command over Spanish and English; many had bilingual relationships (or so envisioned); and all were comfortable expressing what we referred to as a cosmopolitan discourse on sex and gender.

As we suggested, a first reading of their views sounds like another example of the linguistic dichotomy of using one's L1 for emotional concerns and one's L2 for factual declarations (Pavlenko, 2005: 227–247). However, drawing upon the works of Baxter (2003), Kanno and Norton (2003), Lutz (1990) and Pavlenko (2006), we think there is more going on. These students are composing their young adulthood. This involves their own performance of the subjectivities of their gender, sexuality, social class and ethnicity. These performances allow them to move in between their various identity locations and to explore different language practices in the process (Clemente & Higgins, 2008). Because of the style of their English education as well as the personal and social expectations of their Spanish usage, more often than not, they reported that they felt more comfortable expressing their emotions in Spanish and using English to convey information, particularly in terms of sexual issues. But this is because, at this point in their language education, they do not have a command over an emotional discourse in English. Further, their statement that within a Spanish/English relationship they would use English with their partners to discuss safety and prevention issues regarding AIDS is not a non-emotional position. Because they have strong feelings of care and concern about their partners, they want to make sure things are understood. Thus, their choice of English is engendered by their emotional feelings for the other person.

Further, their various models of how they would use the teaching of English to address issues of AIDS in Oaxaca are composed with expressions of their subjective feelings on social issues, sexual diversity, social justice and human dignity. By exploring these issues with the students, we have found that they also want to be able to perform 'English' that will allow them to be able to express the full range of their feelings, hopes and fears. Thus, we humbly suggest that, for these young social actors, talking about sex is safer in either language but only when it is part of the overall multicultural and multilingual context of their everyday lives. This is the arena where they can imagine links between their language education, the performance of their identities particularly in terms of intimacy and sexuality, and the pursuit of social justices. Through the emotional expression of their linguistic praxis, they envision for Oaxaca, an imagined community having social and sexual tolerance for all.

Notes

1. Our methodology involved lengthy dialogues (three to four hours) with each of the students as well as visits to AIDS agencies in Oaxaca.
2. For information on NGOs in Oaxaca dealing with the realities of AIDS, see Higgins and Coen (2008) and Smallman (2007).
3. The information presented here is based on our translations of a set of pamphlets that were given to us by the COESIDA office in the city of Oaxaca.

References

Anderson, B. (1991) *Imagined Communities*. London: Verso Books.
Austin, J.L. (1962) *How to Do Things with Words*. Oxford: Oxford University Press.
Baxter, J. (2003) *Positioning Gender in Discourse*. London: Palgrave.
Butler, J. (1999) Performativity's social magic. In R. Shusterman (ed.) *Bourdieu: A Critical Reader* (pp. 113–129). London: Blackwell Publishers.
Cameron, D. (2007) *Language and Sexual Politics*. London: Routledge.
Clemente, A. and Higgins, M. (2008) *Performing English with a Post-Colonial Accent: Ethnographic Narratives from Mexico*. London: Tufnell Press.
Cruz-Martínez, A. (2007) Debe ser obligatoria la prueba de sida, *La Jornada* (National newspaper of México) 29 November, p. 38.
Gutmann, M. (2007) *Fixing Men: Sex, Birth Control and AIDS in Mexico*. Berkeley: University of California Press.
Hernández Díaz, J. (2007) Dilemas en la construccion de Ciudadanias Diferenciadas e n un Espacio Multicultural: El Caso de Oaxaca. In J. Hernández Díaz (ed.) *Ciudadanías diferenciadas en un estado multicultural: los usos y costumbres en Oaxaca* (pp. 35–86). México, D.F.: Siglo Veintiuno Editores/UABJO.
Higgins, M. and Coen, T. (2008) *Calles, Cuartos y Patios: Lo Cotidiano de la diversidad en el Oaxaca Urbana*. Oaxaca: UABJO.
Kanno, Y. and Norton, B. (2003) Imagined communities and educational possibilities: Introduction. *Journal of Language, Identity, and Education* 2 (4), 241–249.
Lutz, C. (1990) Engendered emotion: Gender, power, and the rhetoric of emotional control in American discourse. In C. Lutz and L. Abu-Lughod (eds) *Language and the Politics of Emotion* (pp. 69–91). Cambridge: Cambridge University Press.
Nelson, C. (2006) Introduction: Special issue on sexuality and language. *The Journal of Language, Identity and Education* 5 (1), 1–16.
Pavlenko, A. (2005) *Emotions and Multilingualism*. Cambridge: Cambridge University Press.
Pavlenko, A. (2006) Bilingual selves. In A. Pavlenko (ed.) *Bilingual Minds: Emotional Experience, Expression and Representation* (pp. 1–33). Clevedon: Multilingual Matters.
Pennycook, A. (2004) Performativity and language studies. *Critical Inquiry in Language Studies: An International Journal* 1 (1), 1–19.

Piller, I. and Takahashi, K. (2006) A passion for English: Desire and the language market. In A. Pavlenko (ed.) *Bilingual Minds: Emotional Experience, Expression and Representation* (pp. 59–83). London: Multilingual Matters.

Scheper-Hughes, N. (1992) *Death without Weeping: The Violence of Everyday Life in Brazil.* Berkeley: University of California Press.

Smallman, S. (2007) *The AIDS Pandemic in Latin America.* Chapel Hill: University of North Carolina Press.

Chapter 4

Safe Sex – Not So Straightforward: Intersubjective Positioning in Gay Men's Accounts of Sexual Exposure to HIV

HENRIKE KÖRNER

Responses to the HIV epidemic have taken two distinct approaches: a 'modern' public health approach and a 'social' public health approach. In a 'modern' public health approach, autonomous individuals receive information from experts, take this information on board, make rational decisions based on this information and change their behavior accordingly. Risk behavior is seen as resulting from a lack of information or from misinformation, and change is achieved by disseminating correct information to the individuals concerned. In contrast, a 'social' public health approach focuses on individuals as members of communities, social relationships and interaction. Individual behavior is seen to be mediated by social relationships; it is contextual and socially embedded. Actions and behaviors are socially and culturally produced in interaction with others. In a 'social' public health approach, prevention information is not passively absorbed by individuals but is actively taken up through interaction in specific social and cultural contexts (Kippax, 2007; Kippax & Race, 2003).

This chapter explores gay men's understanding of 'risk' and 'safe sex', as represented in face-to-face interviews with a social researcher. The data are from the seroconversion[1] study, a Sydney-based study of gay men with recently acquired HIV infection. The aim of this study was to identify the risk of seroconversion in relation to sexual practices and to explore men's understanding of sexual risk. The chapter is specifically concerned with the interpersonal stance men adopted with reference to risk reduction strategies and health promotion messages. Drawing on Bakhtin's notions of heteroglossia and dialogism, and appraisal theory from systemic functional linguistics, the chapter describes the heteroglossic backdrop against which gay men's understandings of 'risk' and 'safe sex' are construed and how they position themselves intersubjectively towards risk reduction strategies and prevention messages.

Background: Approaches to Risk Reduction

In Australia, the vast majority of people infected with and affected by HIV/AIDS are gay men. From the beginning of the epidemic, gay men have been instrumental in developing strategies to protect themselves and each other from HIV infection, and the terms 'safe sex' and 'safer sex' were coined even before the HIV virus was discovered. Early health promotion messages such as 'use a condom every time', 'if it's not on, it's not on' and 'assume everyone is positive' focused on condom use for anal sex. Safe sex was positioned as a community practice, the responsibility of all gay men irrespective of their HIV status (Watney, 1990).

With the availability of the HIV antibody test, antiretroviral therapy (ART), viral load testing and epidemiological knowledge about the likelihood of HIV transmission associated with various sexual practices, gay men in resource-rich countries have developed a repertoire of strategies to manage the risk of HIV infection without necessarily using a condom every time (Kippax, 2002; Kippax & Race, 2003; Rosengarten *et al.*, 2000; Van de Ven *et al.*, 2004).

From an epidemiological perspective, the highest risk of HIV transmission for men is unprotected receptive anal sex with ejaculation (Vittinghoff *et al.*, 1999). However, epidemiology does not take into account the social context in which such a practice occurs. Unprotected anal sex between two HIV-negative men is no risk at all; HIV transmission is simply not possible. Because the HIV antibody test made it possible for individuals to know their serostatus, two HIV-negative men in a regular, committed relationship could avoid using condoms within their relationship and still be safe. With casual partners outside the relationship, condoms were used for anal sex or anal sex was avoided (Kippax *et al.*, 1997). This strategy, termed 'negotiated safety', was translated into a health promotion campaign 'Talk, test, test, trust' (Kippax & Kinder, 2002). Properly applied, negotiated safety has been an effective risk management strategy (Crawford *et al.*, 2001). However, these agreements can and do sometimes break down (Prestage *et al.*, 2006).

'Strategic positioning' describes a risk reduction strategy that incorporates epidemiological knowledge about transmission risk associated with certain sexual practices (e.g. insertive versus receptive anal sex; anal versus oral sex). In serodiscordant[2] regular relationships, a distinct pattern of sexual positioning has been observed whereby most HIV-positive men were receptive and most HIV-negative men were insertive when they had unprotected anal sex. A similar pattern was observed in unprotected anal sex between casual partners (Van de Ven *et al.*, 2002b).

Improved ART suppresses viral replication and boosts the immune system, and has significantly reduced HIV-related illness and death. Viral load tests indicate the amount of HIV particles in a person's blood. 'Undetectable viral load' means the amount of virus in a person's blood is lower than the test is designed to measure – hence 'undetectable'. It does not mean that a person has cleared the virus. HIV is still present but only in very small amounts. HIV transmission from a person with undetectable viral load appears less likely but is still possible (Gray *et al.*, 2001). By combining knowledge about a person's viral load and strategic positioning, gay men have developed new risk minimization strategies other than condom use. Some serodiscordant couples where the HIV-positive partner's viral load is undetectable engage in unprotected anal sex where the negative partner usually takes the insertive and the positive partner the receptive position (Rosengarten *et al.*, 2000; Van de Ven *et al.*, 2002b, 2005).

Furthermore, with improved ART, HIV is no longer a terminal illness but rather a chronic condition. In this context, unprotected anal sex between casual partners has been associated with treatment optimism (Van de Ven *et al.*, 2002a). Two explanations have been offered for this association: Either, gay men are more prepared to engage in unprotected anal sex because perceptions of risk have changed. Alternatively, men who reported having unprotected anal sex may seek to account for their sexual practice in terms of treatment optimism (Van de Ven *et al.*, 1999, 2000).

Knowledge about treatment and clinical markers such as 'viral load' is, however, not widespread among HIV-negative gay men. Furthermore, messages such as 'shared responsibility' and 'assume everyone is positive' can mean different things to HIV-positive and -negative men, with implications for using or not using condoms (Rosengarten *et al.*, 2000). Risk reduction strategies – except for celibacy and masturbation – are not failsafe as they require negotiation and cooperation with sexual partners. Unsafe sex can happen in spite of knowledge about safe sex, not because of a lack of knowledge (Körner *et al.*, 2005a). And sometimes safe sex can fail because a partner does not cooperate (Körner *et al.*, 2005b).

Narratives of gay men about the sexual practices that led to their seroconversion have been found to be highly interdiscursive. They are, on the one hand, informed by the discourses underlying health promotion, with the men presenting themselves as knowledgeable and in control, to make sense of their infection. At the same time, the public health discourses of knowledge and control are recontextualized and enmeshed with the private world of intimate relationships and everyday lives (Kippax *et al.*, 2003; Körner *et al.*, 2004).

In a social public health approach to HIV, health promotion focuses on social relationships, actions, behaviors and meanings as they are produced in social contexts and in interactions with others. In this chapter I am specifically interested in this aspect of health promotion: how health promotion messages are taken up by those for whom they are intended and how they inform their sexual practices. Intersubjective analysis will show how gay men actively engage with risk reduction strategies and prevention messages as individuals, with their partners and as members of their communities.

The Study Context

The seroconversion study was based in Sydney, Australia. It was concerned with an exploration of sexual practices that caused gay men to become infected with HIV, and their understanding of 'risk' in this context. The study started in 1993, with a break between 1997 and 1999 due to practical difficulties with recruitment. It resumed in 2000 and ended in 2001. Because this chapter is concerned with the ways in which gay men engage with the increasingly complex risk reduction strategies that resulted from advances in science and medicine since the mid-1990s, the interviews that were conducted in 2000 and 2001 were chosen for analysis.

Participants were recruited through general practices and specialists with high HIV caseloads. All participants were gay men who had recently seroconverted, that is, had become infected with HIV. Interviews were open-ended. They were conducted in a non-judgemental, conversational style. Participants were asked if they could remember the occasion on which they believed they had become infected and to give a detailed account of the event. Interviews also explored the men's usual sexual practices, whether and how these were different from the seroconversion event, and their understanding and interpretations of 'safe' and 'unsafe' sex. Interviews were audio-recorded and transcribed. To ensure confidentiality, information that could identify participants was removed from the transcripts.

Theoretical Framework: Engagement and Graduation as Resources for Intersubjective Positioning

The theoretical framework for analyzing intersubjective positioning is located within Hallidayan systemic functional linguistics. It is a theory of language that is oriented towards meaning and views language as a social rather than as an individual phenomenon. Discourse analysis in this framework is concerned with, among other things, the role of language in articulating social identities and social relations (Halliday, 1978; Martin & Rose, 2003).

The linguistic resources for adopting an interpersonal stance towards the propositions presented in a text are the systems of engagement and graduation (Martin, 2000; Martin & White, 2005; White, 2000, 2003). The approach is informed by Bakhtin's notions of dialogism and heteroglossia (Bakhtin, 1981, 1986). The essence of dialogism and heteroglossia is that language is not a neutral medium to express an individual's knowledge but rather that all meaning is made against the backdrop of other meanings in a discourse community. Thus, all speech or writing reflects in some way prior speech or writing[3] and anticipates some kind of response from an actual or potential addressee. In other words, all communication occurs against the backdrop of other voices and alternative positions.

A dialogistic perspective attends to the relationship between a speaker's utterances and the utterances of other speakers on the same issue (Martin & White, 2005). Here we ask: What heteroglossic backdrop is construed in a text and how does a speaker engage with this backdrop? Are prior meanings acknowledged? Does a speaker align with them, distance himself or take a neutral stance? And does he expect his position to be shared or is it expected to be resisted or challenged?

Central to this dialogistic perspective is the notion of alignment/ disalignment. This refers to agreement/disagreement with respect to attitudes, beliefs and assumptions about the world as it is or ought to be. A speaker is not seen to simply express himself but to simultaneously invite others to share and endorse these expressions. Thus, a dialogistic perspective focuses on the relationship between speaker and addressee, and speaker and addressee aligning in a community of shared values and beliefs (Martin & White, 2005: 95).

Intersubjective positioning and alignment can be achieved through a variety of lexicogrammatical resources that will be outlined briefly.[4] Those linguistic resources that enable speakers to position themselves with respect to the voices and positions that form the heteroglossic backdrop to a communicative event are grouped together under 'engagement'. They can be divided into two broad categories: those that allow for alternative voices and positions ('dialogistic expansion'), and those that challenge, reject or restrict alternatives ('dialogistic contraction'). The options are shown in Figure 4.1.

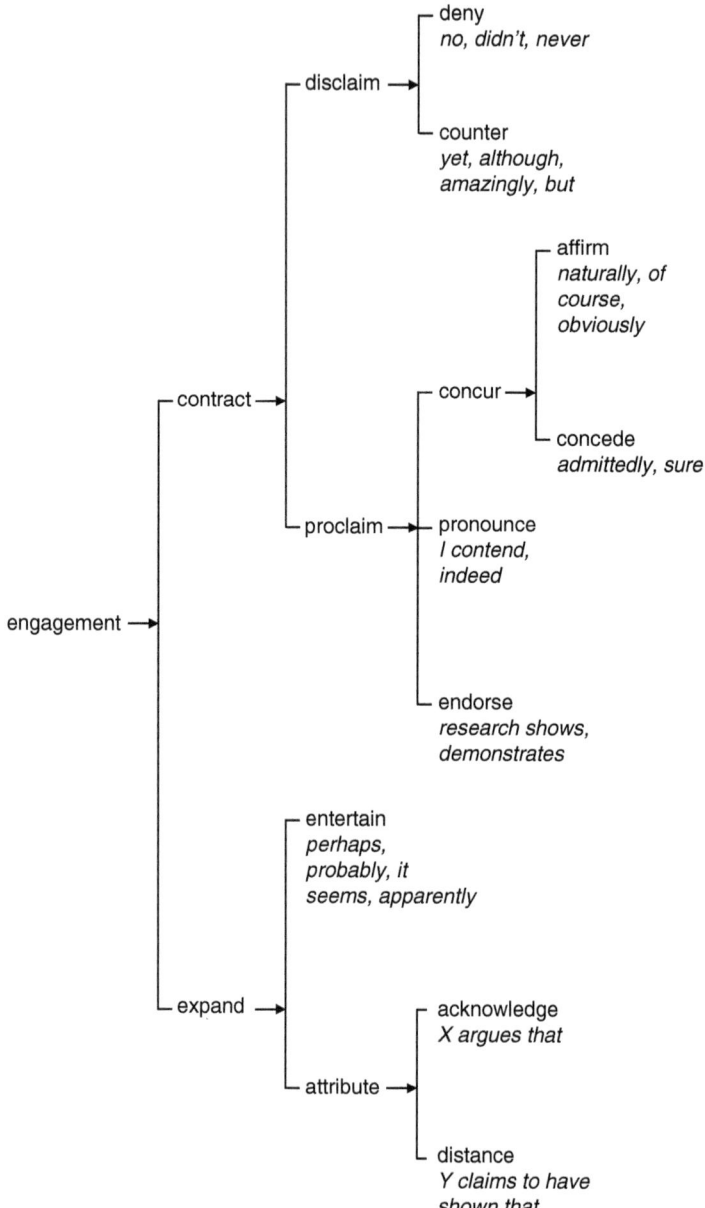

Figure 4.1 Engagement network
Source: Adapted from Martin and White (2005)

Dialogistic expansion can be achieved by bringing an external voice into a text through reporting structures, thereby grounding an alternative position in the subjectivity of an external source ('attribute'), for example 'My partner said kissing was safe'. It can also be achieved through expressions in a speaker's own voice ('entertain'), for example 'Kissing is probably safe'; 'It seems kissing is safe'; 'I think kissing is safe'. In a dialogistic perspective such expressions are not seen as an indication of uncertainty or a lack of commitment to the truth but as an acknowledgement that a position may not be shared by others, and that a position put forward is but one of a range of possible positions that can be taken on an issue.

Dialogistic contraction comprises those expressions that construe a backdrop of other voices and positions by acknowledging alternative positions and challenging, rejecting or restricting these alternatives. Under 'disclaim' are grouped those resources that directly reject alternatives by negating them ('deny'), for example, 'Kissing is not safe', and expressions that counter a position that may have been expected ('counter'), for example 'Although kissing is safe, I'm still worried'.

Under 'proclaim', are grouped expressions that, rather than directly rejecting an alternative position, limit the scope of possible alternatives (e.g. 'Of course kissing is safe'; 'There is evidence that kissing is safe').

'Graduation' comprises the linguistic resources to scale meanings up or down. The options are shown in Figure 4.2.

Graduation operates along two axes: grading according to intensity or amount ('force'), for example 'Kissing is possibly – probably – certainly safe'; 'I always – usually – sometimes – rarely use condoms'. The second axis relates to the grading of prototypicality and preciseness with which category boundaries are drawn ('focus'). Category boundaries can be blurred ('soften') to include marginal members (e.g. 'He kind of penetrated me'), or they can be drawn more precisely ('sharpen') to exclude marginal members (e.g. 'It was full on penetration'). These values allow a speaker to align more or less with the categorization of objects, phenomena and behavior.

As engagement and graduation are oriented towards meaning in context and rhetorical effects rather than towards grammatical form, it is important to consider that the rhetorical potential of individual words may vary in different contexts.

Analysis took a top-down approach. The first question was: What meanings were foregrounded in the men's narratives, that is, what choices from the language system did the men make in relation to the options available; which meanings worked together; and what particular effects were produced by these meanings? The next question was: How did these

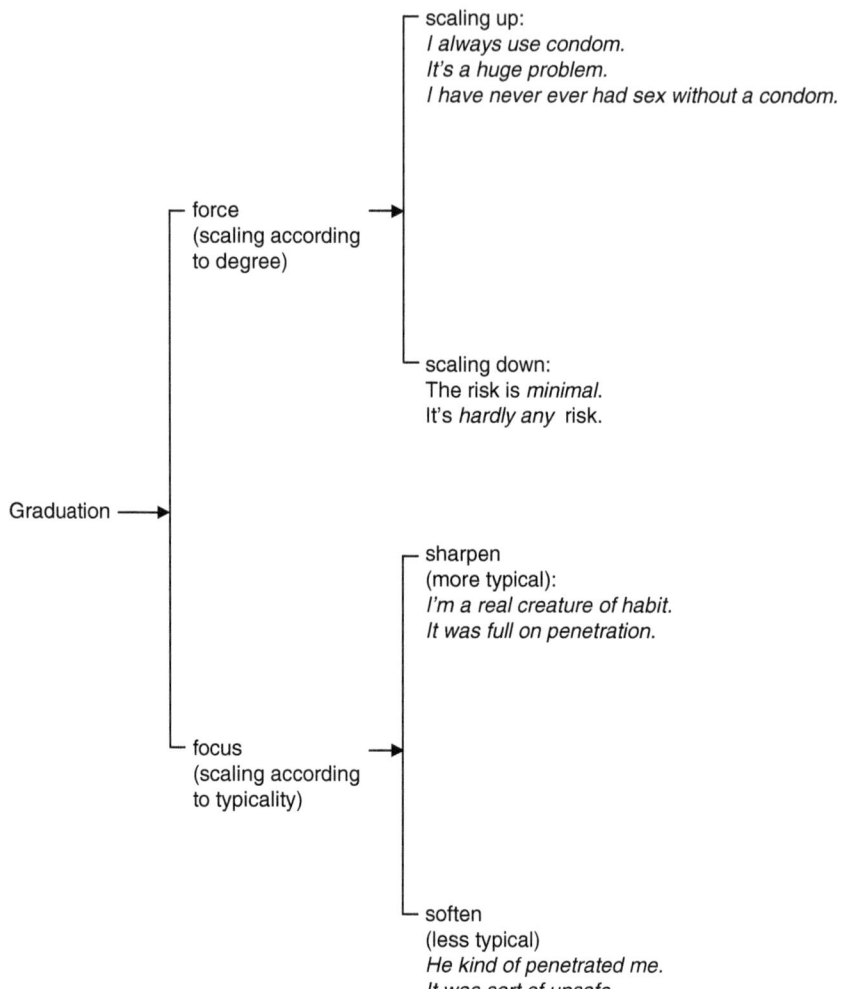

Figure 4.2 Graduation network
Source: Adapted from Martin and White (2005)

choices work to position the men in relation to their own perceptions of safe sex and their own sexual practices, to those of their sexual partners, and to health promotion messages. With what kind of meanings did they align; from what kind of meanings did they distance themselves? And finally: How did these meanings unfold and how did intersubjective positioning change as the narrative progressed (Martin & Rose, 2003)?

Negotiating Risk Reduction Strategies: Intersubjective Alignment and Disalignment

Men's understanding of 'safe sex' is interwoven with health promotion messages of condom use as well as the various alternative risk reduction strategies described above. In addition, the men engage with their partners' understanding of safe sex, including former partners. The following section will discuss engagement and graduation patterns and, where relevant, the way in which they unfold logogenetically.

'Use a condom every time'

Extract 1[5]

(interviewer's questions in *italics*)

Can you tell me what you understand to be safe?

Okay. For me safe sex, I do engage in obviously kissing, oral, fucking, top, bottom. Any kind of penetration is done with a condom and that's that. ... Always. Every time. ... I have never had sex without a condom ever in my life. ... I'm 46 and it – I train and the only reason I train is because it's become a habit. I'm a real creature of habit and I don't change my habit. You know, if I have sex with someone then it's just habit. You just go and put on a condom. There's no heat of the moment situation that occurs for me because it's a habit. It's a clock. It always happens.

This man's understanding of safe sex is grounded in and revolves around health promotion messages such as 'use a condom every time', and the dialogistic space for alternative positions, that is, risk reduction strategies without condoms, is contracted consistently. At the same time, this participant indicates that his position on this issue is but one in a range of alternatives. (Table 4.1; Utterances are numbered. The table should be read following the numbers, if necessary across columns. Values of dialogistic expansion are underlined, dialogistic contraction double underlined, and graduation in SMALL CAPS.)

Where the participant engages with his sexual practices and other activities that he approaches in a similar manner, dialogistic alternatives are constrained ('I do engage in obviously kissing, oral, fucking, top, bottom'). The dialogistic functionality of 'do' and 'obviously' limits the scope of alternatives, that is, sexual activities from which he could refrain ('fucking', 'top', 'bottom'). This rhetorical strategy acknowledges the fact

Table 4.1 'Use a condom every time': Engagement and graduation

| Monogloss | Heterogloss | |
	Expand	Contract
	1. <u>For me</u> [*entertain*], safe sex.	
		2. I <u>do</u> engage [*proclaim: pronounce*] in <u>obviously</u> [*proclaim: concur*] kissing, oral, fucking, top, bottom.
3. Any kind of penetration is done with a condom and that's that.		
	4. <u>ALWAYS</u> [*entertain + intensify: upscale*]. EVERY time [*intensify: upscale*].	
		5. I have <u>NEVER</u> [*disclaim: deny + intensify: upscale*] had sex without a condom <u>EVER</u> [*disclaim: deny + intensify: upscale*] <u>IN MY LIFE</u> [*intensify: upscale*].
6. I'm 46 and it – I train		
		7. and the <u>only</u> reason [*disclaim: counter*] I train is because it's become a habit.
		8. I'm a REAL [*focus: sharpen*] creature of HABIT [*intensify: upscale*] and I <u>don't</u> [*proclaim: deny*] change my HABIT [*intensify: upscale*].
		9. You know, if I have sex with someone then it's <u>just</u> [*disclaim: counter*] HABIT [*intensify: upscale*].
		10. You <u>just</u> [*disclaim: counter*] go and put on a condom.

(Continued)

Table 4.1 *Continued*

| | Heterogloss | |
Monogloss	Expand	Contract
		11. There's <u>no</u> [*disclaim: deny*] heat of the moment situation that occurs for me because it's a HABIT [*intensify: upscale*].
12. It's A CLOCK [*intensify: upscale*].		
	13. It <u>ALWAYS</u> [*entertain + upscale*] happens.	

that some gay men do not engage in anal sex to reduce the risk of HIV transmission but the participant does not apply this alternative to himself. This is followed by a statement that is presented as a proposition for which no dialogistic alternatives need to be considered in this communicative context ('Any kind of penetration is done with a condom'). No alternatives are attributed to an external source, for example, '<u>My partner insists</u> that any kind of penetration is done with a condom', and no alternatives are entertained by the participant himself, for example, 'Any kind of penetration is <u>usually</u> done with a condom'. A series of 'deny' values then overtly reject the possibility of sex without condom ('<u>never</u> had sex without a condom'; '<u>don't</u> change'; '<u>no</u> heat of the moment'). Dialogistic space is further constrained ('<u>just</u> habit'; '<u>just</u> go and put a condom on'); the speaker positions himself in contrast to a position that could be expected in its place, for example, being tired of condom use after so many years, or acting in the heat of passion. Rhetorically this participant distances himself from the reasons that have sometimes been put forward for not using condoms: condom fatigue, passion and the desire for intimacy.

These values that contract the space for dialogistic alternatives to condom use are reinforced by graduation values that intensify these meanings ('<u>never ever in my life</u>') and the repetition of 'habit' ('a real creature of <u>habit</u>'; 'don't change my <u>habit</u>'; 'just <u>habit</u>'; 'it's a <u>habit</u>'; 'it's a <u>clock</u>'). They are further supported by sharpening category boundaries: The participant is not simply 'a creature of habit' but 'a <u>real</u> creature of habit'. Thus, any behavior falling outside the participant's categorization of safe sex through condom use is excluded. By constraining the space for dialogistic alternatives and intensifying these meanings, the participant fully aligns with the health promotion message of 'use a condom every time' disseminated by gay community organizations.

At the same time, however, dialogistic space is expanded; the participant indicates that his position on condom use is but one of a range of possible positions in this matter ('for me'; 'always') and he makes space for these alternatives. The rhetorical effect of 'always' using condoms is that the possibility of an alternative (e.g. to sometimes – usually – rarely – never use condoms) is acknowledged, and the interpersonal investment in this proposition is maximized. Furthermore, while condoms still provide the best protection against HIV, transmission is still possible and this possibility is acknowledged. Risk cannot be eliminated, it can only be reduced.

By expanding dialogistic space, the participant disaligns with those voices among gay men who practice risk reduction without consistent condom use. By contracting dialogistic space, he disaligns with the reasons that are sometimes given for not using condoms: forgetting, condoms not being available, getting carried away by passion or wanting emotional intimacy with a partner (Körner *et al.*, 2005a).

'Negotiated safety' and 'strategic positioning'

Extract 2

In the entire time we've slept together he's [partner] had sex outside the relationship. I haven't. He has confided in me that he has been in about a four-month period before I met him where he'd been unsafe with two people. But he was top and apparently that is a very minimal chance. Whoever plays top has a very minimal chance of contracting HIV. As far as I am concerned that's no excuse. If you have unsafe sex then you shouldn't be telling someone you're negative until you've had a test to prove that. Unsafe sex is unsafe sex and I don't think information like that should be given just because of the less chance of contracting it. It doesn't mean that you're not going to contract it.

This man engages with risk reduction strategies such as negotiated safety in his own relationship, which is however construed as monogamy, and strategic positioning by his partner in casual sexual encounters outside the relationship. He also engages with the way in which these strategies have been taken up by some gay men and the way in which information circulates in the gay community. Through a combination of dialogistically expansive and contractive meanings, and alternating between dialogistic expansion and contraction, a highly heteroglossic backdrop is construed where opinions about risk reduction strategies are divided and contested (Table 4.2).

Table 4.2 'Negotiated safety' and 'strategic positioning': Engagement and graduation

Monogloss	Heterogloss	
	Expand	*Contract*
1. In the ENTIRE time [*intensify: upscale*] we've slept together he's [new partner] had sex outside the relationship.		
		2. I haven't [*disclaim: deny*].
	3. He has confided in me [*attribute*] that he has been in about a four-month period before I met him where he'd been unsafe with two people.	
		4. But [*disclaim: counter*] he was top
	5. and apparently [*entertain*] that is a VERY MINIMAL chance [*intensify: downscale*].	
6. Whoever plays top has a VERY MINIMAL chance [*intensify: downscale*] of contracting HIV.		
	7. As far as I am concerned [*entertain*]	
		8. that's no excuse [*disclaim: deny*].
		9. If you have unsafe sex then you shouldn't [*disclaim: deny*] be telling someone you're negative until you've had a test to prove that.

(*Continued*)

Table 4.2 *Continued*

	Heterogloss	
Monogloss	Expand	Contract
10. Unsafe sex is unsafe sex		
		11. and I <u>don't</u> think [*disclaim: deny*]
	12. <u>information like that</u> [*attribute*] should be given	
		13. <u>just</u> [*disclaim: counter*] because of the LESS chance [*intensify: downscale*] of contracting it.
		14. It <u>doesn't</u> mean [*disclaim: deny*] that you're <u>not</u> going to contract [*disclaim: deny*] it.

'Safe sex' in a regular relationship is construed as monogamy and the alternative is explicitly rejected ('I haven't'). Dialogistic space is then expanded through a proposition that is attributed to an external voice, the partner ('he has confided in me'). But dialogistic space is immediately contracted again by a 'counter' value ('<u>but</u> he was top'). This counter-expectation, in turn, is presented as but one possibility, and dialogistic space is expanded again ('apparently'). Finally, this sequence culminates in a proposition for which alternatives are no longer acknowledged: 'Whoever plays top has a very minimal chance of contracting HIV'.

The participant then explicitly disaligns with this utterance construing risk assessment as it applies to his relationship by explicitly rejecting it ('<u>no</u> excuse'; 'shoul<u>dn't</u>'). However, this rejection is acknowledged as being but one possible position and grounded in the speaker's individual subjectivity ('as far as I am concerned'). And again, this sequence culminates in a proposition without an alternative: 'Unsafe sex is unsafe sex'.

Finally, the speaker engages with epidemiological findings and the way in which they have been taken up to manage risk, deploying the same expand–contract dynamic: Dialogistic space is expanded through attribution to an external source ('information like that'). But this very alternative is rejected by the speaker ('I don't think information like that should be given'), and dialogistic space is further contracted ('it doesn't mean'; 'you're not going to get it').

Graduation here operates separately from engagement. Graduation does not scale the speaker's alignment or disalignment with risk reduction strategies but scales epidemiological models of transmission in non-numerical terms (e.g. 'a very minimal chance').

Overall, this participant aligns with monogamy as a risk reduction strategy; he disaligns with strategic positioning, the research that provides figures about probabilities of transmission, and the way in which these figures have been taken up by some gay men to inform their sexual practices.

'Assume everyone is positive' and 'Talk, test, test, trust'

Extract 3

It would always be a case of, sort of, if you met somebody and you weren't in a relationship, it was like a casual encounter, you met them at a club and went home with them. It would be a case of like, okay, see what it would feel like up there without [condom] for two seconds and then it's got to come out and have something put on it. Do you know what I mean? ... I always had assumed that they were positive. Always had safe sex, always. ... Except when I'd been in past relationships where me and my partner had gone and got tested. Do you know what I mean? And then it would be a case of – even after having the first test – waiting for a few months to have a secondary[6] test sort of thing. And plus you don't meet somebody every day where you kind of have that trust where you know that they're not going to go and have any sort of sexual contact with anybody behind your back. That's very rare, and I really think that's putting your life in somebody's hands.

This participant engages with different kinds of relationships between gay men and different risk reduction strategies for different relationships. 'Assume everyone is positive' promotes condom use as a shared responsibility for all gay men, irrespective of their HIV status. The more recent 'Talk, test, test, trust' was developed out of the phenomenon of negotiated safety, whereby two HIV-negative men in a regular relationship have unprotected anal sex with each other after both of them have had two HIV tests done. Engagement and graduation values are shown in Table 4.3.

Table 4.3 'Assume everyone is positive' and 'Talk, test, test, trust': Engagement and graduation

| | Heterogloss | |
Monogloss	Expand	Contract
	1. It <u>would</u> ALWAYS [*entertain + intensify: upscale*] be a case of SORT OF [*focus: soften*]	
		2. if you met somebody and you <u>weren't</u> [*disclaim: deny*] in a relationship
3. it was LIKE [*focus: soften*] a casual encounter,		
4. you met them at a club and went home with them.		
	5. It <u>would</u> [*entertain*] be a case of like,	
	6. okay, see what it <u>would</u> [*entertain*] feel like up there without [condom] for two seconds	
	7. and then it's <u>got to</u> [*entertain*] come out and have something put on it.	
	8. I <u>ALWAYS</u> [*entertain + intensify: upscale*] had assumed that they were positive.	
	9. <u>Always</u> [*entertain + intensify: upscale*] had safe sex, <u>ALWAYS</u> [*entertain + intensify: upscale*].	

(Continued)

Table 4.3 *Continued*

Monogloss	Heterogloss	
	Expand	*Contract*
		10. Except [*disclaim: counter*] when I'd been in past relationships where me and my partner had gone and got tested.
	11. And then it would [*entertain*] be a case of	
		12. even [*disclaim: counter*] after having the first test – waiting for a few months to have a secondary test SORT OF THING [*focus: soften*].
		13. And plus you don't [*disclaim: deny*] meet somebody EVERY [*intensify: upscale*] day where you KIND OF [*focus: soften*] have that trust where you know that they're not [*disclaim: deny*] going to go and have ANY SORT OF sexual contact [*focus: sharpen*] with anybody behind your back.
	14. That's VERY rare [*entertain + intensify: upscale*]	
	15. and I REALLY think [*entertain + intensify: upscale*] that's putting your life in somebody's hands.	

The heteroglossic backdrop to risk reduction in casual relationships (1–9) is dialogistically expansive and all values are entertained by the participant. He aligns with a risk reduction strategy that has been described as 'nudging' (Richters *et al.*, 2003), that is a brief, shallow or partial penetration without a condom. This strategy is positioned as an alternative to penetration with a condom ('would always'; 'would be a case of'; 'what it would feel like'; 'it's got to come out'). It is entertained by the speaker as one alternative to penetration with a condom that is not shared by all.

Dialogistic expansion is supported by graduation values that soften the boundaries of the relationship categories 'casual' and 'regular'. Types of relationships are positioned as fuzzy, without clear boundaries specifying what counts as, or doesn't count as, as a casual relationship ('a case of sort of'; 'like a casual encounter'; see also Prestage *et al.*, 2001), further opening up semantic space.

The heteroglossic backdrop to risk reduction in regular relationships is dialogistically contractive (10–15). First, risk reduction in regular relationships is positioned as counter ('except') to risk reduction in casual relationships. Other 'disclaim' values engaging with risk reduction in regular relationships don't foreclose alternatives to condom use but alternatives to trust and being faithful, and these are scaled up and the category boundaries are sharpened ('You don't meet someone every day'; 'they're not going to go and have any sort of sexual contact'). This dialogistic contraction, however, is construed as but one possible alternative and this alternative is scaled up for impact ('very rare'; 'I really think').

In summary, this participant aligns with condom use for all, but at the same time this alignment is dialogistically highly expansive. He also aligns with monogamy and trust in a relationship as risk reduction strategies. This is construed by contracting dialogistic space for alternatives.

Treatment optimism

Extract 4

I always knew that I was taking a risk and I'd been seeing a therapist. ... It was like I'd been doing it for so long and I'd been getting regularly tested and I was always fine and I was always thinking that, you know, even if I did become positive it's not a death sentence any more. Now that I have become positive if I had realized the things that, you know, taking the drugs every day, the side effects of the drugs. I used to go to the doctor once a year. In the last three months I think I've been 15 times. ...

Do you think if you'd seen anyone with AIDS –?

Oh for sure. And on top of that, like, also the fact that even if I knew if I became positive that there were the drugs there that would make like, you know, pretty much as normal. I probably looked at it like something similar to diabetes. That was kind of how I looked at it.

This participant negotiates, firstly, his perceptions and sexual practices before he became infected and the role of ART in this and, secondly, his actual experience of treatment after infection in contrast to his perception of HIV infection as a chronic illness (Table 4.4).

Table 4.4 Treatment optimism: Engagement and graduation

Monogloss	*Heterogloss*	
	Expand	*Contract*
	1. I ALWAYS [*entertain + intensify: upscale*] knew that I was taking a risk	
2. and I'd been seeing a therapist		
3. it was like I'd been doing it for SO LONG [*quantify: upscale*]		
4. and I'd been getting regularly tested		
	5. and I was ALWAYS [*entertain + intensify: upscale*] fine	
	6. and I was ALWAYS [*entertain + intensify: upscale*] thinking	
		7. that even [*disclaim: counter*] if I did [*disclaim: counter*] become positive
		8. it's not [*disclaim: deny*] a death sentence anymore.
9. Now that I have become positive if I had realized the things that, you know, taking the drugs EVERY day [*intensify: upscale*], the side effects of the drugs.		

(Continued)

Table 4.4 *Continued*

| Monogloss | Heterogloss | |
	Expand	Contract
10. I used to go to the doctor once a year.		
	11. In the last three months <u>I think</u> [*entertain*] I've been 15 times.	
12. Interviewer: Do you think if you'd seen anyone with AIDS –?		
13. Oh FOR SURE [*intensify: upscale*].		
		14. And on top of that, like, also the fact that <u>even</u> [*disclaim: counter*] if I knew if I became positive that there were the drugs there
	15. that <u>would</u> [*entertain*] make, like, you know, PRETTY MUCH [*focus: soften*] as normal.	
	16. I <u>probably</u> [*entertain*] looked at it like SOMETHING SIMILAR [*focus: soften*] to diabetes.	
17. That was KIND OF [*focus: soften*] how I looked at it.		

In his risk perception (1–8), values of dialogistic expansion are entertained by the speaker and intensified through repetition ('<u>always</u> knew'; 'was <u>always</u> fine'; 'was <u>always</u> thinking'). By acknowledging that his position of knowing about risk and knowingly engaging in risk practices is but one alternative, he disaligns with those men who attribute their HIV infection to being uninformed or being taken advantage of by others. This position is rhetorically supported by two monoglossic utterances ('I'd been doing it for so long'; 'I'd been getting tested regularly'). No alternatives to the speaker's risk management strategies are acknowledged; a negative test result seems to be taken for granted.

Dialogistic contraction in this section first counters the position that might be expected from someone who knows that he has taken risks for a long time ('even if I did become positive'), and then rejects the consequences of HIV infection prior to ART ('not a death sentence any more').

In the second section (9–17), the reality of being HIV-positive and taking ART is being negotiated. Dialogistic expansion ('In the last three months I think I've been 15 times') construes the difficulties associated with ART: regular monitoring of blood counts, the difficulty of getting the right regimen and the need to manage side effects. Dialogistic expansion is still entertained by the speaker and explicitly grounded in his own subjectivity ('I think'). Another thread in the heteroglossic backdrop here is the participant's perception of HIV as a chronic condition rather than a terminal illness. Dialogistic expansion is rhetorically supported by graduation values blurring the category 'HIV chronic illness' ('pretty much as normal'; 'something similar to diabetes'; 'kind of how I looked at it').

Negotiating risk reduction trajectories

Extract 5

Can you tell me what you consider is a risk for HIV?

I'll get to that. The first person I had sex with overseas I didn't know at the time was actually positive. So it was quite a shock to me then and I was giving – and I had no knowledge of HIV or transmission or anything at all. I was quite innocent about it all, and hadn't had sex much with guys. We went to his doctor and got tested and got quite a bit of information. That was the first person I had sex with over there. So, after that I sort of got a bit of a shock and was a lot better for a while.

What do you mean you were a lot better?

In terms of safer sex, like protected sex and using condoms, but there was more discussion with him. This was when the first drugs – He was actually undetectable levels then and so we actually talked again about having sex without condoms and he said a lot of his friends do things like that and we grew apart. . . . After that I was having a lot of sex but only fucking, not getting fucked. I obviously didn't like using condoms and my idea was always – became like that I got regularly tested and that I never got fucked. . . . By the time until recently I had that much unprotected sex only being the active partner that I had pretty much believed in my own mind that I wasn't going to catch it for that very reason. That it was safe enough to be top but not a bottom.

This extract represents probably the most complex heteroglossic backdrop in this sample. It engages with the participant's HIV-positive partner, his partner's doctor and friends. It also engages with the participant's life trajectory from coming out as a gay man, his homosexual debut in a sero-discordant relationship, casual encounters after the break-up with his partner, and the trajectory from no 'safe sex' knowledge to incorporating complex risk reduction strategies into his repertoire (Table 4.5).

Table 4.5 Negotiating risk reduction trajectories: Engagement and graduation

| Monogloss | Heterogloss | |
	Expand	Contract
1. I'll get to that.		
		2. The first person I had sex with overseas I didn't [disclaim: deny] know at the time was actually positive.
3. So it was QUITE a shock [intensify: upscale] to me then		
4. and I was giving		
		5. and I had no knowledge [disclaim: deny] of HIV or transmission or anything AT ALL [intensify: upscale].
6. I was QUITE innocent [intensify: upscale] about it ALL [intensify: upscale],		
		7. and hadn't had [disclaim: deny] sex much with guys.

(Continued)

Table 4.5 *Continued*

| Monogloss | Heterogloss | |
	Expand	Contract
	8. We went to his doctor and got tested and got QUITE A BIT [*quantify: upscale*] of information.	
9. That was the first person I had sex with over there.		
10. So, after that I SORT OF [*focus: soften*] got A BIT of a shock [*intensify: downscale*] and was A LOT better [*intensify: upscale*] for a while.		
11. (interviewer): What do you mean you were A LOT better [*intensify: upscale*]?		
12. In terms of safer sex, like protected sex and using condoms,		
		13. but [*disclaim: counter*]
	14. there was MORE discussion [*attribute + quantify upscale*] with him.	
15. This was when the first drugs –		
16. He was actually undetectable levels then		
	17. and so we actually talked again about [*attribute*] having sex without condoms	

(Continued)

Table 4.5 *Continued*

Monogloss	Heterogloss	
	Expand	*Contract*
	18. and <u>he said</u> [*attribute*] A LOT [*quantify: upscale*] of his friends do things LIKE THAT [*focus: soften*]	
19. and we grew apart.		
20. After that I was having A LOT of sex [*quantify: upscale*]		
		21. <u>but only</u> [disclaim: counter] fucking, <u>not</u> [*disclaim: deny*] getting fucked.
		22. By the time until recently I had THAT MUCH [*quantify: upscale*] unprotected sex <u>only</u> [*disclaim: counter*] being the active partner
	23. that I had PRETTY MUCH [*intensify: upscale*] <u>believed</u> [*entertain*] in my own mind	
		24. that I <u>wasn't</u> going to catch it [*disclaim: deny*] for THAT VERY reason [*focus: sharpen*].
25. That it was safe ENOUGH [*focus: soften*] to be top		
		26. <u>but</u> [*disclaim: counter*] <u>not</u> [*disclaim: deny*] a bottom.

The first three disclaim values ('<u>didn't</u> know'; '<u>no</u> knowledge'; '<u>hadn't</u> had sex much with guys') reject the alternative of the speaker being knowledgeable about HIV and, in fact, him being homosexually active as someone who came out quite late in life. He thus construes himself as being apart from the gay community, which promoted knowledge about HIV transmission and risk reduction through condoms. These dialogistically contractive utterances alternate with monoglossic utterances in describing his emotional reaction when first coming into sexual contact with an HIV-positive man, and these are intensified ('<u>quite</u> a shock'; '<u>quite</u> innocent about it all').

This prosody of monoglossic utterances with intensification continues through the next five utterances (8–12). The communicative values intensified are information ('<u>quite a bit</u> of information') and concomitant risk reduction through condom use ('<u>a lot</u> better'). These monoglossic utterances are then countered ('but') and dialogistic space is now expanded, bringing the partner's voice into the text ('<u>discussion</u> with him').

Dialogistic expansion in this extract is typically attributed to other voices: the doctor who provides information about HIV, and the partner who brings his (presumably HIV-positive) friends into the discussion ('we <u>talked about</u> having sex without condoms'; '<u>he said</u> a lot of his friends did things like that'). This thread of the heteroglossic backdrop hinges on the partner's undetectable viral load, which is represented by the participant in a monoglossic utterance, as if taken for granted ('He was actually undetectable levels'), when there are really two external sources involved: '<u>My partner said</u> that <u>his doctor had told</u> him that he was undetectable levels'.

In the last phase of this extract (20–24), the participant negotiates his risk management post-breakup: dialogistic space is contracted by excluding the alternative that carries the highest risk of transmitting HIV ('<u>only</u> fucking'; '<u>not</u> getting fucked'; '<u>only</u> being the active partner'; '<u>but not</u> a bottom') and the concomitant expectation of being safe ('<u>wasn't</u> going to catch it'). This last utterance, however, hinges on a dialogistic expansive utterance ('<u>I ... believed</u>'), which positions the expectation of not becoming infected with HIV as but one possible outcome.

This participant initially disaligns with homosexual activities generally, the gay community and the risk reduction advocated by the community. But then he aligns fully with the complex risk reduction strategies without condoms that have been developed by gay men, to the extent that the alternative of condom use is now foreclosed.

The Heteroglossic Nature of 'Safe Sex' Knowledge

'Safe sex' and 'safer sex', as represented in semi-structured, in-depth social research interviews with gay men who seroconverted, are not a phenomenon that can be defined in the way that, for example, scientific terms can be defined. Rather, gay men present a rich tapestry of knowledge where numerous threads are interwoven with each other: individual knowledge, community knowledge, biomedical knowledge, and the knowledge of friends, partners and doctors. Furthermore, accounts of knowledge are dialogistically interwoven with accounts of enacting this knowledge in specific contexts of sexual relationships, past and present. Accounts of knowledge are also interwoven with accounts of partners enacting their respective understandings of safe sex in sexual relationships with other men.

Intersubjective analysis identifies not only the voices that constitute the heteroglossic backdrop to participants' safe sex knowledge, but also how these voices interact with each other, and how individual players respond to, engage with, and converge or diverge with these voices. Medical technologies such as HIV testing, viral load tests and ART have become part of prevention. However, the relationship between biomedical technologies and risk reduction is not a straightforward one. Some risk reduction strategies such as negotiated safety, as they are presented by the participants, are neither 'safe' nor 'negotiated'. Intersubjective analysis shows just how dialogistically expansive some accounts of these strategies are and the extent to which heteroglossic alternatives are acknowledged and invited.

While this chapter does not attempt to measure or quantify heteroglossic choices and intersubjective positionings, the amount of heteroglossic utterances does stand out. In a dialogistic framework, monoglossic utterances (or 'bare assertions') are understood to represent social subject positions that are unproblematic and uncontested in a particular communicative context (White, 2003). Intersubjective analysis shows that there is actually very little in the men's accounts that is uncontested and commonly accepted. For most positions, alternatives are acknowledged.

A further observation is that (except for extract 5) most dialogistic expansion is entertained by the participants. Thus, heteroglossic alternatives are construed by invoking participants' individual subjectivity rather than attributing alternatives to external sources.

Heteroglossia, Dialogism and Social Public Health

Social public health focuses on social relationships, the social glue, so to speak, between individuals and their communities. A heteroglossic, dialogistic framework stresses the interaction between broader social positions rather than the interactions between autonomous, self-determining individuals (White, 2000, 2003). The interconnected notions of heteroglossia and dialogism, and linguistic microanalysis enable us to describe some of the complexity of this social glue in a specific social context. This approach makes it evident how knowledge about safe sex and acting on this knowledge are socially produced by individuals in interactions with others: knowledge is multiply constructed, contextualized and recontextualized through active engagement with scientific information, with other men, with health professionals and with the gay community.

The notions of heteroglossia and dialogism also challenge the dichotomy between what is 'objective' or 'subjective', 'fact' or 'opinion'. A dialogistic approach emphasizes that utterances enter into relationships with other, convergent or divergent, utterances. Thus 'objective facts' such as 'His viral load was undetectable' are interpersonally charged because they are seen as one utterance in a relationship with alternative and potentially contradictory utterances. Thus, the difference between 'objective' and 'subjective' is not one between 'fact' and 'opinion' but the degree to which the dialogistic context in which an utterance operates is acknowledged (White, 2000).

Australia has adopted a social public health approach in its response to the HIV epidemic (Kippax, 2007). Critical to its success has been a partnership between the communities most affected by HIV/AIDS, the non-government organizations who represent and advocate for these communities, governments, clinicians and researchers. This cooperation has not only contained the spread of the epidemic, it has also produced a range of new risk reduction strategies that have been taken up by gay men to varying degrees. It has been argued that risk reduction strategies without condoms post-1996 should not be seen as a return to the 'old ways' but as a post-crisis position with its own dynamic (Race, 2001). With the success of new therapies in 1996 that turned HIV infection into a chronic, controllable condition, gay men have developed alternative ways of thinking about and acting in relation to risk (Kippax & Race, 2003).

Another crucial element in Australia's response to the HIV epidemic has been critical reflexive practice in the collaboration between social researchers and health educators (Kippax & Kinder, 2002). Reflexive practice examines the respective relationships between researchers and research participants, and between health educators and the targets of health promotion. Essentially, it involves taking up an epistemological stance that recognizes multiple social subject positions; 'to be (critically) reflexive one has to know that one can think differently than one thinks, and perceive differently than one sees' (Kippax & Kinder, 2002: 94). Critical reflexivity acknowledges the 'subjective', multi-voiced nature of knowledge. It acknowledges alternative forms of knowledge and interpretations. It acknowledges that meanings are made against a backdrop of other meanings and attends to relationships between meanings in a discourse community. Thus, the critical reflexive stance of a social public health approach resonates strongly with Bakhtin's notions of heteroglossia and dialogism, and with the multi-voiced nature of discourse. 'Safe sex', both as a practice and as a discourse, is indeed anything but straightforward and rather a choice between alternative technologies and subjectivities, acknowledging some and rejecting others in different social and sexual contexts.

Acknowledgment

The interviews were conducted and transcribed by Olympia Hendry, National Centre in HIV Epidemiology and Clinical Research.

Notes

1. Approximately two to three months after infection, the body begins to produce antibodies against HIV, that is seroconvert.
2. One partner is HIV positive, and one partner is HIV negative.
3. Because this chapter deals with spoken language data, the terms 'speaker' and 'listener' will be used from now on, even though the theory applies to both spoken and written texts.
4. For a detailed account, including reasoning and theoretical underpinnings, see Martin and White (2005: chap. 3).
5. For reasons of space and readability, clarification questions and feedback utterances such as 'okay', 'right', etc. have been omitted.
6. A second test after three months to account for the window period.

References

Bakhtin, M. (1981) Discourse in the novel (C. Emerson and M. Holquist, trans.). In M. Holquist (ed.) *The Dialogic Imagination* (pp. 259–522). Austin: University of Texas Press.
Bakhtin, M. (1986) The problem of speech genres (V.W. McGee, trans.). In D. Emerson and M. Holquist (eds) *Speech Genres and Other Late Essays* (pp. 60–102). Austin: University of Texas Press.
Crawford, J., Rodden, P., Kippax, S. and Van de Ven, P. (2001) Negotiated safety and other agreements between men in relationships: Risk practice redefined. *International Journal of STD & AIDS* 12, 164–170.
Gray, R.H., Wawer, M.J., Brookmeyer, R., Sewankambo, N.K., Serwadda, D., Wabwire-Mangen, F., Lutalo, T., Li, X., van Cott, T., Quinn, T.C. and the Rakai

Project Team (2001) Probability of HIV-1 transmission per coital act in monoga-
mous, heterosexual, HIV-1-discordant couples in Rakai, Uganda. *Lancet* 357,
1149–1153.
Halliday, M.A.K. (1978) *Language as Social Semiotic. The Social Interpretation of
Language and Meaning*. London: Edward Arnold.
Kippax, S. (2002) Negotiated safety agreements among gay men. In A. O'Leary
(ed.) *Beyond Condoms. Alternative Approaches to HIV Prevention* (pp. 1–15). New
York: Kluwer Academic/Plenum Publishers.
Kippax, S. (2007) *Reflections of a Social Scientist on Doing HIV Social Research*.
Retrieved 15 November 2007, from http://nchsr.arts.unsw.edu.au/presenta-
tions/KippaxIHHR.doc.
Kippax, S. and Kinder, P. (2002) Reflexive practice: The relationship between social
research and health promotion in HIV prevention. *Sex Education* 2, 91–104.
Kippax, S., Noble, J., Prestage, G., Crawford, J., Campbell, D., Baxter, D. and
Cooper, D. (1997) Sexual negotiation in the AIDS era: Negotiated safety revis-
ited. *AIDS* 11, 191–197.
Kippax, S. and Race, K. (2003) Sustaining safe practice: Twenty years on. *Social
Science & Medicine* 57, 1–12.
Kippax, S., Slavin, S., Hendry, O., Ellard, J., Richters, J., Grulich, A. and Kaldor, J.
(2003) Seroconversion in context. *AIDS Care* 15 (6), 839–852.
Körner, H., Hendry, O. and Kippax, S. (2004) 'I didn't think I was at risk':
Interdiscursive relations in narratives of sexual practices and exposure to HIV.
Communication and Medicine 1 (2), 131–143.
Körner, H., Hendry, O. and Kippax, S. (2005a) It's not just condoms: Social contexts
of unsafe sex in gay men's narratives of post-exposure prophylaxis for HIV.
Health, Risk & Society 7 (1), 47–62.
Körner, H., Hendry, O. and Kippax, S. (2005b) Negotiating risk and social relations
in the context of post-exposure prophylaxis for HIV: Narratives of gay men.
Health, Risk & Society 7 (4), 349–360.
Martin, J.R. (2000) Beyond exchange: Appraisal systems in English. In S. Hunston
and J. Thompson (eds) *Evaluation in Text: Authorial Stance and the Construction of
Discourse* (pp. 142–175). Oxford: Oxford University Press.
Martin, J.R. and White, P.R.R. (2005) *The Language of Evaluation. Appraisal in English*.
New York: Palgrave Macmillan.
Martin, J.R. and Rose, D. (2003) *Working with Discourse*. London: Continuum.
Prestage, G., Mao, L., McGuigan, D., Crawford, J., Kippax, S., Kaldor, J. and
Grulich, A. (2006) HIV risk and communication between regular partners in a
cohort of HIV-negative gay men. *AIDS Care* 18 (2), 166–172.
Prestage, G., Van de Ven, P., Grulich, A., Kippax, S., McInnes, D. and Hendry, O.
(2001) Gay men's casual sexual encounters: Discussing HIV and using condoms.
AIDS Care 13 (3), 277–284.
Race, K. (2001) The undetectable crisis: Changing technologies of risk. *Sexualities* 4
(2), 167–189.
Richters, J., Hendry, O. and Kippax, S. (2003) When safe sex isn't safe. *Culture,
Health & Sexuality* 5 (1), 37–52.
Rosengarten, M., Race, K. and Kippax, S. (2000) *'Touch Wood, Everything Will Be
Ok.' Gay Men's Understandings of Clinical Markers in Sexual Practice (Monograph
7/2000)*. Sydney: National Centre in HIV Social Research, University of New
South Wales.

Van de Ven, P., Kippax, S., Crawford, J., Rawstorne, P., Prestage, G., Grulich, A. and Murphy, D. (2002b) In a minority of gay men, sexual risk practices indicate strategic positioning for perceived risk reduction rather than unbridled sex. *AIDS Care* 14, 471–480.

Van de Ven, P., Kippax, S., Knox, S., Prestage, G. and Crawford, J. (1999) HIV treatment optimism and sexual behavior among gay men in Sydney and Melbourne. *AIDS* 13, 2289–2294.

Van de Ven, P., Mao, L., Fogarty, A., Rawstorne, P., Crawford, J., Prestage, G., Grulich, A., Kaldor, J. and Kippax, S. (2005) Undetectable viral load is associated with sexual risk taking in HIV serodiscordant couples in Sydney. *AIDS* 19, 179–184.

Van de Ven, P., Murphy, D., Hull, P., Prestage, G., Batrouney, C. and Kippax, S. (2004) Risk management and harm reduction among gay men in Sydney. *Critical Public Health* 14 (4), 361–376.

Van de Ven, P., Prestage, G., Crawford, J., Grulich, A. and Kippax, S. (2000) Sexual risk behavior increases and is associated with HIV optimism among HIV-negative and HIV-positive gay men in Sydney over the 4 year period to February 2000. *AIDS* 14 (18), 2951–2953.

Van de Ven, P., Rawstorne, P., Nakamura, T., Crawford, J. and Kippax, S. (2002a) HIV treatments optimism is associated with unprotected anal intercourse with regular and with casual partners among Australian gay and homosexually active men. *International Journal of STD & AIDS* 13, 181–183.

Vittinghoff, E., Douglas, J., Judson, F., McKirnan, D., MacQueen, K. and Buchbinder, S.P. (1999) Per-contact risk of human immunodeficiency virus transmission between male sexual partners. *American Journal of Epidemiology* 150 (3), 306–311.

Watney, S. (1990) Safer sex as community practice. In P. Aggleton, P. Davies and G. Hart (eds) *AIDS: Individual, Cultural and Policy Dimensions* (pp. 19–23). London: The Falmer Press.

White, P.R.R. (2000) Dialogue and inter-subjectivity: Reinterpreting the semantics of modality and hedging. In M. Coulthard, J. Cotterill and F. Rock (eds) *Dialogue Analysis VII: Working with Dialogue* (pp. 67–80). Tübingen: Max Niemeyer Verlag.

White, P.R.R. (2003) Beyond modality and hedging: A dialogic view of the language of intersubjective stance. *Text* 23 (2), 269–284.

Chapter 5

Dangerous Dogmas: AIDS, Discourse and the Rakhel System in India

NOUSHIN KHUSHRUSHAHI

> *AIDS does not exist apart from the practices that conceptualize it,*
> *represent it, and respond to it. We know AIDS only in and through*
> *those practices ... If we recognize that AIDS exists only in and through*
> *[these constructions of an underlying reality], then hopefully we can*
> *also recognize the imperative to know them, analyse them, and wrest*
> *control of them*
> Crimp (1988: 3)

Introduction

More than 20 years have now passed since Douglas Crimp (1988) put forward his landmark contribution on AIDS activism, arguing against the discursive constructions of homosexuality and promiscuity as essential 'facts' driving the AIDS epidemic. Such conceptualizations, he argued, are cultural representations, shaped and reshaped by the dogmas of a particular society. In India, the HIV/AIDS epidemic is formed in the context of specific cultural dogmas that intersect the discourses of gender, sexuality and responsibility. At the heart of this overlap is a gap between professional health care messages and local knowledge and practices that emphasize the importance of language, image and discourse in shaping ideologies about sex and sexuality.

Although linguistic analysis of professional health care discourses has been relatively rare in the Indian context, recent work focusing on other contexts has been particularly useful in providing a framework for conceptualizing the epidemic in India as well (Faria, 2008; Gee, 1996, 1999; Jones, 1997, 1999, 2002; Norris & Jones, 2005; Scollon, 1997). Current scholarship in India has largely focused on the structural vulnerabilities of brothel-based sex-workers, and there are many rich accounts examining the effectiveness of top-down prevention programmes, the constraints faced by these women, their health beliefs and norms, and their different modes of resistance (Amin, 2004; Bhattacharya, 2004; Dandona *et al.*, 2005; Evans & Lambert, 1997; Majumdar, 2000; Mooney & Sarangi, 2005; Nag, 1996; Nagelkerke *et al.*, 2002; Nath, 2000; Panda *et al.*, 2002; Pande, 2003; Rao *et al.*, 1994; Rao & Walton, 2004; Sarkar *et al.*, 2006; Verma *et al.*, 2004).

In this chapter, I examine the discursive context that shapes the manner in which some sex workers[1] in India conceive and respond to HIV/AIDS intervention messages. In particular, I explore how these women engage with, decode and respond to the information given in three government-sponsored pamphlets. I follow Cicourel's (quoted in Candlin, 2001: 187) emphasis that

> Verbal interaction is related to the task in hand. Language and other social practices are interdependent. Knowing something about the ethnographic setting, the perception of and characteristics attributed to others, and broader and local social organisational conditions becomes imperative for an understanding of linguistic and non-linguistic aspects of communicative events.

My analysis shows that women's responses to the pamphlets reveal the pervasiveness and significance of the *rakhel*[2] system – an oft ignored (in) formal marriage system incorporating sex workers and their long-term partners – in the spread of HIV/AIDS in India. My focus in this chapter is quite specific, as I explore why sex workers, who are both *knowledgeable about* and *able to* demand safe sex, engage in unprotected intercourse with regular patrons while insisting on condom use with less intimate clients. My broader aim, therefore, is to problematize the all-too-predictable assumption that information acquisition and increased capacity are the only two factors determining whether or not women (and specifically sex workers) engage in safe-sex practices. My argument is essentially this: the sex workers' engagement with government-produced awareness pamphlets reveals much about how they position themselves within wider discourses of gender and responsibility, and that these practices often shift depending on their self identification as sex workers, on the one hand, and as women/wives, on the other.

Discourse, Interpellation and Decoding: Conceptual Points of Entry

In order to better understand the reception of the discourses in the HIV prevention/intervention pamphlets and their broader implications, it is crucial to recognize that the words and images in these pamphlets do not invoke 'abstract ideas ... but rather ... individual actions within the semiotic aggregates that institutions and ideologies produce' (Norris & Jones, 2005: 11). As a result, discussions surrounding these HIV prevention/intervention pamphlets will inadvertently reveal social actions undertaken by sex workers, each of which are shaped and influenced by local discourse. Here, I use 'discourse' to refer to the 'characteristic ways of talking, acting, interacting, thinking, believing and valuing ... writing, reading and/or interpreting' (Gee, 1992: 20), which in relation to HIV prevention refers to understanding what constitutes 'appropriate' sexual behavior for both men and women. Locating the nexus of appropriate prevention practice requires an understanding of broader discourses dealing with how norms, social practices and behavior interrelate. It is here that Foucault's (1991) notion of 'governmentality', Gramci's (Williams, 1997) discussion of 'hegemony' and Althusser's (1971) theory of interpellation become particularly relevant.

Using the metaphor of pastoral power to describe the technique of modern statecraft, Foucault (2000) argued that self-rule requires that individual 'sheep' is led down the right (and in this case 'righteous') path by controlling potentially crippling deviance in order to preserve the societal 'herd' as a whole. Since 'the disciplines of the body and the regulations of the population [constitute] the two poles around which the organization of power over life [is] deployed' (Foucault, 1990: 139), sexuality, the most intimate facet of personal life, becomes the focus of a state's power. In India, gender and sexuality are mutually exclusive, and severe restraints on women's sexual behavior are part of everyday life. Any woman who contradicts the hegemonic edict of the 'pure', modest, virtuous and virginal unmarried female – either through her actions or perceived actions – is automatically targeted for her deviant ways.

Here, the Gramscian conceptualization of hegemonic culture, 'which has to be seen as *the lived dominance and subordination of particular classes*' (Williams, 1997: 100; emphasis added), becomes especially relevant. Since female sex-workers are effectively marginalized by this re-packaging of concerns as general concerns, they continue to be subordinated in the name of national interest. Ideology, therefore, '"acts" or functions in such a way that it "recruits" subjects ... [by a] very precise operation called interpellation or hailing' (Althusser, 1971: 162–163), whereby subjects involuntarily respond to this calling by virtue of a set of ingrained beliefs. Since female sex-workers are stigmatized as the deviant harbingers of AIDS by much of the Indian society, they are no longer mediated through the simple hailing of a 'Hey, you there!' but a 'Hey, you there ... no, not you ... YOU!' (Mazzarella, 2004).

Interpellated by hegemonic, context-specific practices and narratives, sex workers then become members of a very specific 'community of practice', through their 'participation in an activity system about which participants share understandings' in which they are identified by and identify with particular gendered literacies and practices (Lave & Wenger, 1991: 98). Since their historically and culturally situated literacy practices are 'almost always fully integrated with, interwoven into, [and] constituted [as] part of the very texture of wider practices that involve, talk, interaction, values, and beliefs' (Gee, 1996: 41), understanding the literacy practices of female sex-workers requires the decoding of relevant social practices according to the textual moments that resonate with them (Hall, 2001). When encountering HIV prevention/intervention pamphlets, the meanings that resonate most and the ideologies that are retained are situated in a particular cultural model, 'a totally or partially unconscious explanatory theory or "storyline" connected to a word – bits and pieces of which are distributed across different people in a social group' (Gee, 1999: 44).

This chapter marks a preliminary effort to understand the literacy practices of sex workers who choose not to use condoms with regular patrons. I concurrently show how their discursive responses reflect the widespread practice of the *rakhel* system, thereby revealing how sex workers engage the larger discourse of gender, sexuality and responsibility. Of particular relevance to my study are the following questions:

- What cultural models are relevant to the identification, interpellation and textual decoding of pamphlets as a form of literacy?
- Whose interests are these models representing?
- Are there differences here between the cultural models that are affecting espoused beliefs and those that are affecting actions and practices?
- How are the relevant cultural models (Gee, 1999: 78) here helping to reproduce, transform or create social, cultural, institutional and/or political relationships?

Selling Sex, Selling AIDS: Background, Study Setting and Methodology

'See', she urged, thrusting forth the paper. 'See how they make women look?'

I was entering the administrative office of Saheli HIV/AIDS Karyarta Sangh, the only sex-workers' collective in the Indian city of Pune, when Mira (not her real name), a history student and volunteer, pointed indignantly to a folded newspaper on the table. It was a section from one of the country's leading English language newspapers, the *Times of India*.

"What happened?" I asked as I greeted the other two women in the room. Mira paused, looked entreatingly at the object of attention, and motioned for me to sit next to her.

"All these reports look at the women only", she continued, ignoring my interruption. "What about men? They say the husbands gave them AIDS, so why even ask these women if they did sex-work".

It was the summer of 2007 and I was just beginning to engage the complicated world of HIV/AIDS prevention on the ground. As I sat there listening to the ongoing debate, I zeroed in on the report's sombre admonition: 'AIDS: HOW IT'S CREEPING INTO OUR LIVES'. According to the article, which reported on the spread of HIV in married Indian women, *'women who denied any history of commercial sex work [CSW] ... but attended clinics for treatment of sexually transmitted infection* (STI), have now been found to have a high prevalence of ... AIDS' (Kashyap, 2007; emphasis added). Despite acquiring the virus from their 'high-risk' husbands, these women, the majority of whom 'reported only one lifetime sexual partner and no condom use', are denounced for their lack of education and early 'initiation' of sexual intercourse. Finally, by quoting the deputy director of the National Aids Research Institute (NARI), it is asserted that the infected women 'are *clearly* not representative of the general population of women, who have a significantly lower HIV prevalence rate' (quoted in Kashyap, 2007; emphasis added).

By all accounts, this report follows the standard format of 'reliable' commentary on the virus in present-day India: it informs the reader of the epidemic's increasing reach, dismisses its urgency in the same breath and tacitly directs the blame almost wholly at the women. Two working assumptions motivate this gender-based condemnation: sexually transmitted infections in women must be due to inappropriate sexual relations on their part and, if not, the fault lies in the source of men's 'high-risk' sexual behavior – the female sex-workers they frequent. In this way, and despite urging the expansion of current risk-reduction efforts to include marital relationships, the article reiterates the 'common perception, mostly propagated through distorted media reports, that AIDS is a disease primarily confined to female sex-workers and their clients' (Nag, 1996: 51). Such representations are further reflected in popular discourses, as Pande (2003: 94) discovered during her journey across India researching women's health. She comments, 'there is an awkwardness and embarrassment in the eyes of ... women seeking treatment for their sex-related problems' due to 'countless doctors and midwives who look at women articulating sexual problems and see a whore' (Pande, 2003: 94).

This scene, together with the internal construction of judgment in the newspaper article, is offered as available context for showcasing how female sex-workers continue to be the reference point of blame in the Indian AIDS epidemic, despite official messages emphasizing the indiscriminate nature of the disease. This relationship between sex work and HIV began when the virus was first detected in 1986, after serological testing found 10 out of 102 female prostitutes in Chennai to be HIV positive (Verma *et al.*, 2004: 21). Today, and with an estimate of 2.5 million people living with HIV,[3] India is the third-worst-affected country after South Africa and Nigeria (Sinha, 2007). Heterosexual contact[4] is the dominant mode of HIV transmission (Amin, 2004: 5; Dandona *et al.*, 2005: 2) and mathematical modelling (Nagelkerke *et al.*, 2002) is often used to support prevention interventions heavily focused on (female) sex workers as a 'deviant' group and 'important driver of the epidemic' (O'Neil *et al.*, 2004: 852). This logic is based on the observation that HIV heterosexual epidemics have one central feature in common: unprotected sex with female sex-workers who 'rapidly acquire HIV and infect their male clients, who then infect other female partners, who then infect their children' (Jha *et al.*, 2001: 224).

Accordingly, India's National AIDS Control Organization's (NACO) HIV Sentinel Surveillance reported that as of 2005, 8.44% of sex workers examined across 83 sites were HIV positive (NACO, 2006: 2). In its 2006 report, NACO discovered that 556 out of 2498 female sex-workers examined across 10 sites carried the virus – 22.26% of the women examined; and during NACO's most recent examination of female sex-workers in Maharashtra, 126 out of 250 women – almost 50% – were infected. Not surprisingly then, sex workers are on the receiving end of rigorous HIV/AIDS prevention information. Although movies, posters, public service announcements and newspaper commentaries are media forms that are increasingly used in the battle against ignorance about HIV/AIDS, pamphlets are the primary educational texts that are disseminated to these women.

The present analysis uses a gender perspective to assess the reception and broader implications of pamphlet-based prevention messages for sex workers in Budhwar Peth, Pune's oldest and best-established red light area. Data were collected in June 2007 and July 2007. As India's eighth largest city, Pune provides the ideal context for this study because of its dynamic brothel-based business and sizable reduction in HIV/AIDS prevalence. There are 394 active brothels in the area, each of which houses anywhere between 10 and 12 sex workers per room (personal interview).

Ethnographic methods inform my study, much of which was conducted during near daily visits to the administrative office of Saheli HIV/AIDS Karyarta Sangh (literally 'Female Friends HIV/AIDS Co-operative Union'), one of the most prolific HIV/AIDS prevention programmes in Pune. Data were gathered through field-based ethnographic research, informal discussions and observation. Reports and policy documents of Saheli Sangh were also reviewed in order to adequately understand the background to and development of certain programmes. Additionally, data from sentinel sites, especially yet-to-be published material from 2007, and pilot studies were examined to gauge the mechanisms through which HIV/AIDS continues to spread in some regions but decline in others. The *sangh* uses peer-education strategies to achieve high levels of infection-reduction in Budhwar Peth; it also works on the goals identified by the women themselves, and focuses predominantly on the needs of individual sex-workers in the course of achieving collective empowerment. It covers over 70 brothel-lodges in the district and works with approximately 6000 non-brothel-based sex-workers to provide adequate support and information concerning their health and basic rights.

Several factors limit the scope and detail of my study. First, numerous police-initiated brothel raids at the time prevented me from engaging with sex workers who did not frequent the administrative office, and my conversational findings are based on discussions with the older and more powerful *tais* (peer educators). Moreover, I focus almost wholly on these women, not on their live-in patrons, because of the relative impossibility I faced in gaining access to them. Secondly, the bulk of my research is based on the casual conversations I enjoyed with the various *tais* in an informal setting. Although the *tais* and I engaged varying topics, there was a mutual unwillingness to discuss their sexual lives beyond their professional worker–client relationship. When I asked a *sangh* worker if most *tais* still lived and worked in the brothels, she responded,

> We don't know how many *tais* still do sex work. We don't ask, and they don't tell. We don't ask what they do with their husbands. They don't want to tell.

While reproducing conversations without participant consent might go beyond the ethical boundaries of field research, the *sangh* worker's response reflects the impossibility of conducting consensual official interviews or of asking direct questions about the *tais'* private (intimate) lives. It also disallowed me from using a tape recorder or jotting down conversations verbatim; instead, I kept detailed notes about these discussions once the informal conversations were over. Secondly, our exchanges were mostly in Hindi with the occasional sprinkle of broken English; but often, when the women engaged in furious Marathi[5] among themselves, I required a *sangh* member's help for translation. Finally, I must acknowledge that this research is exploratory at this stage and is only an initial attempt to understand the reasoning – beyond statistical findings – of the literacy practices of women engaged in the *rakhel* system.

Pamphlets as a Site of Engagement: Data Analysis

If wall posters and handouts are anything to go by, people living with or at risk for acquiring HIV are happy-looking people. Just as Jones (1997) discovered in his analysis of advertisements targeting the virus, pamphlets and leaflets handed out in Budhwar Peth are steeped in a sense of visual optimism. Unlike the newspaper example discussed in the previous section, these pamphlets evoke a sense of power through confident-looking people and words of encouragement and hope. Especially striking is the reinforcing narrative of a woman being supported by a loving male partner, and vice versa.

I acquired the pamphlets discussed below from the offices of Saheli HIV/AIDS Karyakarta Sangh, each of which are recent attempts by the Indian government – and the state of Maharashtra in particular – to deal with the fear, stigmatization and ignorance about HIV/AIDS prevention methods. My reason for choosing these pamphlets is twofold: first, they were the most readily available for reference as there were numerous copies either stacked up on desks or blown up into wall posters, and second, because they generated a lot of conversation without me having to probe too deeply. My analysis is organized into three areas of interest:

- The classification of the pamphlet (type, produced by).
- The nature of the content, both narrative and visual.
- The central themes picked upon by respondents based on the content they identify with.

Pamphlet 1: Locating the *rakhel* system as a social practice

The first pamphlet (no figure shown) comes from the government-sponsored *Female Condom Programme*, part of a country-wide effort to encourage protection among women, especially sex workers who are often faced with uncompromising, unwilling and violent clients. It is informative in nature, colourful and glossy in appearance, and works like a mini-booklet informing women about the use of the female condom. The front page of the booklet displays two separate images, each of which represent a storyline. On the left end of the cover, a happy-looking woman is consulting a female sex-educator about the female condom while her supportive male partner stands behind her. In the background, a group of women are seated on the ground, implying that they are in an information session that is promoting the female condom and educating them about safer sex practices. On the right end of the cover is the silhouette of a man and a woman embracing each other. The two images are placed in such a manner so as to suggest that the couple consulting with the female sex-educator are the same couple in the silhouette. The implication here is that the couple are not only embracing one another – they have also embraced the information and education that they have received. Entitled 'Yours or mine, either is fine!' and 'Power, Protection, and Pleasure', the titles were the only aspect of the pamphlets (along with the names of the programme's affiliated sponsors) that was written in English – the rest of the text in both pamphlets is in Marathi.

In one of the meetings I attended where female condoms were discussed, the general consensus was that the product was too uncomfortable and too complicated for regular use. Most women acknowledged its value and wanted another instructional demonstration so as to be prepared for 'difficult' customers, and although many supported it during the meeting, many had casually commented that they would take a chance and not use the female condom with their male partners.

Personally impressed by the expensive-looking pamphlet, I asked some *tais* whether they enjoyed reading such handouts. After passing a cursory glance at the stack of pamphlets, many of the women indicated how the dense written material served no real purpose since none of them could effectively read and write Marathi. They started to reflect on how the admittedly beautiful images were completely disconnected from their lives. For the women gathered in that room, then, the visual material had yet to reflect their reality. The rows of seated women in the pamphlet is key to the interpellation of the sex workers as the identifiable and intended recipients of the information, as the scene describes the typical components of information sessions normally held for sex workers: rows of women, an educator and a product directly related to HIV/AIDS prevention. Nonetheless, it was the image of a man attending a meeting session as a supportive partner that provoked discussions about their relationships with men and the role of these men in negotiating condom use.

One *tai* pointed out how the presence of a supportive male partner was virtually unheard of at these meetings as they are not co-held with *babus* and no *mard* has attended such sessions. I overheard another *tai* telling her peer that even though she did not like the female condom, she felt it was a good option when compared with the embarrassment of asking her *babu* to use a condom. Protecting herself was her own responsibility, she suggested, as women could only count on themselves. None of the women were talking about 'clients' per se; their use of the terms *babu* and *mard* specifically pointed to a certain sub-sector of men they considered to be their partners. Male partners, as is suggested by the larger dogmas of gender and sexuality, are exempt from worrying about HIV because social and prevention discourses continue to heap the burden of safe-sex practices onto women.

Indeed, in every supervised trip around the area, every meeting and every informal conversation I had with and about the area's sex workers, reference was made to a *mard* (man), *gharwala* (man of the house), *baba* (respectful term for man) or *babu* (endearing term for man) indicating that most women, be they sex workers or brothel keepers, were either legally married through a formal union or metaphorically bonded to a long-term partner. This *rakhel* system is far from unique in Budhwar Peth. Evans and Lambert (1997: 1792), for example, discovered that out of the 27 sex workers interviewed for their Calcutta-based study, 85% were in a long-term relationship with a *babu*. Sleightholme and Sinha (1997: 115) showed that out of 27 sex workers in the Sett Bagan red light area in Calcutta, over 60% had been in a relationship with the same *babu* for periods ranging from 6 to 20 years; and similarly, in her study of brothel clients in Pune city, Bhattacharya (2004) discovered that out of 100 clients interviewed, over 30 had ongoing relationships with particular sex workers in a brothel.

Still, however, client-focused Indian AIDS discourse is surprisingly bereft of critical analysis of the *rakhel* system. Significant recent research is either limited to descriptive narratives focused on the nature of said relationships or ethnographic studies for the purpose of biomedical, epidemiological and statistical investigation (e.g. Bhattacharya, 2004; Evans & Lambert, 1997; Sleightholme & Sinha, 1997). A lack of critical research on the system relates to the fact that *babus* are categorized by 'low-risk' professional occupations that range anywhere between being wealthy businessman, young students or lower-middle-class bus drivers, salesmen, rickshaw pullers, factory workers and/or small shopkeepers.

Two essential findings emerge from the women's reflections about the pamphlet. First, despite recent successes in educating and empowering sex workers to negotiate condom use, there is a relative dearth of safe-sex practices exercised by *rakhels* and their *babus*. Put more concretely, according to Nath (2000: 105), in 1997, only 51.5% of the *babus* in the Sonagachi brothel in Calcutta had ever heard of AIDS and only 1.5% used condoms. Despite greater information over the years, 2004 statistics reveal that only 13.3% of *babus* in Pune's brothels consistently use condoms (Bhattacharya, 2004: 192); and, in a recent pilot study conducted in Budhwar Peth, only 12% of the female sex-workers interviewed admitted to using condoms with their husbands. This number is particularly shocking since over 98% of sex workers in this sample readily admitted to consistently using condoms with other customers.

Second, and on the descriptive front, *rakhels* are engaged in two types of relationships with their *babus*, the first of which is a form of exploitation. In the Immoral Traffic (Prevention) Act of India, 1956 (recently amended in 2006), these *babus* are identified as

> Live in ... lovers [who] are committing an offence by living off the earnings of prostitution. If any *babu* who is proved to be living with a sex-worker is arrested under these charges, he is assumed to be living off her earnings unless he can prove otherwise. (As cited in Sleightholme & Sinha, 1997: 56)

The second category of *babus* live with their wives and children. They regularly visit the same woman for several months or years, develop emotional attachments to them, pay them fixed monthly sums and engage in what 'becomes like a husband–wife relationship' (Sleightholme & Sinha, 1997: 115). Such polarized categorizations between 'good' and 'bad' *babus*, I came to understand, are neither unfair nor limited in their scope – a fact further noted when Evans and Lambert's (1997: 1792) sample of sex workers defined *babus* in terms of *khane vale* (those who eat[from]) and *dhene vale* (those who give).

Pamphlet 2: Self-identification through the gendered cultural model of a 'wife'

The second pamphlet considered is a widely spread promotional handbill from the same *Female Condom Programme*. Rani *tai* (not her real name), a peer educator whom I often relied on to take me into and around the brothels of Budhwar Peth, had frequently and proudly mentioned the fact that she was 'married' and had thus achieved some sort of status among her peers. Often, when she mentioned her *mard*, I tried to engage her about the nature of her relationship without much success. She did, however, repeatedly reveal that she was pleased to have had a 'good' *mard* for so

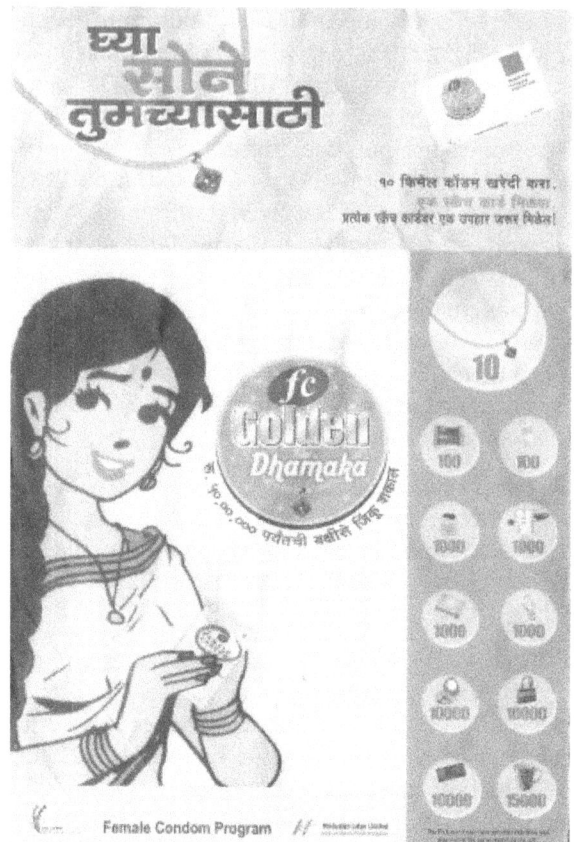

Figure 5.1 Handbill for female condom programme

long and that she felt that her life was happy and stable, 'just like the lady in the picture'. This image (Figure 5.1) of a smiling woman holding the female condom was hung as a large blow-up poster in the *sangh*'s administrative office. The front cover informs us about this 'fc Golden Dhamaka' in Marathi by telling us to

- Take GOLD for yourself.
- Buy 10 female condoms.
- Receive one scratch card.
- Every scratch card has a guaranteed gift!

The use of the term '*dhamaka*' here is quite deliberate. Although literally translated as 'explosion', the term *dhamaka* is often used in a promotional context to refer to dance competitions, film shows and presentations, as well as hugely popular lotteries and raffles. Protection, profit and happiness therefore go hand in hand.

On a separate occasion, after the *tais* had gathered around to scratch booklets upon booklets of such cards they received from the *sangh*, I began to talk to them about the woman in the picture. One glaring cultural marker identified her as a wife to the women: the necklace she sports is a *mangal sutra*, the Hindu symbol of marriage. Moreover, the handbill's instruction to 'Take GOLD for yourself' is a distinctive reference to being married, as gold is often given to and by a woman in a marriage context. Most *rakhels* (and all of the women in the room) wore their marriage on their body: marital symbols such as *sindhoor, mangalsutras*, toe-rings and *tillis* were worn in great numbers so as to emphasize their status in the sex-working community. I had encountered few such markers during my rounds around the brothels where the younger sex-workers sat out to work. Being a wife meant earning respect, I learnt, especially in society where knowledge of their profession was unknown. The image of woman on the pamphlet resonated well with the women who could 'understand' why she was smiling. It was not a mere question of winning a purse or a pair of gold earrings – it had everything to do with her stable position as a happy and respectable wife.

Such interpretations are directly related to Indian sexual discourses that have generally focused on the natural quality of sexual relations on the one hand, and the unforgivable sin of pre-marital or extra-marital sexual relations on the other. M. Banerjee's (2003: 1) definition of 'prostitution' as immoral 'promiscuous sexual intercourse' and corrupt 'intercourse for hire whether in money or in kind' is often used to describe any and every form of sexual trade in India. Indeed, the sex worker is condemned as 'a woman who sells herself for sexual purposes to a great number of men in succession and with little or no choice among them' (Banerjee, 2003: 1). This promiscuity is measured against normative Indian female sexuality, often defined as 'heterosexual, marital, [and] chaste' (Kapur, 2005: 56). Women who engage in the sex trade are, therefore, obvious outsiders to this categorization and are accordingly outcast to bear the burdensome social and legal stigmas. In order to be happy, therefore, married sex-workers did not want to embarrass their *babus* by asking them to put on a condom – often against their better judgment. Self-sacrifice, marriage and happiness, it seems, are intrinsically linked with the identification of what 'role' these women take on.

Pamphlet 3: Engaging literacy practices

The third pamphlet provides information on how to access local HIV/AIDS tests and resources, how to understand blood test results, what to do if one is infected and general precautions for people at potential risk for HIV. Although it is not aimed specifically at sex workers, it has been widely distributed in Budhwar Peth in order to provide basic information about the then relatively new Volunteer Confidential Counselling and Testing Centre (VCCTC). The pamphlet is sponsored by the Maharashtra AIDS Control Society (MSACS).

In this pamphlet, the dominating image is the silhouette of a couple standing against a solid purple background (Figure 5.2). Although their faces cannot be seen, this 'modern' couple stares straight at the reader while holding each other's hands in solidarity. Once again, light shines through from behind the couple's image as if illuminating the darkness that has consumed their lives.

> SPEAK OUT! REMOVE THE DARKNESS FROM YOUR MIND
> HIV/AIDS SCARING YOU?
> DO YOU HAVE ANY SUSPICIONS OR DOUBTS?
> MEET FEARLESSLY AND WITH AN OPEN MIND
> CONTACT YOUR NEAREST AIDS CLINIC

In another part of the text (not seen in figure), the following text appears in Marathi:

> BLOOD TESTS: WHAT DO THEY MEAN!
> There can be only two results of the blood tests taken: either the patient has tested HIV positive or HIV negative. Even if the patient has tested negative, he shall still be given advice to take care and precaution for the future. For example, men who regularly visit brothels shall be advised that they run the risk of getting HIV and hence should take all possible precautions. Even if the patient has tested negative, he shall be advised that he may still be having the HIV virus as the virus has the tendency to come back again after three months for another HIV blood test.

This pamphlet, and particularly the preceding excerpt, struck a chord with the one and only *babu* I got to officially interview:

> I never wear condoms. Why is it necessary? My lover *tells* me it's not necessary. Condoms are only to protect with other men. If she is protected when doing work, why should I wear a condom when I'm with her? I will not get anything, and she will not get anything. And there is no problem of her getting baby because I will take care. So why wear condom?

He was adamant that he was not at risk of AIDS and that the pamphlet might be useful for a few of his friends who frequented Budhwar Peth

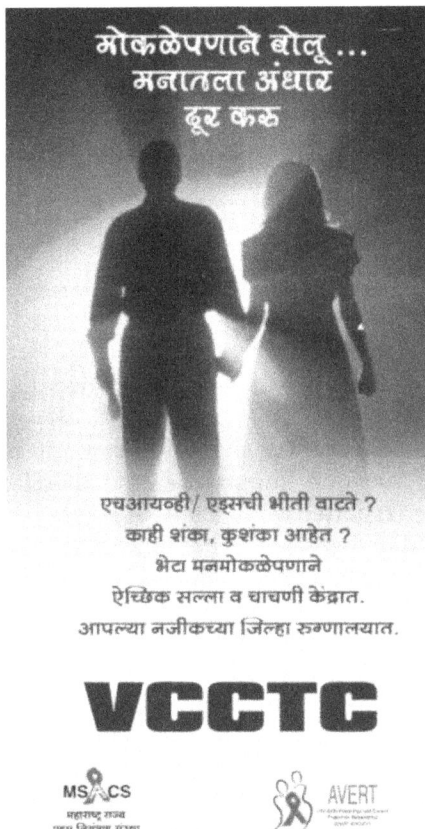

मोकळेपणाने बोलू ...
मनातला अंधार
दूर करू

एचआयव्ही / एड्सची भीती वाटते ?
काही शंका, कुशंका आहेत ?
भेटा मनमोकळेपणाने
ऐच्छिक सल्ला व चाचणी केंद्रात.
आपल्या नजीकच्या जिल्हा रुग्णालयात.

VCCTC

MS/\CS   AVERT
महाराष्ट्र राज्य
एड्स निवारण संस्था

Figure 5.2 VCCTC pamphlet

without a 'favourite', but not for him and a woman like his lover. They never used condoms, he continued, but that was no cause to worry – she was experienced and educated when it came to disease prevention and if she was not worried with her 'favourite', then he need not be. They were committed to each other insofar as she protected herself 'at work'. If there was no chance she could get infected from other men, then there was no reason to sacrifice pleasure and comfort – feelings associated with a marital relationship and not brothel-based sex work. Since she was confident that there was no 'need', he was confident that condoms were unnecessary.

This reasoning is further reflected in Bhattacharya's (2004) work, which is one of the few studies taking a closer look at the *rakhel* system. Mr. M,

Table 5.1 Condom use in *rakhel* and non-*rakhel* clients

	Rakhel clients, N = 30 (percentage)	Non-rakhel clients, N = 70 (percentage)
Condom use		
Always used	4(13.3)	34(48.6)
Sometimes used	14(46.7)	30(42.9)
Never used	12(40.0)	6(8.5)

Source: Bhattacharya (2004: 192).

a *babu* she interviewed, believed 'that he is not at risk of AIDS as his *rakhel* is 'like his wife' (Bhattacharya, 2004: 189). Since *babus* often consider their relationships with sex workers as marital in essence, condom use is not considered to be of pressing importance, and therefore lower rates of condom use have been reported in Pune's brothels (see Table 5.1). Normative sexuality, as indicated in the previous pamphlet analysis, implies that only women who engage in unacceptable, immoral sexual behavior are susceptible to infection. However, since *babus* do not engage in sexual relations with sex workers other than their *rakhels*, many men deny that their relationships involve any risk of infection.

Since their relationship resembles the intimacy between husband and wife, these *babus* do not consider the numerous avenues for infection, especially since many of their *rakhels* continue to engage in sexual activity with other men in order to financially support themselves and their families. The danger of such beliefs is reflected in another case study, noted below:

> Mr. K is a 36 year old auto-rickshaw driver, who had his first contact with sex-workers at the age of 16. After having multiple sex partners, he developed a relationship with one woman in the brothel, whom he supported financially for four to five years. Subsequently his *rakhel* developed AIDS and died. According to his account, he has been supporting her two children, a boy and a girl, for the past five years. He now has another *rakhel*. . . . (Bhattacharya, 2004: 189)

Implications of the *Rakhel* System

Returning to Gee's (1999) concept of cultural models, it is clear that sex workers decode the overall structure and messages of the pamphlets in accordance with two competing public discourses – both of which represent the dual interests of the Indian government to quell the epidemic on the one hand, and to promote an idealized agenda of what a 'good' woman should do and be on the other. These women reflect such dangerous dogmas when they focus their attention on certain situated meanings in the pamphlet that help guide them 'in selecting which patterns and sub-patterns to focus on' (Gee, 1999: 52). The *rakhel* system, therefore, is a cultural model in itself that guides the choices, meanings and identities of many of these women who wish to integrate into the dominant cultural model of 'woman' and 'wife', despite the fact that this model discriminates against them. Their literacy practices are heavily influenced by how they position themselves within these models: sex workers must insist on protection whereas wife and partner need not. In this way, gender, sexuality and responsibility are constructed and consumed as synonymous entities. Their reflections demonstrate three implicit beliefs and realities: the responsibility women face in protecting themselves is dependent on what identity they take on; there is a low risk-perception associated with marriage and the *rakhel* identity and there is a certain amount of stability, happiness and status that comes with being in such a relationship.

In developing such an account, I hope to show that a critical conception of ideology and hegemonic norms is not passively received by the audience of media texts. Although cultural norms differ around the world, the *rakhel* system is one such example of how embodied local beliefs and practices play out in the face of the HIV/AIDS epidemic. Incorporating the meanings, experiences and impacts of discourse on sex workers is crucial for effective HIV/AIDS messages, not just for women in the trade who can still protect themselves from irregular clients, but also for women and men across the country who associate risk with unmarried, casual intercourse.

Acknowledgments

I would like to express my gratitude to the Hung Hing Ying and Leu Hau Ling Charitable Foundation for graduate students in the Master of Arts in Asia Pacific Policy Studies, the Shastri Indo-Canadian Institute and the Centre for South Asian Studies at the University of British Columbia for their financial assistance in making my research possible. I am extremely grateful to Tejaswi, Aditya, Sarika, and Latika for showing me the ropes around Saheli Sangh. I am also especially grateful to all the *tais* and sangh members for taking me out into the field, answering my questions, and allowing me to sit in on their meetings. Their compassion and kindness when I hurt my leg and their ability to cook a mean *daal* and rice will never be forgotten.

Notes

1. Throughout this chapter, I use 'sex workers' to refer specifically to brothel-based sex-workers.
2. Hindi for 'mistress' or 'kept woman', the term *rakhel* is used as a derogatory address towards women in most social situations. I follow Bhattacharya's (2004) use of the term to describe such bonds, placing no judgment whatsoever on the men and women who engage in such relationships.
3. At 5.7 million people in 2005, India was recently considered to be the leading country with HIV/AIDS. In July 2007, however, UNAIDS/WHO as well as a host of other international and grassroots organizations endorsed India's new estimate of 2.5 million people living with the HIV/AIDS based on arguably more 'reliable' data compiled from records available from the NACO sentinel sites as well as the National Family Health Survey – III. Yet, 'despite the new survey bringing down the number of infected people', as union health minister A. Ramadoss rightfully argued, 'there is no room for complacency as India is still home to [3 million] people living with HIV' (Sinha, 2007). Moreover, as a recent Bharat *et al.* (2001) study concluded, 'weaknesses in the serosurveillance system, bias in targeting groups for testing, and the lack of availability of testing services in several parts of the country suggest a significant element of underreporting'.
4. Conventional intercourse or normative (heterosexual) intercourse refers specifically to the missionary position. Oral, anal and intercourse with a 'woman initiating sexual activity is in some respect indecent and outside the purview of prevailing cultural norms' (Kapur, 2005: 63). Although a fairly substantial group of male sex-workers have been identified as 'high risk' due to inconsistent condom use with male clients, the focus almost always falls on their female counterparts for being a highly visible symbol of 'anti-Indian' values and behavior. Much more research needs to be conducted on the virus's spread among men who have sex with men (MSMs), male sex-workers and *hijras* (eunuchs) engaged in unprotected intercourse.
5. Hindi is the official language of India and Marathi is a regional language most widely spoken in the Indian state of Maharasthra.

References

Althusser, L. (1971) *Lenin and Philosophy and Other Essays*. London: New Left Books.

Amin, A. (2004) *Risk, Morality, and Blame: A Critical Government and US Donor Responses to HIV Infections in Sex Workers in India*. Tacoma Park, MD: Centre for Health and Gender Equity.

Banerjee, M. (2003) Introduction: On the prostitutes in early India. In S.N. Sinha and N.K. Bose (eds) *History of Prostitution in Ancient India: Upto 3rd cen. A.D.* (pp. 1–22). Kolkata: Shree Balaram Prakasani.

Bharat, S., Aggleton, P. and Tyrer, P. (2001) *India: HIV and AIDS-Related Discrimination, Stigmatization, and Denial*. Geneva: UNAIDS.

Bhattacharya, S. (2004) Brothels and brothel clients in Pune city. In R.K. Verma, P. Pelto, S. Schensul and A. Joshi (eds) *Sexuality in the Time of AIDS: Contemporary Perspectives from Communities in India* (pp. 179–194). New Delhi: Sage.

Candlin, C. (2001) Medical discourse as professional and institutional action: Challenges to teaching and researching languages for special purposes. In M. Bax and C. Zwart (eds) *Reflections on Language and Language Learning: In Honour of Arthur Van Essen* (pp. 185–208). Amsterdam: John Benjamins Publishing Co.

Crimp, D. (1988) AIDS: Cultural analysis, cultural activism. In D. Crimp (ed.) *AIDS: Cultural Analysis, Cultural Activism* (p. 3016). Cambridge, MA: MIT Press.

Dandona, R., Dandona, L., Guiterrez, J.P., Kumar, A., McPherson, S., Samuels, F., Bertozzi, S. and the ASCI FPP Study Team. (2005) High risk of HIV in non-brothel based female sex workers in India. *BMC Public Health* 5 (87), 1–10.

Evans, C. and Lambert, H. (1997) Health-seeking strategies and sexual health among female sex workers in urban India: Implications for research and service provision. *Social Science & Medicine* 4 (12), 1791–1803.

Faria, C. (2008). Privileging prevention, gendering responsibility: An analysis of the Ghanaian campaign against HIV/AIDS. *Social & Cultural Geography* 9 (1), 41–73.

Foucault, M. (1990) *The History of Sexuality, Volume One.* London: Vintage Books.

Foucault, M. (1991) Governmentality. In G. Burchell, C. Gordon and P. Miller (eds) *The Foucault Effect: Studies in Governmentality, with Two Lectures by and an Interview with Michel Foucault* (pp. 87–104). London: Harvester Wheatsheaf.

Foucault, M. (2000) Subject and power. In J. Faubion (ed.) *Power* (pp. 326–348). New York: New York Press.

Gee, J. (1992) *The Social Mind: Language, Ideology, and Social Practice.* New York: Bergin and Garvey.

Gee, J. (1996) *Social Linguistics and Literacies: Ideology in Discourses* (2nd edn). London: Taylor & Francis Ltd.

Gee, J. (1999) *An Introduction to Discourse Analysis.* London: Routledge.

Hall, S. (2001) Encoding/decoding. In M. Gigi and D. Keller (eds) *Media and Cultural Studies: Key Works* (pp. 166–176). Malden, MA: Blackwell Publishers.

Jha, P., Nagelkerke, N.J.D., Ngugi, E.N., Prasada Rao, J.V.R., Willbond, B., Moses, S. and Plummer, F.A. (2001) Reducing HIV transmission in developing countries. *Science* 292 (5515), 224–225.

Jones, R.H. (1997) Marketing the damaged self: The construction of identity in advertisements directed towards people with HIV/AIDS. *Journal of Sociolinguistics* 1 (3), 393–418.

Jones, R.H. (1999) Mediated action and sexual risk: Searching for "culture" in discourses of homosexuality and AIDS prevention in China. *Culture, Health & Sexuality* 1 (2), 161–180.

Jones, R.H. (2002) A walk in the park: Frames and positions in AIDS prevention outreach among gay men in China. *Journal of Sociolinguistics* 6 (4), 575–588.

Kapur, R. (2005) *Erotic Justice: Law and the New Politics of Postcolonialism.* Norfolk: Biddles Ltd.

Kashyap, S. (2007) AIDS: How it's creeping into our lives. *Times of India,* June 13, Times City, Pune edition.

Lave, J. and Wenger, E. (1991) *Situated Learning: Legitimate Peripheral Participation.* Cambridge: Cambridge University Press.

Majumdar, A. (2000) Halting AIDS on the highway. In S. Raju and A. Leonard (eds) *Men as Supportive Partners in Reproductive Health: Moving from Rhetoric to Reality* (pp. 38–39). New Delhi: The Population Council.

Mazzarella, W. (2004) Culture, globalization, and mediation. *Annual Review of Anthropology* 33, 345–367.

Mooney, A. and Sarangi, S. (2005) An ecological framework of HIV preventive intervention: A case study of non-government organizational work in the developing world. *Health* 9 (3), 275–296.

Nag, M. (1996) *Sexual Behavior and AIDS in India.* New Delhi: Vikas Publishing House, Ltd.

Nagelkerke, N.J.D, Jha, P., de Vlas, S.J., Korenromp, E.L., Moses, S., Blanchard, J.F and Plummer, F.A. (2002) Modelling HIV/AIDS epidemics in Botswana and India: Impact of interventions to prevent transmission. *Bulletin of the World Health Organization* 80 (2), 89–96.

Nath, M. (2000) Women's health and HIV: Experiences from a sex-workers perspective in Calcutta. *Gender and Development* 8 (1), 100–108.

Norris, S. and Jones, R. (2005) Discourse as action/discourse in action. In S. Norris and R. Jones (eds) *Discourse in Action: Introducing Mediated Discourse Analysis* (pp. 3–13). London: Routledge.

O'Neil, J., Orchard, T., Swarankar, R.C., Blanchard, J., Gurav, K. and Moses, S. (2004) Dhanda, dharma, disease: Traditional sex work and HIV/AIDS in India. *Social Science & Medicine* 4 (59), 851–860.

Panda, S., Chatterjee, A. and Abdul-Quader, A.S. (eds) (2002) *Living with the AIDS Virus: The Epidemic and the Response in India.* New Delhi: Sage.

Pande, M. (2003) *Stepping Out: Life and Sexuality in Rural India.* New Delhi: Penguin Books.

Rao, V. and Walton, M. (2004) Culture and public action: Relationality, equality of agency, and development. In V. Rao and M. Walton (eds) *Culture and Public Action.* Stanford, CA: Stanford University Press.

Rao, A.M., Nag, K. and Dey, A. (1994) Sexual behavior pattern of truck drivers and their helpers in relation to female sex workers. *The Indian Journal of Social Work* 55 (4), 603–616.

Sarkar, K., Bal, B., Mukherjee, R., Saha, M.K., Chakraborty, S., Niyogi, S.K. and Bhattacharya, S.K. (2006) Young age is a risk factor for HIV among female sex workers – An experience from India. *Journal of Infection* 53 (4), 225–259.

Scollon, R. (1997) Handbills, tissues, and condoms: A site of engagement for the construction of identity in public discourse. *Journal of Sociolinguistics* 1 (1), 39–61.

Sinha, K. (2007) HIV figures down 50% to 2.5 million. *Times of India*, July 7, Times Nation, Mumbai edition.

Sleightholme, C. and Sinha. I. (1997) *Guilty Without Trial: Women in the Sex Trade in Calcutta.* New Brunswick, NJ: Rutgers University Press.

Verma, R.K., Pelto, P.J., Schensul, S.L. and Joshi, A. (2004) Introduction: The time of AIDS in India. In R.K. Verma, P. Pelto, S. Schensul and A. Joshi (eds) *Sexuality in the Time of IDS: Contemporary Perspectives from Communities in India* (pp. 21–41). New Delhi: Sage Publications.

Williams, R. (1977) *Marxism and Literature.* Oxford: Oxford University Press.

Chapter 6
Discursive Constructions of Responsibility in HIV/AIDS Prevention: Re-entextualization Practices in Tanzania

Introduction

In 1998, Peter Piot, Executive Director of UNAIDS, described AIDS as a 'woman's epidemic' (cited in Baylies, 2000: 4). His characterization of the disease aptly portrays the focus of most prevention efforts in sub-Saharan Africa since the 1990s, as increasing attention has been given to women's experiences in contracting, and also preventing, the spread of the disease. In Tanzania, the National Policy on HIV/AIDS recognizes the power of societal structures such as gender inequality, declaring 'Girls and women in our social and cultural environment are more vulnerable to HIV infection as they do not have control over their sexuality' (National Policy on HIV/AIDS, 2001: 10). Women are indeed at a higher risk of infection due to their physiology, their economic dependence on men, their lower status at home and their collectively lower education levels, which in turn make them more vulnerable in the economic realm. Accordingly, a great deal of HIV/AIDS prevention targets women in their conventional roles as caretakers and mothers through parent-to-child communication and mother-to-child-transmission prevention campaigns (Akeroyd, 2004; Baylies, 2000). Prevention campaigns have also been directed at lowering sexually transmitted infections among female sex workers as an indirect way of harnessing the transmission of HIV.

While these campaigns have made some progress in reducing the risk of contracting HIV among women in sub-Saharan Africa, such efforts result in a strongly *gender-specific* approach to HIV/AIDS prevention (Akeroyd, 2004; Baylies, 2000; WHO, 2003). In the field of international development, gender-specific approaches characterize the *Women in Development* (WID) framework[1], an approach established in the 1970s in order to formally create pathways for women in developing nations to participate more fully in liberalized market economies. WID projects target activities and skills women already perform and are concerned with getting women involved in economic activity. Though it is still a dominant approach to development (cf. Brown, 2007), the WID framework has been criticized for treating western liberal understandings of development as value-free and for myopically focusing on women's capacity to contribute to economic growth while failing to consider social aspects of development (Marchand & Parpart, 1995; Parpart, 2000). Furthermore, by treating men and women as separate groups with isolated problem sets, gender-specific approaches fail to address the problem of communication *between* men and women in terms of making decisions together about their shared sexual health (Akeroyd, 2004; Baylies, 2000). The same problem applies to the more recent approaches that specifically target men. For example, the 2000 World AIDS Campaign focused on men and boys explicitly (UNAIDS, 2000) with the 'men make a difference' slogan. Other efforts have included marketing condoms as a way to enhance one's masculinity through the branding of condoms with very masculine names such as *Dume* (literally 'maleness') in Tanzania or HIV/AIDS campaigns that used male soccer players to give public service announcements in Lesotho (Akeroyd, 2004).

In sum, a great deal of HIV/AIDS education and prevention efforts take a *gender-specific* approach by targeting men and women separately as groups who have their own unique needs. Much of the rationale behind this approach is premised on the existence of clearly defined gender roles at home and in most aspects of social life. However, as Baylies (2000) explains, any approach that focuses on women or on men as separate agendas assumes a particularly western, individualistic model of public health that will ultimately fail to transform the social and economic inequality that women experience. What is needed instead are prevention strategies that recognize the role of *gender relations* in the spread of HIV/AIDS, as articulated in the *Gender and Development* framework (GAD), an approach that emerged in the 1980s as the outcome of meetings and writings among Third World feminists (Sen & Grown, 1987). The GAD approach calls for investigations of women's material conditions and patriarchal structures that maintain women's subordination across social spheres. A focus on gender relations also examines how men and women negotiate their sexual relationships, and it is concerned with how parents discuss sexual health with their children (Baylies, 2000; Boler & Aggleton, 2005; Bujra & Mokake, 2000).

In this chapter, I explore educational sessions sponsored by a large NGO in Dar es Salaam, Tanzania, to identify whether and to what degree community awareness campaigns address gender relations. I analyze a variety of interactions at education sessions to understand how discourses of gendered responsibility are discursively constructed in role plays, street performances and community-based education classes. Employing an ethnographically informed approach to critical discourse analysis (Blommaert, 2005), I investigate the discursive positioning of men and women in regard to discourses of responsibility about the spread and prevention of HIV. The data show that women and girls are often discursively constructed as the target of NGO-sponsored educational efforts, and, yet, these efforts do little to distribute the discourses of gender and responsibility more equitably among male and female Tanzanians. To conclude, I discuss how raising awareness of these discourses among NGOs is a first step towards reframing the ways gender is treated in HIV/AIDS education.

Before turning to the details of the study, I briefly examine the relevance of a GAD framework for HIV/AIDS education in Tanzania. While the WID model has been critiqued as neo-colonialist and as ultimately detrimental to women in developing nations, I will argue that a GAD approach provides spaces for more bottom-up, grassroots negotiations of gender relations, which also makes space for local constructions of gender.

Local Knowledge and Gender

Many scholars of gender in sub-Saharan Africa have argued that present-day gender roles and gender relations are in large part legacies of the colonial period (e.g. Amediume, 1987; Oyewùmí, 1997; Snyder, 2006; Stambach, 2000). For example, Snyder (2006) examines how under German and British rule, the Iraqw people of central Tanzania experienced new forms of governance which had an enduring impact on gender relations. The colonial government followed European models and hence excluded women from positions of authority. At the same time, Iraqw women's work in the domestic sphere, once the source of women's authority, was increasingly devalued. A cash crop economy was put in place by the colonists, and taxation, wage labor and the introduction of education followed;

however, all were aimed at men. The result was a 'reformulation of the public sphere' in which women had less power after colonial contact (Snyder, 2006: 89).

In spite of such examples, WID development discourses have perpetuated neo-colonial depictions of women in developing countries like Tanzania as victims who have long been in need of western forms of modernization and emancipation (e.g. Chowdhry, 1995; Mohanty *et al.*, 2001). This victimization has been exacerbated by the World Bank's structural adjustment programs that have impacted negatively on most poor women who now experience increased workloads and a higher cost of living (Chowdhry, 1995: 33). In response to these problems, feminist scholars have argued that development efforts which embody the GAD framework and its focus on the social construction of gender are more likely to promote the inclusion of local knowledge and empowerment for women (Connelly *et al.*, 2000: 58). The GAD framework calls for policies that recognize that women in developing nations are affected not only by their sex, but also by their class, their role in the domestic and public spheres, their access to education and economic opportunity, and, in most cases, multiple forms of patriarchy. Importantly, the GAD framework calls for the deconstruction of WID development discourses that often reduce women to victims, and for the inclusion of women's voices in development policy and practice.

The example of the Iraqw people is one among many that shows how colonialism and development have perpetuated west-based, rather than African, discourses of gender (Callaway, 1987; Oyewùmí, 1997). Consequently, gender and gender relations in Tanzania cannot be thought of as purely 'local' since local conceptualizations of gender have adapted over time with reference to colonial west-based knowledge (cf. Canagarajah, 2002). Nevertheless, a feminist GAD framework provides new ways of thinking about ways forward in development because it welcomes diversity and acknowledges previously subjugated voices and forms of knowledge. Moreover, it questions the demarcation between the (outsider) policy 'experts' and the target populations. Parpart and Marchand (1995: 19) argue that a feminist GAD framework 'can lead to development policies that foster self-reliance and self-esteem, rather than ignoring women's knowledge and creating policies and projects that increase patriarchal control over women's bodies and labor'. Accordingly, in my exploration of the presence of WID or GAD frameworks in HIV/AIDS education, I seek to establish to what degree current educational approaches offer Tanzanians the opportunities to move past gender-specific approaches in order to contribute to policies and practices that decrease oppressive forms of patriarchy.

The Context

The research I report here is based on fieldwork in the Kinondoni district[2] of Dar es Salaam, which contains some of the most densely populated and poverty-stricken wards in the city. Since my first visit to Dar es Salaam in 2001, I had noticed that the media often presented the idea that prostitution is caused by women, and that the clothing which women wear causes sexual promiscuity and sexual desire among men. My initial observations of NGO education sessions also revealed a strongly gendered pattern. While equal numbers of boys and girls attended the community-based education classes, community events organized by NGOs frequently failed to draw adult men. This was alarming since the 2003–2004 Tanzania HIV/AIDS Indicator Survey shows that men aged 40–49 years have higher infection rates than women of this age group, and it is often these men who act as 'sugar daddies' for younger women who have sexual relations in return for financial support (Tanzania Commission for AIDS, 2005: 15).

The emphasis on women as the target group for behavior change and responsible sexual practices was most evident to me in 2006 when the city commissioner of Dar es Salaam made a media spectacle in a poverty-stricken part of the city where prostitution, heavy drinking and drug use was rampant, a place known as *Uwanja wa Fisi* ('field of hyenas', named for a local soccer team). With the cameras rolling, the commissioner cleared out pay-by-the-hour guesthouses where prostitutes were working. Members of the media then forced prostitutes to be interviewed on television where they were interrogated for all to see. Practically no attention was paid to the male customers of these prostitutes during this time. Instead, the discourses about responsibility were heavily placed on young women's shoulders, women who typically had few choices for how to support themselves financially. They were asked a range of obtuse questions such as 'Why do you have sex for money'? and 'Are you a prostitute because you enjoy the work'?

The presence of discourses such as these pushed me to investigate the relationship between gender and education at NGO-sponsored events to which I eventually gained access. I became particularly interested to see how women (and men) were positioned at these sessions, and to see if the discourses of education cast them in roles that challenged the unequal degrees of responsibility that I observed in the public discourses in the media. In short, I wanted to see whether these sessions challenged the WID framework's 'continuing tendency to focus on women rather than on gender relations, and in spite of apparently adopting a gender discourse, to continue to treat women as merely victims' and as perpetrators of the spread of HIV (Bujra & Baylies, 2000: 48).

The data in this chapter come from a larger ethnographic study on language in HIV/AIDS education in Dar es Salaam, Tanzania, which I initiated in the summer of 2005. My research is the result of my affiliation with a non-governmental organization called the African Medical and Research Foundation (AMREF), a non-profit organization that has worked for over 40 years in sub-Saharan Africa to improve public health. AMREF is funded mostly by outside donors including the United States Agency for International Development (USAID), Family Health International, the Swedish International Development Agency and the European Union. AMREF identifies itself as the largest indigenous NGO in Africa, with projects and offices in seven countries. Notably, in 2005, AMREF received the Gates Award for Global Health, a million-dollar award given by the Bill and Melinda Gates Foundation in recognition of AMREF's contributions to the improvement of public health in Eastern and Southern Africa.

In 2006, I collaborated with 18 community-based organizations (CBOs) that had received training from AMREF and which then had the responsibility of teaching their friends and neighbors and organizing community bonanzas which took an 'edutainment'[3] approach to HIV/AIDS awareness. Large NGOs with substantial budgets like AMREF offer many resources such as clinics for voluntary counseling and testing, and they also usually offer training and teaching materials for volunteers from CBOs who receive short-term training and then take the messages of the NGOs to their home communities to educate their neighbors. This transmission of information is meant to create 'capacity building' for NGOs, an increasingly important criterion for receiving funding from donor agencies such as USAID and the World Bank.

A unique aspect of the youth-oriented CBOs I worked with was that they were all led by young men. Mbilinyi and Mwabuki (1996) point out that small, grassroots organizations are typically staffed by unpaid female workers, and Bujra and Mokake (2000) note that the paid positions at NGOs are typically occupied by males, while female volunteers do much of the hands-on work 'on the frontline' (p. 168). A possible explanation for the male-dominated leadership of the CBOs I worked with is that they were affiliated with AMREF, an internationally recognized NGO with a great deal of resources. In spite of these circumstances, though, these male CBO leaders were not remunerated very well. They were given 30,000 Tanzanian shillings (approximately $30) a month to facilitate the work of the entire organization, which included coverage of any travel expenses, purchasing notebooks and pens for their community-based education classes, typing and printing monthly reports for AMREF and organizing community bonanzas. Most of the CBO organizers I got to know over the course of my research were remarkably generous human beings who often used their own money to carry out their work, even though all of them struggled financially at a personal level in making ends meet.

The purpose of offering community classes and bonanzas was to spread the life skills education (LSE) curriculum into the community, using a 'ripple effect' approach. This curriculum for HIV/AIDS prevention has been developed by the World Health Organization (WHO) in order to provide people with the necessary skills that are supposed to reduce the risk of HIV/AIDS transmission. These skills have been standardized into a set of 10 skills, and they are used in most Tanzanian NGOs' training materials without any alteration. The training materials produced by AMREF list these life skills as: (1) self-awareness (*kujitambua*), (2) relationship skills (*mahusiano*), (3) communication skills (*mawasiliano*), (4) problem-solving skills (*kutatua matatizo*), (5) decision-making skills (*kufanya maamuzi*), (6) self-control (*kuhimili mihemko*), (7) stress management (*kuhimili msongo*), (8) creative thinking (*fikra bunifu*), (9) critical thinking (*fikra yakinifu*) and (10) empathy (*ushirikeli*). These skills do not explicitly encompass discussions of sexuality or HIV/AIDS in particular, but focus on more general skills that are supposed to provide individuals with the capacity to govern their daily interactions with others. These skills are highly decontextualized from the local constraints and challenges faced by particular communities, but their generic quality also allow educators to localize them in culturally appropriate ways.

Using techniques they learned from AMREF, all of the CBOs organized role plays and street shows involving theatrical performances to inspire audiences to attend their sessions and to transmit the messages of prevention in culturally relevant ways. Such innovative approaches are used in other educational contexts in sub-Saharan Africa as well and have been found to provide more comfortable environments for talking about HIV/AIDS (cf. Norton & Mutonyi, 2007). In the sessions that I observed, gender relations almost always became relevant, but unequal gender relations were not typically challenged or problematized. Instead, gender-specific aspects of the AIDS epidemic were depicted, and more often than not, women and girls were the primary focus of the LSE in two ways: (1) the audiences who attended the community bonanzas and street shows were largely comprised of females, and (2) the themes of the role plays used to teach the LSE typically starred a female character as the protagonist who became HIV positive or experienced other problematic consequences resulting from unprotected sex. While the choice to focus on the harsh realities that women and girls face is worthwhile since it focuses on a high-risk group who generally lack full control over their sexual health, in all of the performances I observed, gender relations remained radically under-problematized.

For the purpose of this chapter, I discuss the activities I observed among three CBOs which were the most active. The data I gathered for the larger study include video and audio recordings of 35 educational sessions (seminars, life skills classes, community street shows, bonanzas), interviews with educators and their audiences, document collection, and field notes. I spent a total of four months researching AMREF's Adolescent Sexual and Reproductive Health project in this district, interviewing AMREF staff, collecting training materials, observing workshops and recording educational sessions carried out by the different AMREF-trained CBOs.

Re-entexualization of Responsibility

To examine how responsibility is discoursed in educational events, I turn to the concept of *re-entextualization* (Bauman & Briggs, 1990; Blommaert, 2005; Silverstein & Urban, 1996). This concept borrows theoretically from Bakhtin's (1981) notions of intertextuality and polyphony in that speakers' utterances are never uniquely authored, as each word has its own social history, imbued with the many meanings acquired from previous speakers and listeners. In the process of re-entextualization, speakers may 'take some fragment of discourse and quote it anew, making it seem to carry a meaning independent of its situation within two now distinct co(n)texts', or, alternatively, they can take a text and 'reanimate it through a performance that, being *a* (mere) performance of *the* text, suggests various dimensions of contextualized "interpretive meaning" added on to those seemingly inherent in the text' (Silverstein & Urban 1996: 2). Importantly, performances such as role plays can be understood as 'verbal art ... [that] can transform, rather than simply reflect, social life' (Bauman & Briggs, 1990: 69). In spite of the contexts of their production, which may seem riddled with gender inequality, and a lack of agency, verbal performances can be decentered from these material conditions and can attempt to shift a hegemonic discourse through re-entextualization. In considering the value of role play performances in education sessions, it is important to recognize that such performances may raise critical awareness by virtue of drawing public attention to the topic of HIV/AIDS, a typically very private matter. As Bauman and Briggs explain, 'performance puts the act of speaking on display – objectifies it, lifts it to a degree from its interactional setting and opens it to scrutiny by the audience' (Bauman & Briggs, 1990: 73). Of course, whether critical awareness is raised depends on what the audience does with the messages being presented to them, and whether they interpret the performance as mere entertainment or something more profound.

My analysis focuses on whether the discourses of female responsibility are re-entextualized in ways that draw attention to gender relations, rather than to women's responsibilities in HIV prevention. I am especially interested in how the role plays and performances might produce local perspectives on gender relations, and whether such local viewpoints can be transformative as well. After recording and transcribing the educational sessions, I selected relevant data by locating episodes in the transcripts where gender roles or gender relations were made relevant.

In focusing on language in HIV/AIDS education, I do not mean to disregard the importance of structural factors such as economic opportunity and access to education among women. These factors clearly contribute to women's ability to control their sexual lives, and to control their own bodies. The study of discourse here, rather than social structures, should not be taken as an alignment with the rationalist approach to HIV/AIDS prevention (Boler & Aggleton, 2005) which treats the solution to the pandemic as filling knowledge gaps. In addition to structural challenges, I believe that discourse is part of all social practices that contribute to the reproduction of social structures. As Fairclough (2001) argues, if changes can be made in discourses and in the social relationships enacted within these discourses, then we can expect to see effects on the knowledge and beliefs of individuals, institutions and societies. Through addressing discourses, then, we can raise awareness and potentially transform social practices about HIV/AIDS.

Data Analysis

The analysis of my data is driven by three general questions.

(1) Are the messages of educational sessions *gender-specific* in nature, or is there evidence that *gender relations* are a pedagogical focus?
(2) How is local knowledge about gender roles and gender relations discoursed?
(3) To what degree are hegemonic discourses of gender reproduced (i.e. women are responsible for societal ills) and/or re-entextualized (i.e. relationships among men and women are where transformation can begin)?

First I look at the messages of prevention that were created at educational sessions. The first example illustrates a typical session run by a CBO in Manzese, the same part of town where prostitutes were expelled by the district commissioner in 2006. This session began with drumming and dancing, followed by a performance, which is the focus of analysis. Approximately 30 people stopped to listen to the music and watch the play, though many more came and went during the hour-long event. In this play, we see discourses of females as the group targeted for behavior change, discourses of females as promiscuous and the positioning of women as those responsible for sexual morality. The data come from a play performed by a CBO on the unpaved streets of the city. In the play, Adia's mother ('MamaAdia') has discovered birth control pills in her daughter's school bag. She confronts Adia and ultimately throws her out of the house for having sexual relations. The data are translated from Swahili.

Street show in Manzese: Adia's story

MamaAdia:	So, Adia has gotten into these things. She goes to school but also gets into other things. Birth control pills. Adia! Adia!
Adia:	Yes, mother.
MamaAdia:	Come here, come here right now.
Adia:	I'm coming mother.
MamaAdia:	Explain these to me right now. What is this?
Adia:	One of my friends who I took pictures with at school during a party, at school,
MamaAdia:	Uh huh, and these birth control pills?
Adia:	Ah mother let me tell you. Now my friend gave me these pills when I had a headache.
MamaAdia:	You know, you youth, I don't want you to torment me. Do you hear?
Adia:	Mother, these pills were given to me by my friend.
MamaAdia:	Stop tormenting me. Do you hear? What kind of friend? I mean, do you go to school to do this kind of foolishness?
Adia:	No, mother.
MamaAdia:	You take pictures with men?
Adia:	No, mother.
MamaAdia:	You young people, this is what you do. ((mimicking a young person)) 'If I take birth control pills.' Today, you'll be the end of me today!
Adia:	Mother, I beg forgiveness mother!

MamaAdia: ((yelling)) You monkey! You dog. I don't want dogs like
that. If I look at you these days, you've become like a
monkey to me. You're like a dog. ((audience laughter))
Don't say anything to me, and if your father comes you
will be the end of him. You, we've lost so much money
on your for your studies and now there's no forgiveness.
((audience laughter continues))
Adia: Forgive me mother. I made a mistake. ((begging))
MamaAdia: There is no 'mother' here.
((audience laughter and extended applause for
MamaAdia's performance))

In this play, mothers and daughters are presented as the primary characters who are affected by decisions about sex. Adia's mother takes on the role of determining sexual morality, and Adia is presented as a 'bad' daughter for not listening to her mother and not being grateful for her parents' financial support for her school fees. The father is only briefly mentioned in the play, and no mention is made of why Adia chose to become sexually active with men; her sexual partner does not even appear as a character in the play. At the end of the performance, Adia is cast away by her mother, who insults her with a string of verbal abuse. Judging by the audience's reaction, it was clear that the play was very entertaining. The audience laughed throughout the play and applauded with enthusiasm for the animated performance by the actress portraying MamaAdia.

The play highlights a recurrent theme in many conversations among the older generation in Tanzania when discussing changes in society that they have witnessed over their lifetimes. In conversations about the younger generation, there is a strong tendency to construct modernity as the source of societal problems and as an external force that corrupts local values. In his anthropological study of the Chagga, Setel noted that AIDS is 'one of the many diseases of development' (Setel, 1999: 196), and that Tanzanians associated the disease with a range of behaviors involving desire, greed and a lack of self-control. Likewise, Becker (2007: 31) writes of 'a tendency to reify the past, especially regarding its supposedly higher moral standards' among Muslims who express high levels of discontent over the current state of *maendeleo* ('development') in the Lindi region of Tanzania. These themes are also present in Dilger's (2003) research on the Luo in Northwestern Tanzania, who often cited advanced schooling as a main factor in the decreasing importance of the African family in imparting moral teachings. With many temptations surrounding them, and with higher degrees of independence due to schooling, Dilger's participants expressed that young people are freer to spend time away from their parents. This theme is echoed in Adia's story as well when her mother questions whether she attends school in order to be sexually active.

When I interviewed people who watched this performance, many onlookers thought that the play pointed out the need for greater communication between parents and children. All three of the interviewees I include below were women, and their views are representative of the perspectives I found among the audience. Below are some of their responses to 'what they learned from the play'.

(1) 'I've learned that communication of parents and children makes for good child-rearing. We shouldn't cut our children off from our families, this kind of parenting isn't what we need.'
(2) 'I learned that we should educate our children, and together with that, we shouldn't castigate our children.'
(3) 'If parents talk to their children, they can prevent these kinds of problems, like using birth control pills.'

These comments are not surprising since many CBOs focus on the topic of parent-to-child communication as part of the life skill of 'communication'. While they may achieve some awareness raising through modeling poor parent-to-child communication in plays (and exaggerating it for humorous effect, even), such performances fail to address the issues of gender relations and the forces that act upon young women such as Adia. Plays almost never star a male protagonist, nor do they represent mothers discussing sexual education with their daughters.

Role Play in the *madrassa*: Munira's story

A similar set of discourses was present in a role play that was done after a LSE class at a *madrassa*, an Islamic school. Since it was the first LSE class, the lesson was on the first skill, 'self-awareness' (*kujitambua*). Approximately 15 children between 9 and 15 years were in attendance, and the educator was a 25-year-old Muslim CBO leader who had arranged the class with the help of the local *imam*. The educator had asked a group of children to develop a play illustrating their understanding of 'self-awareness', and they developed an impromptu performance that focused on Munira, a young girl who is lured into having unsafe sexual relations with Sele, a boy who has been approaching her on her way to school. Here again, we see that the primary female character is targeted as promiscuous because of her decision to agree to sexual relations.

Scene 1

Sele:	How's it going?
Munira:	Good.
Sele:	Come closer. Why are you this way (so far away)?
Munira:	I'm afraid of my mom.
Sele:	You're afraid of your mom! Will your mom come here?
Munira:	What if she sees me?
Sele:	How can your mother find us? Your house is far away. She won't come here, don't worry. Okay? Don't worry at all. You're with me, okay?
Munira:	Okay.
Sele:	Don't be so afraid of your mom. ((Sele's friend Felix enters the scene))
Felix:	Hey Sele, my friend ((gives him a high-five, then they move off to the side so Munira cannot hear)). Give her money for a drink, even juice from the street or something.
Sele:	((To Felix)) I'll see you later. ((Sele gives Munira money))
Munira:	Well, I'm leaving for home.
Sele:	Okay, see you tomorrow.

Scene 2

Sele:	How's it going?
Munira:	Good.
Sele:	What's new?
Munira:	I went to the hospital.
Sele:	Mhm. Malaria? ((audience laughter))
Munira:	No. The problem is … that I'm pregnant with your baby.
Sele:	((cries out)) Hey now, speak the truth. My baby, oh no! It's not my baby, you. It's not my baby, you. You shouldn't try to mess with my head, I'm a grown person. The idea of you with my baby, you, no way. ((Sele leaves))

Scene 3

Munira:	Hello, mother.
MamaMunira:	Hello. Now come here so I can see you.
Munira:	Today I didn't go to school because my stomach hurt.

MamaMunira:	When did the stomachache start? Since when? Now tell me clearly. Be straight with me.
Munira:	It's not that my stomach hurts, mother. I went to the hospital and found out that I'm pregnant.
MamaMunira:	You're what?!
Munira:	I'm pregnant.
MamaMunira:	You're pregnant. Ehe! ((starts to push Munira away))
Munira:	No, mother!
MamaMunira:	If you are pregnant I don't even want to see you with my eyes. Get out, get out, get out! ((pushes Munira out of the house)) ((audience laughter))

As was the case in Adia's story above, Munira's mother is presented as the character responsible for determining sexual morality (rather than any male character) when Munira invokes her mother as a reason for avoiding physical contact with Sele. Instead of taking the opportunity to model a discussion between Munira and Sele that shows how young people might talk about their choices, the students enacting this role play depict Munira as a 'bad' daughter since she did not listen to her mother. Moreover, Sele is presented as an easily corruptible boy who listens to his male friends, rather than a young man who can talk to his romantic partners about safe sex. Like Adia, Munira is characterized as a young girl who can be corrupted by desire for material things (in this case, money, drinks and food).

In the end, Munira is the one to suffer the consequences, as she, like Adia, is thrown out of her home. The moral of the role play seems to be that Munira should have made different decisions, rather than being swayed by Sele's efforts. The role play does not depict Sele as responsible for the consequences of unprotected sex, and at the end of the play, the audience expects that Munira has to find a way to take care of herself and her baby on her own.

After the role play, the CBO facilitator engaged the students in a discussion of what they had learned, which provided me with the chance to see how they interpreted the performance they had just witnessed. The children worked together in groups to write the lessons of what they had learned on large pieces of paper. From their answers (presented here in translated form only), it was clear that they focused on gender-specific aspects of the play, rather than noticing that the gender relations between Sele and Munira could have also been important. The children also highlighted the theme of temptation in the film, a factor that highlights the failings of Munira and Sele as individuals rather than addressing the unequal gender relations in Tanzanian society which often constrain the degree of individual agency women and girls can experience.

Educator: Now you've had the chance to talk together. So, can you explain what you've learned, what have you learned in your group? From this play of ours.

Student (f):   We learned that temptations aren't good. And that if a person has a friend, you should really critically look at that friend. I mean that, Sele, he had a friend who was persuading him to do bad things. So, we- you have to check out your friends. If this one has good character, then you go along with him or her. Then, also, girls shouldn't be fearful. They need to be assertive. In this way, Munira wasn't assertive. When she was called by Sele, she just went with him. She didn't assert herself; she didn't respect herself. So, in addition, we also need to respect ourselves.

The next group was asked to report on what they had learned by reading from their poster-sized paper. This group highlighted the relationship between Munira and her mother and also the relationship between Sele and Felix. No discussion of the relationship between Sele and Munira was raised.

Educator: Yes, now the next group. Number two.

Student(m):   Well in the play we learned that there is self-protection and there is temptation. And if a person doesn't listen to her parents, she gets pregnant. And protecting oneself from sexual diseases like AIDS and chlamydia and others. Not to be persuaded by temptations of any kind. Getting pregnant without wanting to, being kicked out of your home, and being rejected by a man who got her pregnant, like Sele.

Another group reported what they learned in the class, pointing out the importance of the relationship between Munira and her mother, and MamaMunira's responsibility towards her daughter's well-being. This group ended by citing a well-known proverb about the need to teach the young while they are still willing to be taught, which clearly points to the group's focus on the mother–daughter relationship, rather than that between Munira and Sele.

Student(f):   We learned about MamaMunira, when she was teaching her child at home. But she didn't follow up Munira's progress at school. The result is that she didn't know what

she was doing at school or if she went to school. Every day
she could have told Munira to give a report, or something.
It wasn't a happy story. And Munira didn't care about
school. She was only caring about romance. She didn't
know, let's say, she didn't know the importance of school –
and romance and sex, these things don't have importance.
Because she is very young she didn't know. Her mother
didn't even tell her.

Educator: Yes,

Student(f):   And then this guy (Felix) here tempted his friend, and Sele
proceeded to deceive Munira. Sele followed Felix, thinking
this is my friend, maybe he'll teach me something good.
But he didn't learn anything. Afterward, his friend
corrupted him. When that happened, he didn't know what
to do, so he rejected Munira. And her mother kicked her
out of the house. Let's say, there's a saying about this.
'*Samaki mkunje angali mbichi*' ('bend a fish while it is still
wet', i.e., teach a child while s/he is young).

In sum, the discussion in the *madrassa* focused on how Munira and Sele
should have been stronger individuals who were capable of thinking for
themselves and taking responsibility for their own actions. The GAD focus
on gender relations was absent in the role play and in the class discussion,
as no attention was paid to why boys and men offer girls and women
material goods such as drinks and money, and no strategies for how to
reject such an offer were mentioned.

Interview with all-male focus group

A final set of data comes from interviews I carried out with a group of
vocational students aged 18–25 years who had just sat through a
co-educational life skills class in which they learned about effective
communication strategies as part of the LSE curriculum. In the class,
several students were asked to perform a role play in which a teen-aged
boy would approach a teen-aged girl and ask her to become his girlfriend,
a theme also present in Munira's story above. The students were instructed
to show how the girl might refuse the offer, which gave the class the
opportunity to re-entextualize the discourses of HIV/AIDS prevention
with female agency, and also to highlight the importance of negotiating
gender relations. The role play appeared to succeed in this, as the female
student-actor quickly rejected the male student-actor's offer to buy
her food in a very straightforward manner. She simply said '*mimi sitaki*'

('I don't want to'), and the boy went on his way. As we saw in Munira's story, in Tanzania, the offer to buy a girl food, or even a soda, is often interpreted as a sexual invitation (also see Bujra & Baylies, 2000). In this brief role play, however, the male character immediately accepted the female character's rejection without further comment. In my interviews with the male students after the class ended, I suggested that such a rejection might not be so realistic. The students discussed how 'real-life' interaction was typically much more complicated. Here the English translation is provided with relevant Swahili words and phrases included.

C: Okay, we saw that the girl was able to say she wasn't interested (*mimi sitaki*), and then the boy left her alone. But I've seen here at NGOs with CBO groups that they really emphasize *uthubutu* ('assertiveness'), do you understand *uthubutu*? Especially for girls, so that they can say *'Mimi sitaki'* and be listened to. But I'm not sure that they can really say it once and then have success. What do you think?

M1:   It's possible since it happens a lot. It's happened to me like three times where a girl has said *sitaki* and she doesn't want to talk and so she leaves.

M2:   The thing is, it depends on the attitude of the person. … For example if someone says *sitaki* and their heart really says it too, and there are others who say *sitaki* and it's that they are analyzing you to see what kind of person you are, if you seem like you have money, if you have the ability to enjoy the nightlife by going out, 'What's this person like? Does he have the ability to buy me things, clothes, what might I wear?' Then she agrees.

C: How do you all differentiate these different *sitaki*s?

M2:   There is the sincere *sitaki*,

M3:   The *sitaki* of *kukutega* (setting a trap for you).

M2:   Then there's the *sitaki* of looking you over,

M3:   Meaning, to look you over, like – do you have the courage to keep trying or what. Because you can keep trying to get a girl for like a whole month while being rejected, but she's assessing you the whole time, checking out your personality and character. Now if you increase your efforts, she sees, 'Oh, this guy, he really likes me.'

To compare the male perspective with the views of the female students at this education session, I also interviewed the female students separately. They offered rather different views, which points to the urgency of attending to gender relations at these education sessions.

F1:   If you decide to say *sitaki*, then you need to really refuse for real. In other words, you must refuse beginning with your face, and then your whole body. But if you refuse here ((points at face)) and if you agree here ((points at body)), it shows that you want more. But if you say *Mimi sitaki*, then you must refuse with a voice that shows that you really aren't interested. So, your body, your hands, I mean, you say you don't want it but then, you're surprised because your suitor thinks you want more, and he pursues you.

F2:   He knows that this one wants me but still she refuses. Maybe if I bring her something, she'll agree. So he keeps trying until you agree. That's how it works.

These comments reveal that even though some education sessions offer the opportunity to re-entextualize education with GAD discourses, these discourses often require deeper discussion. The example of the multiple kinds of *sitaki*s illustrates the necessity of drawing on life experience of the participants in order to uncover how unequal gender relations govern everyday interactions. The women's comments above reveal their perceived need to formulate their behavior with regard to a male perspective, rather than being able to engage in a negotiation that involves both male and female points of view. Notably, they do not argue that the young men are the one who need to alter their understandings of women's perspectives. These comments suggest that further discussion of how such conversations actually unfold in educational settings could encourage young people to delve into the area of gender relations. More frank discussions about cross-gender interactions could be a promising way to provide young men in particular with ideas about how to share the responsibility of safe sexual relations with young women.

Discussion

In these three examples, we see that the models offered in the education sessions generally are not highly successful at re-entextualizing gendered discourses of HIV/AIDS responsibility among males and females towards a focus on gender relations. These examples show the predominant trend of reproducing a focus on women and girls as those responsible for making decisions about their sexual relationships, rather than including men and boys as equally responsible agents. The examples also show how a great deal of LSE does not encourage a focus on gender relations, at least as it is currently being carried out in practice by CBOs. If a greater focus on gender relations is to come to fruition, it will be necessary for LSE educators to emphasize this approach in HIV/AIDS education. However, since the educational practices of most NGOs and CBOs are driven by international policies produced by the WHO and the World Bank, change will have to come from above if gender relations are to be a focus of prevention efforts. At the same time, awareness of how LSE is connected to transformative practices can be initiated from the ground up. If more research is carried out on actual educational practices, local educators can have a better sense of the messages that they are producing in their education efforts. Unfortunately, very little attention (and funding) has been given to qualitative research on HIV/AIDS that could shed light on the discourses which circulate in educational practices.

One of the central messages that calls for greater attention in current educational efforts is the tendency to link potentially risky or harmful sexual behavior with modernization and lifestyle changes among the younger generation, changes that are often associated with schooling and urbanization. In many role plays and LSE classes I observed, this 'modern living' is often castigated by Tanzanian elders as the source of social ills and is targeted as the cause of the loss of a 'local' sensibility with an externally 'modern' (and corrupt) way of life. In the role plays starring Munira and Adia, schooling practices were treated as opportunities for girls to become sexually active, and the desire for recreational pleasures was depicted as the cause of moral corruption in Munira's story and in the interviews with the vocational students. In addition to many other role plays and street shows that I have observed, these three performances illustrate how young Tanzanians usually treat the choice to live a modern life as a morally questionable one that is full of risks, rather than one that can be challenged by re-appraising gender relations in an increasingly modernizing Tanzania. Realistically, there are no signs of change on the horizon in regard to this modernizing project, because many young Tanzanians continue to leave their families in order to attend secondary schools in distant places, and the desire for material goods continues to grow, particularly among the younger generations. These changes in lifestyle seem to have outpaced the way that many Tanzanians manage their social relationships and how they conceive of responsibility in their gender relations.

Conclusion

At the end of my two months of research, I shared my findings with AMREF regarding discourses of gender as well as several other themes. NGOs such as AMREF do not do such research on their own educational practices, as they are typically staffed by medical doctors and public health experts who value large-scale quantitative research over and above qualitative studies of educational discourse. In spite of our different orientations to research, however, I am happy to report that AMREF was very interested in my research. The project manager for the Kinondoni district project expressed sincere disappointment that the responsibility for safe sexual practices was being targeted at girls and women, and he agreed that more needs to be done to address this issue in particular.

Although AMREF staff are required to attend seminars that examine the role of gender and HIV/AIDS, it was clear to me that without closely analyzing their own educational practices, NGO workers are often not able to see the discourses of gender that are being reproduced in their own work. Many of the staff reported to me that they had never thought about the role of language from the perspective of discourse, and that my research offered them the opportunity to see their work from a new angle. They were especially enthusiastic about my transcripts, and they wanted to use them for future training of educators.

For many reasons linked to policy initiatives and funding constraints, institutions like AMREF are not able to mandate a wholesale shift from gender-specific HIV/AIDS education to an approach that focuses on gender relations. However, if international agencies such as the WHO advocate for more attention to the GAD framework, it is highly likely that NGOs will implement these policies in order to align with policy and to qualify for the funding opportunities. In the meantime, I continue to work with AMREF to address these concerns through materials development that will train peer educators to more deeply consider the ways that language and discourses operate in their educational practices.

Acknowledgments

I am grateful to Paul Waibale, Tanzanian Director of the African Medical and Research Foundation (AMREF) for granting me permission to study AMREF's educational practices, and to the Tanzanian Commission for Science and Technology for permission to carry out research on this topic. My research would not have been possible without the assistance of George Kanga, project manager of the Adolescent Sexual Reproductive Health (ASRH) project in Kinondoni, and the warm assistance and tremendous perseverance of the many educators running the CBOs in Sinza (WASTAMASI), Manzese (MWANGAZA) and Mwananyamala (YOP) in Dar es Salaam.

Notes

1. The WID framework was formulated as a policy statement in the Percy Amendment to the US Foreign Assistance Act of 1973.
2. The Kinondoni district houses Manzese, Mwananyamala, Tandale and Kigogo, four wards that are notorious for high rates of crime, prostitution, illicit drinking, drug use and harsh living conditions (Kinondoni Municipality, 2007). The research I report on here comes from Mwananyamala and Kigogo. Other parts of the district are distinctly middle and upper class (e.g. Mikocheni, Msasani and Sinza).
3. Edutainment combines education and entertainment in the forms of plays, singing and dancing in order to disseminate messages of prevention at public events.

References

Akeroyd, A. (2004) Coercion, constraints and 'cultural entrapments': A further look at gendered and occupational factors pertinent to the transmission of HIV in Africa. In E. Kalipeni, S. Craddock, J.R. Oppong and J. Ghosh (eds) *HIV & AIDS in Africa: Beyond Epidemiology* (pp. 89–103). Malden, MA: Blackwell.

Amediume, I. (1987) *Male Daughters, Female Husbands*. London and New York: Zed.

Bakhtin, M. (1981) *The Dialogic Imagination* (M. Holquist, ed. and C. Emerson and M. Holquist, trans.). Austin: University of Texas Press.

Bauman, R. and Briggs, C. (1990) Poetics and performance as critical perspectives on language and social life. *Annual Review of Anthropology* 19, 59–88.

Baylies, C. (2000) Perspectives on gender and AIDS in Africa. In C. Baylies and J. Bujra (eds) *AIDS, Sexuality and Gender in Africa: Collective Strategies and Struggles in Tanzania and Zambia* (pp. 1–24). London: Routledge.

Becker, F. (2007) The virus and the scriptures: Muslims and AIDS in Tanzania. *Journal of Religion in Africa* 37 (1), 16–40.

Blommaert, J. (2005) *Discourse*. Cambridge: Cambridge University Press.

Boler, T. and Aggleton, P. (2005) *Life Skills Education for HIV Prevention: A Critical Analysis*. London: Save the Children and ActionAid International.

Brown, A. (2007) WID and GAD in Dar es Salaam, Tanzania: Reappraising gender planning approaches in theory and practice. *Journal of Women, Politics, & Policy* 28, 57–83.

Bujra, J. and Baylies, C. (2000) Responses to the AIDS epidemic in Tanzania and Zambia. In C. Baylies and J. Bujra (eds) *AIDS, Sexuality and Gender in Africa: Collective Strategies and Struggles in Tanzania and Zambia* (pp. 25–59). London: Routledge.

Bujra, J. and Mokake, S. (2000) AIDS activism in Dar es Salaam: Many struggles; a single goal. In C. Baylies and J. Bujra (eds) *AIDS, Sexuality and Gender in Africa: Collective Strategies and Struggles in Tanzania and Zambia* (pp. 154–174). London: Routledge.

Callaway, H. (1987) *Gender, Culture, Empire: European Women in Colonial Nigeria*. Oxford: MacMillan/St. Anthony's College.

Canagarajah, S. (2002) Reconstructing local knowledge. *Journal of Language, Identity, and Education* 1, 243–259.

Chowdhry, G. (1995) Engendering development? Women in development (WID) in international development regimes. In M.M. Marchand and J.L. Parpart (eds) *Feminism/Postmodernism/Development* (pp. 26–41). New York: Routledge.

Connelly, M.P., Li, T.M., MacDonald, M. and Parpart, J.L. (2000) Feminism and development: Theoretical perspectives. In J.L. Parpart (ed.) *Theoretical Perspectives on Gender and Development* (pp. 51–160). Ottawa: IDRC Books.

Dilger, H. (2003) Sexuality, AIDS, and the lures of modernity: Reflexivity and morality among young people in rural Tanzania. *Medical Anthropology* 22, 23–52.

Fairclough, N. (2001) *Language and Power* (2nd edn). London: Longman.

Marchand, M. and Parpart, J. (eds) (1995) *Feminism Postmodernism Development*. New York: Routledge.

Mbilinyi, M. and Mwabuki. J. (1996) NGOs and the struggle against HIV/AIDS. Paper presented at the Annual Gender Studies Conference, Dar es Salaam, 5–8 December.

Mohanty, C., Russo, A. and Torres, L. (eds) (2001) *Third World Women and Politics of Feminism*. Bloomington: Indiana University Press.

National policy on HIV/AIDS (2001) The United Republic of Tanzania Prime Minister's Office. Dar es Salaam.

Norton, B. and Mutonyi, H. (2007) 'Talk what others think you can't talk': HIV/AIDS clubs as peer education in Ugandan schools. *Compare* 37, 479–492.

Oyewùmí, O. (1997) *The Invention of Women: Making an African Sense of Western Gender Discourses*. Minneapolis: University of Minnesota Press.

Parpart, J.L. (ed.) (2000) *Theoretical Perspectives on Gender and Development*. Ottawa: IDRC Books.

Parpart, J.L. and Marchand, M.H. (1995) Exploding the canon: An introduction/conclusion. In J.L. Parpart and M.H. Marchand (eds) *Feminism/Postmodernism/Development* (pp. 1–22). New York: Routledge.

Sen, G. and Grown, C. (1987) *Development, Crisis and Alternative Visions: Third World Women's Perspectives*. New York: Monthly Review Press.

Setel, P.W. (1999) *A Plague of Paradoxes: AIDS, Culture, and Demography in Northern Tanzania*. Chicago: University of Chicago Press.

Silverstein, M. and Urban, G. (1996) The natural history of discourse. In M. Silverstein and G. Urban (eds) *Natural Histories of Discourse* (pp. 1–17). Chicago: University of Chicago Press.

Snyder, K. (2006) Mothers on the march: Iraqw women negotiating the public sphere in Tanzania. *Africa Today* 53, 79–99.

Stambach, A. (2000) *Lessons from Mount Kilimanjaro: Schooling, Community, and Gender in East Africa*. New York: Routledge.

Tanzania Commission for AIDS (2005) *A New Look at the HIV and AIDS Epidemic in Tanzania*. Dar es Salaam, Tanzania.

World Health Organization (2003) *Integrating Gender into HIV/AIDS Programmes: A Review Paper*. Geneva: WHO.

Chapter 7
Uganda's ABC Program on HIV/AIDS Prevention: A Discursive Site of Struggle

SHELLEY JONES and BONNY NORTON

Introduction

In Uganda, what began as a national war against HIV/AIDS has become a battle for ownership of the discourse on HIV/AIDS, with life and death implications for Ugandan people, and young women in particular. One such battleground is Uganda's ABC program on HIV/AIDS prevention (A for abstinence, B for be faithful, C for condoms), in which diverse stakeholders are implicated in struggles over the policy and its implementation. This chapter will address three of the primary stakeholders in this battle, namely policy-makers at the macro level, teachers at the institutional level and female students at the micro level, respectively.

At the macro level of policy, we consider the genesis of the ABC policy, and its relationship to national and international agendas of development. We demonstrate that the discourse of the ABC program, particularly with reference to condom usage, is a site of struggle in which national and global agendas take precedence over the daily challenges of those most affected by policy initiatives. At the institutional level, we consider how policy at macro level impacts health education in schools. At the micro level, we investigate the challenges young rural Ugandan women face in negotiating the principles of ABC on a daily basis, demonstrating how the ABC program inadequately addresses what is being called the increasing 'feminization of AIDS' (Dworkin & Ehrhardt, 2007: 13).

We frame our argument with reference to poststructuralist theories of language as 'discourse' (Bourdieu, 1977; Foucault, 1980; Weedon, 1987), in which language is conceptualized as the complexes of signs and practices that organize social existence and social reproduction. By extension, the discourse of HIV/AIDS is theorized as constituted in and by language and other sign systems, which serve to organize meaning-making practices associated with HIV/AIDS. In this view, discourses on HIV/AIDS construct and are constructed by a wide variety of social relationships, ranging from the most intimate, such as those between client and sex worker, to the more abstract, such as those between wealthy and poor nations. In poststructuralist theory, then, the social meaning of HIV/AIDS is a site of struggle, with conflicting claims to the truth about the origins, spread and control of the disease. Our analysis of Uganda's ABC program provides a window on this site of struggle.

The Discourse of the ABC Program: From ABC to PEPFAR

In Uganda, the high rate of HIV infections in the early 1990s led the government to strengthen its ABC education campaign. Condom use had been minimal up to this time for reasons of limited access and awareness, as well as resistance from various religious and political groups who believed that promoting condoms would undermine the prevention messages of abstinence and be faithful (Okware *et al.*, 2005). However, it became increasingly clear that condom use was extremely effective in preventing HIV transmission, and in 1991, the government promoted a policy of 'quiet promotion and responsible use of condoms with appropriate education' (Okware *et al.*, 2005: 627).

Condom use increased immediately and dramatically from 5% use between non-cohabiting partners in 1987 to over 60% by 2002, with the procurement of condoms rising concomitantly from 10 million in 1994, to 30 million in 1997, to 120 million in 2003 (Okware *et al.*, 2005: 627). According to Dr. Alex Coutinho, Executive Director of The Aids Support Organization in Uganda (TASO), quoted in Garbus and Marseille, critical has been

> [t]he gradual buildup and social acceptability of interventions like condom promotion in the media and public places without hindrances from religious groups. A key to this acceptance has been the A, B, C campaign where condoms are seen as an alternative to abstinence and faithfulness. Social marketing of condoms has been very successful allowing especially the youth to accept that safe sex can be fun sex. (Garbus & Marseille, 2003: 28)

Uganda, however, is donor reliant for most of its HIV/AIDS programming and therefore must acquiesce to donor priorities to receive much of this funding (Stewart, 2006). It has been observed that Uganda's official waning support for the promotion of condom use coincided with funding priorities in the United States under the Bush administration, where the overwhelming focus of its PEPFAR program (President's Emergency Plan For AIDS Relief) was on abstinence (Schoepf, 2003: 555). Clearly, powerful interests at policy level were imposing a highly adverse meaning to the 'C' in the ABC program. For example, over 50% of the monies received from 2004 to 2006 by Uganda through US funding were spent on abstinence/be faithful programmes and not on condom use (Berry & Noble, 2006; Buonocore, n.d.; Cohen, 2005; Cohen & Tate, 2005; Das, 2005). ABC bill-boards, once ubiquitous throughout Uganda, were replaced with adver-tisements promoting abstinence (Berry & Noble, 2006; Cohen, 2005).

It was also at about this time (2004) that the Ugandan national brand of condoms, *Engabu*, distributed for free by the government to health clinics and other public sources, were recalled due to issues of quality. The valid-ity of this recall is contentious, as it has been claimed that there were no problems with these condoms other than an unpleasant odor (Wakabi, 2006), and that the retraction of condoms, and the ensuing delay in repleni-shing the supply of condoms, coincided with the onset of US funding priorities (Stewart, 2006). Ambassador Stephen Lewis, the former United Nations Secretary General's Special Envoy for HIV/AIDS in Africa, said 'there is no question that the condom crisis in Uganda is being driven and exacerbated by PEPFAR and by the extreme policies that the administra-tion in the United States is now pursuing' (Altman, 2005). The resulting shortage of condoms, and the high price of condoms that were available, put large numbers of the population, especially the poor, at risk. Many working in the area of HIV/AIDS were worried that the years spent promoting condom use to the general population would be severely undermined by this struggle over the ownership of the ABC discourse:

> "We're almost back to square one," one of the organization's staff members said, adding: [B]ecause of our culture, it was very difficult for us to get people to use condoms. Now, trying to promote absti-nence in this social environment is very difficult. If you tell people to abstain, they'll say, "You were the people telling us to use condoms, and now you're telling us to abstain. Does this mean condoms weren't effective and you were lying to us?" (Cohen & Tate, 2005)

What was once a discourse that reflected patriotism, solidarity and community mobilization around the battle against HIV/AIDS evolved into a raging debate on what constituted the truth about condom effective-ness. One side of the debate included researchers, health workers and public representatives who feared that the recent 'war against condoms' spelt disaster (Berry & Noble, 2006; International Community of Women Living With HIV/AIDS, 2004; Schoepf, 2003). On the other side of the debate were those such as global policy-makers, policy analysts, senior advisors and some researchers who rallied behind PEPFAR, and were often involved in PEPFAR policy and implementation. They minimized the importance of condoms in HIV/AIDS prevention, and sought to make the case that abstinence and partner reduction *and not condom use* were the key reasons for the decline in HIV/AIDS prevalence in the 1990s (Allen, 2006; Green & Witte, 2006; Shelton, 2006; Wilson, 2004). These tactics were used to justify PEPFAR's lack of support for condom use (Allen, 2006; Green & Witte, 2006; Shelton, 2006; Wilson, 2004).

Clearly, PEPFAR was closely aligned with the conservative, religious fundamentalism that had lodged itself firmly within the sexual health discourse in the US and Uganda (Berry & Noble, 2006; Cohen, 2005; Roberts, 2006; Schoepf, 2003; Wakabi, 2006). For example, Uganda's First Lady, Janet Museveni, herself an evangelical Christian and whose office received funding from the PEPFAR program, became an outspoken supporter of abstinence. Her claim that 'The young person who is trained to be disciplined will, in the final analysis, survive better than the one who has been instructed to wear a piece of rubber and continue with "business as usual"' has served to undermine HIV/AIDS prevention measures involving condom-related education (Roberts, 2006).

Further, those who oppose mainstream promotion of condom use claim that 'condomcentric' approaches to combating HIV/AIDS promote promiscuity, immorality and sexual colonization. They argue, specifically, that Northern countries are imposing their sexual practices – specifically condom use – on Southern countries, and that condoms are not conducive to general HIV/AIDS educational programs, unless targeting 'high-risk' groups such as sex trade workers (Genuis & Genuis, 2008; Green & Witte, 2006; Wilson, 2004). For example, Edward Green, then a member of President Bush's AIDS Advisory Council, pronounced to the US Congress that condoms were a 'western, technological solution, inappropriately exported to Africa' and that abstinence and partner reduction should be acknowledged as the most important factor in the decline of HIV/AIDS infection rates (Schoepf, 2003: 555).

The view represented by Green clearly conflicted with those of many prominent Ugandans. Ugandan Vice President, Gilbert Bukenya, openly challenged the way in which the ABC discourse had been hijacked by ideology linked to US funding: 'The use of condoms was politicized. Much as the religious sector is against it, I feel there are people who can't be left out' (Wakabi, 2006: 1387). Other notable individuals who had worked extensively with HIV/AIDS organizations, such as Sophie Wacasa-Monico, a former director of the world-respected TASO, publicly expressed their dismay about assertions such as Green's. Addressing the US Congress, Wacasa-Monico, quoted in Schoepf (2003: 555) stated, 'I am deeply concerned when I hear people taking a single element of our successful national program – for instance abstinence – out of context and ascribe all our achievements to that one element. They must all be implemented together in order for prevention to work'. In a similar spirit, David Serwadda, a leading HIV/AIDS researcher and Director of the Institute of Public Health at Makerere University in Kampala, Uganda, noted as follows:

> As a physician who has been involved in Uganda's response to AIDS for 20 years, I fear that one small part of what led to Uganda's success – promoting sexual abstinence [and faithfulness] – is being overemphasized in policy debates. Abstinence is not always possible for people at risk. Many women simply do not have the option to delay initiation of sex or to limit their number of sexual partners. (Serwadda, 2003: A29)

From PEPFAR to PIASCY

The battle over the ownership of the ABC discourse also seriously and negatively impacted sexual health education at institutional levels in Uganda. Although education is a foundational pillar of the ABC program, the polarized arguments around the promotion of condom use led to instructions for health providers and public spokespersons to refrain from discussing condom usage as an HIV/AIDS preventative strategy, and to promote abstinence only (Berry & Noble, 2006; Cohen, 2005; Cohen & Tate, 2005). Cohen (2005) describes how President Museveni's progressive and innovative President's Initiative on HIV/AIDS Strategy on Communication to Youth (PIASCY), initially developed in 2001 to provide comprehensive sexual health information for every student in Uganda, was later revised in a way that accorded with PEPFAR priorities. The original PIASCY text covered a wide range of topics, such as how to prevent oneself from becoming infected (including through the use of condoms), sexual negotiations (e.g. how to 'say no') and sexual hygiene. However, when the original texts were launched in 2003, there was a huge outcry from the evangelical community, claiming that the textbooks were pornographic and encouraged youth to become sexually active. This took place at about the same time that the PEPFAR initiative required that one-third of its HIV/AIDS prevention funding be spent on abstinence programs.

The revised texts emphasized abstinence and characterized sexual intercourse as an act that should be confined to marriage; they omitted information about condom use and sexual hygiene and instead inserted messages intended to scare students away from having sex (Cohen, 2005). For example, a draft of the revised PIASCY text claims that 'condoms are not 100% perfect protective gear against STDs and HIV infection. This is because condoms have small pores that could still allow the virus through' (Cohen & Tate, 2005: 5).

In 2004, USAID hired the Uganda Program for Human and Holistic Development (UPHOLD) to provide training for 40,000 teachers on the use of these PIASCY materials. Teachers were explicitly instructed not to talk about condoms with their students. One teacher said, 'At the PIASCY training, we were told not to show (pupils) how to use condoms and not to talk about them at our school. In the past, we used to show them to our upper primary classes. Now we can't do that'. Another commented: 'President Museveni said there is no use teaching young people about condom use ... because then children will go and experiment with them'. Some teachers said they taught their pupils about condoms anyway because, as one put it, 'people don't buy this idea of abstinence, because in Uganda, many girls are using sex to buy their daily bread' (Cohen, 2005).

The Discourse of the ABC Program: The Micro Level of Practice

While policy-makers and teachers were debating the merits and limitations of the ABC program, young girls in rural Uganda were anxiously wondering how they could afford their next semester of schooling. To illustrate the severity of their situation, we draw on data collected in a longitudinal study we conducted with a group of secondary school girls of approximately 17 years of age in Kyato Secondary School (KSS)[1] in Kyato Village in rural Uganda. While the aim of the larger study was to better understand the challenges young rural women face in securing a quality education, the data provided much insight into the limitations of the ABC policy on HIV/AIDS prevention.

The ethnographic study used a number of qualitative data collection methods over the course of two years (August 2004–September 2006). Participants were 15 girls from KSS who, over this period, were in the process of completing their secondary school education. Data were collected through interviews, observations, questionnaires, journals and document analysis. Fieldwork was conducted primarily by Jones from August 2004 to August 2005, during which time she lived full-time in Kyato Village. Jones and Norton had made an initial visit to the site in August 2003, and Norton returned to the site in October 2004 and February 2006, during which time she participated in data collection.

Kyato Village borders a trading centre that is approximately seven miles from the nearest town centre, Masaka, in southwestern Uganda. Poverty in this rural area of the country is endemic and acute. Most of the students' families survive by subsistence-level farming, with small incomes sometimes earned through men's employment (e.g. as labourers or in other occupations, such as tailoring or driving taxis), the sale of crafts such as mats and baskets made by women, or the sale of extra food grown in the family gardens. The official per capita income is less than US$1 per day, although it is likely that many families live on less than US$1 per day. Malnutrition, disease and poor living conditions are widespread, and it has been one of the areas in the world hardest hit by the HIV/AIDS pandemic.

Two questionnaires were particularly important for data collection with respect to HIV/AIDS prevention, one administered in May 2005 by Jones and a second administered in September 2006 by a local research assistant, Daniel Ahimbisibwe. Thirteen girls completed the first questionnaire, referred to as Q1, and 12 girls completed the second questionnaire, referred to as Q2.

Examples of questions from Q1 include the following:

- Many girls have talked about the problems of girls having sex for money – to pay for school fees, supplies, etc. Do you think this is a general problem in Uganda?
- Do you know of any girls who have had sex to pay for school fees/books/supplies?
- Have you ever had sex in order to raise money for your own school fees/supplies/books? If yes, how do you feel about that experience?
- Do you know any male teachers that have had sex with their female students?
- Do you know of any parents who have encouraged girls to have sex in order to pay for school fees?

Examples of questions from Q2 include the following:

- Do you think that most girls are aware that condoms prevent the transmission of AIDS?
- Do you know of any young women or men who have become infected with HIV/AIDS? If yes, how many girls? boys?

- Are you sexually active? If yes, at what age did you first have sex? Have your partners used condoms?
- Have you received gifts or money for sex? If yes, what have you received? If you have received money, what have you used that money for?
- Do you have any concerns about having unprotected sex? If yes, what are these concerns?
- Have you ever been afraid to refuse a request for sex? [If yes] Why were you afraid?
- Are you worried about becoming infected with HIV/AIDS?

The central argument we make, drawing on data from this study, is that the ABC approach has limited resonance with the lived experiences of the young women in our study (Jones & Norton, 2007). As we argue, to abstain from transactional sex, to be faithful to only one person, or to access resources such as condoms are untenable luxuries for many young rural Ugandan women. Further, even if condoms are available, young women have great difficulty insisting that their partners use them. Poverty and gender inequities rendered the ABC policy meaningless for many of the participants in our study. Drawing on our data, we now turn to a closer analysis of the discourses of abstinence, be faithful and condom use.

The discourse on abstinence and be faithful

We begin by contrasting assertions about abstinence within the pro-PEPFAR rhetoric with these young women's voices. James Shelton, of the Bureau for Global Health, US Agency for International Development, based in Washington, DC, makes the following claim:

> Abstinence efforts provide an opportunity to promote personal self-efficacy more broadly among young people, as well as fidelity and partner limitation once sexual activity commences. (James Shelton, 2006: 1948)

All of the girls in our study knew that abstinence was the greatest protection against HIV/AIDS, and most advocated abstinence until marriage. Comments in this regard include the following:

- Please young girls abstain from sex till you grow up.
- The comment I would like to share is with those who are not engaged in sex is to abstain until they get married.
- I would like to comment about girls because they are most affective with HIV/AIDS. So they should use this method: A – abstinence from sex; B – being faithful; C – condom use.

However, although the girls generally believed in the virtue of absti-nence, 10 of the 12 girls in Q2 noted that they were sexually active, having begun sexual activity at the average age of 16. While five girls had had only one sexual partner, five had had multiple partners, mostly with adolescent boys, but also with 'sugar daddies', teachers and boda-boda men.[2] Such disconnect between publicly expressed views by youth concerning sexual relationships and their actual, lived sexual experiences are documented in other studies, as well. Agyei *et al.* (1994) report: '[t]here were contradictions between behavior and attitudes, with many more young people reporting that they engaged in sexual behavior than report-ing that they approved of premarital sex' (Agyei *et al.*, 1994: 1).

Pressures against abstinence

Pressure from the partner was cited most commonly as the reason why the girls in our study engaged in sexual activity, though the need for money was almost equally important. In Q1, 12 of 13 girls noted that the problem of girls having sex to pay for school fees and supplies was a common one in Uganda, and four of the girls said that they had had sex to raise money for their own school fees and supplies. When asked how they felt about those sexual experiences, their responses were as follows:

- It's bad because of many problems in it. But I do it because I want to buy books and to pay some school fees.
- I feel bad … about that action.
- It because male can tell you to have sex to pay for your school fees.
- I felt very happy because of that money.

In Q2, 9 of the 10 sexually active girls noted that they had received gifts or money for sex. The money received was used to buy books, stationery, clothing, food and toiletries. As one girl said, 'I used that money to buy things that helped me to stay at school because I was at home lacking things to use'. Another said, 'It is true that girls usually expect money or gifts in exchange for sex because some parents failed to pay school fees for girls and then she decide to exchange sex in order to get money'. Their sexual partners, however, had not always given money to the girls, but rather services in kind. Thus while the sugar daddy generally gave the girl cash, the teacher gave 'high marks in the teacher's subject', 'good results' and 'guideline in studying', while the boda-boda man provided 'easy transport', 'taking you to school' and 'lifts'.

Our study also suggests that some parents are complicit in encouraging the transactional sex of their daughters. In answer to the Q1 question, 'Do you know of any parents who have encouraged girls to have sex in order to pay school fees'?, 12 of 13 girls answered yes. Further, in a focus group interview in January 2005, one of the girls noted as follows:

> Our mother can force us to, to go and practice fornication. If you say at home, 'Mum, I want books, pencils. I don't have a uniform', she can tell you that 'I don't have money. What can you do? You can go and practice fornication in order to get money.'

For many of these girls, then, sex has become an exchangeable commodity, a resource that the girls, some with the encouragement of parents, can use to cover costs of schooling and basic necessities. These transactional sexual relationships are generally intergenerational – young women with older men as sexual partners – as older men have more financial resources than male students (Vavrus, 2005). Alarmingly, these intergenerational sexual relationships are believed to account largely for the reason that young women are up to six times more likely to contract HIV/AIDS than are their male counterparts (Hallett *et al.*, 2007; Leach *et al.*, 2003; Luke, 2003).

Young women's 'choices' about their sexual behavior are also often compromised by forced sex and various kinds of abuse, which are alarmingly common in Uganda and other sub-Saharan countries (Hulton *et al.*, 2000; Leach *et al.*, 2003; Luke, 2003; Nyanzi *et al.*, 2001). Hulton *et al.*'s study (2000) of a group of adolescent girls elicited from them a wide spectrum of abuse, including 'rape', 'abuse from boys', 'boys trying grope you', being 'strongly convinced' (Hulton *et al.*, 2000: 43). Luke (2003) uncovered similar findings: 'The research offers numerous examples of older partners, such as teachers and relatives, and peers (and sometimes groups of peers) who forced girls to have sex' (Luke, 2003: 74–75).

In our study, 11 of 12 girls in Q2 said that they had been afraid to refuse a request for sex, the consequences of which included the following:

- When I refused he forced me until I get sex with him.
- You can abused and punished by these people.
- The teacher had started beating me at school without any reason.
- The person hates you until death.

Tragically, the context of the school, in which adolescent girls should be receiving support and encouragement to develop autonomy, self-confidence and strength in negotiating equality, is the very environment in which girls are often at risk of sexual, physical and emotional abuse. Exploitative sexual relations between teachers and students are, in fact, considered a widespread problem in Uganda (see, e.g. Lacey, 2003; Luke, 2003; Nyanzi *et al.*, 2001.) In Nyanzi *et al.*'s research, 54% of the students mentioned teachers among the three most common types of 'sugar daddy'.

Our research corroborates this finding. In Q1, all 13 girls said they knew of girls who had had sex with teachers. In a questionnaire administered to teachers at both the secondary school and two primary schools in Kyato village, 17 out of 30 teachers knew of teachers who had had sexual relationships with their students, and 20 out of 30 teachers believe this to be a general problem in Uganda. The girls in our study indicated that having sex with a teacher might help a girl receive 'money and … marks'; 'being graded [more] highly than the others'; 'status'; and 'high marks in class during examination period'. In Q2, three girls said that they had been afraid to refuse sexual advances made by teachers: one girl (who had sex with her teacher) said 'I was fearing him … he would have beaten [me] in class and punished me every time'; another girl said she 'fear[ed being] mistreated at school'.

Discourses on condoms

Our findings with respect to condom use are equally significant. We found that while 9 of the 10 sexually active girls indicated that they asked their partners to use condoms to prevent both pregnancy and HIV/AIDS transmission, power differentials in terms of gender and age, combined with the financially dependent position of the girl, often made it impossible for the girl to insist on protected sex. As Stromquist (1990: 98) notes, '[a] key element in the subordination of women has been men's control over women's sexuality and … norms such as virginity, limited physical mobility, the penalization of abortion, and the association of the use of contraceptives [or barrier methods] with sexual promiscuity' (see also Schoepf, 2003). Indeed, as Kuate-Defoe (2004) argues, the more financially dependent girls are, the less scope they have to protect themselves.

In our study, although the vast majority of girls asked their partners to use condoms, five said that males usually do not use condoms when they have sex with adolescent girls. Reasons given include the following:

* because some of them want to impregnate them and stop them from school;
* they say that sex with condoms are not interesting to them and they do not get satisfaction. They said that having sex with condom is like eating packed sweet;
* the majority do not use condoms. They are affected and they say why do we use condoms for what … They say 'Do AIDS cost money'.

In sum, at the micro level of practice, we have demonstrated that the ABC policy on HIV/AIDS prevention has severe limitations. Extreme poverty, gender power imbalances, sexual abuse and exploitation limit the ability of young women to exercise agency in their sexual encounters. Notwithstanding the discourses of policy-makers at the macro level, and teachers at institutional level, young Ugandan women remain highly vulnerable to HIV/AIDS.

Conclusion

In this chapter, we have made the case that the discourse on the ABC program of HIV/AIDS prevention in Uganda is a site of struggle, in which diverse stakeholders have vested claims to the 'truth' about the disease. While the mid-1980s to early 1990s saw an emphasis on A and B in the ABC program, due to reluctance by religious and other leaders in society to promote condom use, the years 1992–2002 included C, condom use, as a result of research that provided convincing evidence of the effectiveness of condoms in HIV/AIDS prevention. The pendulum swung again with the introduction of PEPFAR in 2004, with increasing opposition to condom use. These changes in policy reflect shifts in discourses of power with respect to HIV/AIDS prevention, which in turn impacts important institutional discourses in homes, schools, hospitals and community centres.

Significantly, the struggle over HIV/AIDS discourse has a formidable impact on the lives of people, young and old, consequences that are no less serious than a war fought with guns and tanks. It is a battle that is waged in boardrooms, classrooms and bedrooms, and is constituted in and by language. Of central interest, as Bourdieu (1977) asks, is whose voice has greater value? Who can impose reception on others, and to what extent is accessibility to resources implicated in claims to truth? Clearly, the discourse of the Ugandan ABC program provides insight into the ways in which policies on HIV/AIDS in developing countries are vulnerable to shifts in global policies and local economies.

Controversy about the ABC policy, as outlined in this chapter, has caused pedagogical paralysis for many HIV/AIDS educators, as they fear reprisals for promoting any kind of prevention other than abstinence and faithfulness (Berry & Noble, 2006; Cohen & Tate, 2005). This shift in HIV/AIDS education emphasis from ABC to AB(c) has serious repercussions for effective sexual health education for youth and, as we have argued, is not a viable option for many girls (Cohen, 2005; Jones & Norton, 2007; Lacey, 2003; Roberts, 2006). Our study demonstrates that despite the girls' recognition that abstinence and faithfulness were the best methods of HIV/AIDS prevention, as well as their stated desire to abstain or be faithful, their actual life circumstances made healthy sexual behaviour difficult to maintain. Extreme poverty limited their ability to exercise choice, and thus abstinence policies on HIV/AIDS prevention had limited relevance for them. As Ugandan research assistant, Daniel Ahimbisibwe said:

> These girls know. They are smart. They know abstinence is the only guarantee against AIDS. But – what can they do? They need the money. They don't need more education about abstinence.

We challenge policy-makers, funding bodies and health educators to listen to the voices of the young women in our study, as well as those of other young women whose lives are at risk. These young women need to be involved not only in the design and implementation of HIV/AIDS education programmes, but in policy-making initiatives that address the root causes of their vulnerability: the poverty and gender inequity in their daily lives. HIV/AIDS prevention will only be effective if those who are most vulnerable in Ugandan society help to shape the discourse on ABC.

Acknowledgments

We would like to express our deep gratitude to the girls who so generously and willingly shared with us their life experiences. We would also like to thank the Ugandan research assistant, Daniel Ahimbisibwe, who was an integral part of the data collection for our research. We gratefully acknowledge funding support for this research from the Social Sciences and Humanities Research Council of Canada (SSHRC), the International Development Research Centre of Canada (IDRC) and the University of British Columbia Hampton Foundation.

Notes

1. Pseudonyms are used for the names of the school, village and research participants to protect the identities of those who participated in, and those who were associated with, this study.
2. The original boda-bodas were bicycle taxis that operated in eastern Uganda and took people over the border to Kenya; the etymological origin of the boda-boda is 'border-to-border', the call of bicycle owners seeking customers.

References

Agyei, W.K., Mukiza-Gapere, J. and Epema, E.J. (1994) Sexual behavior, reproductive health and contraceptive use among adolescents and young adults in Mbale District, Uganda. [Electronic version]. *Journal of Tropical Medical Hygeine* 4, 219–227.

Allen, T. (2006) AIDS and evidence: Interrogating some Ugandan myths. *Journal of Biosocial Science* 38, 7–28.

Altman, L.K. (2005) U.S. blamed for condom shortage in fighting AIDS in Uganda. [Electronic version]. *New York Times*, 20 August.

Berry, S. and Noble, R. (2006) *Why is Uganda Interesting?* Avert.org. Retrieved on 8 August 2006, from http://www.avert.org/aidsuganda.htm.

Bourdieu, P. (1977) The economics of linguistic exchanges. *Social Science Information* 16 (6), 645–668.

Buonocore, D. (n.d.) HIV/AIDS education in Uganda. [Electronic version]. *Future Leaders Summit*. Retrieved on 6 August 2006, from http://www.org.elon.edu/summit/essays/essay12.pdf.

Cohen, J. (2005) *A Tale of Two Presidential Initiatives: Changes in an HIV Prevention Program in Uganda*. GlobalAIDSLink. Retrieved on 14 July 2006, from http://www.hrw.org/english/docs/2006/02/01/uganda12591.htm.

Cohen, J. and Tate, T. (2005) The less they know the better. Abstinence-only HIV/AIDS programs in Uganda. [Electronic version]. *Human Rights Watch* 17 (4), 1–79. Retrieved on 9 October 2006, from http://www.popline.org/docs/290913.

Das, P. (2005) Condom crisis in Uganda. [Electronic version]. *The Lancet* 5, 601–602. Retrieved on 14 March 2007 from http://www.thelancet.com/journals/laninf/article/PIIS1473309905702279/abstract.

Dworkin, S.L. and Ehrhardt, A.A. (2007) Going beyond "ABC" to include "GEM": Critical reflections on progress in the HIV/AIDS epidemic. [Electronic version]. *American Journal of Public Health* 97 (1), 13–18. Retrieved on 9 January 2008, from http://www.ajph.org/cgi/content/abstract/97/1/13.

Foucault, M. (1980) *Power/Knowledge: Selected Interviews and Other Writings 1972 – 1977*. (C. Gordon, trans.). New York: Pantheon Books.

Garbus, L. and Marseille, E.M. (2003) HIV/AIDS in Uganda. *Country AIDS Policy Analysis Project*. [Electronic version]. San Francisco, CA: Aids Policy Research Center, University of California. Retrieved on 16 January 2008, from http://www.popline.org/docs/274984.

Genuis, S.J. and Genuis, S.K. (2008) HIV/AIDS prevention in Uganda: Why has it worked? [Electronic version]. *Postgraduate Medical Journal* 81, 615–617. Retrieved on 9 January 2008, from http://pmj.bmj.com/content/vol81/issue960/.

Green, E.C. and Witte, K. (2006) Can fear arousal in public health campaigns contribute to the decline of HIV prevalence? [Electronic version]. *Journal of Health Communication* 11 (3), 245–259. Retrieved on 17 January 2008, from http://www.informaworld.com/smpp/content~content=a742066536.

Hallett, T.B., Gregson, S., Lewis, J.J.C., Lopman, B.A. and Garnett, G.P. (2007) Behavior change in generalized HIV epidemics: Impact of reducing cross-generational sex and delaying age at sexual debut. *Sexually Transmitted Infections* 83, 50–54. [Electronic version]. Retrieved on 17 January 2008, from http://sti.bmj.com/cgi/reprint/83/suppl_1/i50?maxtoshow=&HITS=10&hits=10&RESULTFORMAT=1&author1=Hallett&author2=Gregson&title=Behaviour+change&andorexacttitle=and&andorexacttitleabs=and&andorexactfulltext=and&searchid=1&FIRSTINDEX=0&sortspec=relevance&volume=83&firstpage=50&fdate=1/1/2004&resourcetype=HWCIT,HWELTR.

Hulton, L.A., Cullen, R. and Khalokho, S.W. (2000) Perceptions of the risks of sexual activity and their consequences among Ugandan adolescents. [Electronic version]. *Studies in Family Planning* 31 (1), 35–46. Retrieved on 14 November 2006, from http://links.jstor.org/sici?sici=0039-3665(200003)31%3A1%3C35% 3APOTROS%3E2.0.CO%3B2-R.

International Community of Women Living With HIV/AIDS (2004) *Newsletter*. On WWW at http://www.icw.org/node/100, 2004.

Jones, S. and Norton, B. (2007) On the limits of sexual health literacy: Insights from Ugandan schoolgirls. *Journal of Diaspora, Indigenous and Minority Education* 1 (4), 285–305.

Kuate-Defo, B. (2004) Young people's relationships with sugar daddies and sugar mummies: What do we know and what do we need to know? [Electronic version]. *African Journal of Reproductive Health* 8 (2), 13–37. Retrieved on 8 July 2006, from http://www.bioline.org.br/request?rh04023.

Lacey, M. (2003) For Ugandan girls, delaying sex has economic cost. [Electronic version]. *New York Times*, 18 August. Retrieved on 5 July 2006, from http://query.nytimes.com/gst/fullpage.html?sec=health&res=9507EFDB1330 F93BA2575BC0A9659C8B63.

Leach, F., Fiscian, V., Kadzamira, E., Lemani, E. and Machakanja, P. (2003) *An Investigative Study of the Abuse of African Girls in School*. London: DFID.

Luke, N. (2003) Age and economic asymmetries in the sexual relationships of adolescent girls in Sub-Saharan Africa. *Studies in Family Planning* 34 (2), 67–86.

Nyanzi, S., Pool, R. and Kinsman, J. (2001) The negotiation of sexual relationships among school pupils in south-western Uganda. *AIDS Care* 13 (1) 83–98.

Okware, S., Kinsman, J., Onyango, S., Oplo, A. and Kaggwa, P. (2005) Revisiting the ABC strategy: HIV prevention in Uganda in the era of antiretroviral therapy. [Electronic version]. *Postgraduate Medical Journal* 81, 625–28. Retrieved on 14 January 2008, from http://pmj.bmj.com/cgi/content/abstract/81/960/625.

Roberts, K.M. (2006) The AIDS pandemic in Uganda: Social capital and the role of NGSs in alleviating the impact. Unpublished doctoral dissertation, University of Bergen.

Schoepf, B.G. (2003) Uganda: Lessons for AIDS control in Africa. [Electronic version]. *Review of African Political Economy* 30 (98), 553–72. Retrieved on 11 January 2008, from http://www.ingentaconnect.com/content/routledg/crea/ 2003/00000030/00000098/art00003.

Serwadda, D. (2003) Beyond Abstinence. [Electronic version]. *Washington Post*, 16 May, p. A29. Retrieved on 3 January 2008, from http://www.washingtonpost. com.

Shelton, J.D. (2006) Confessions of a condom lover. *The Lancet* 368, 1947–1949.

Stewart, K.A. (2006) Can a human rights framework improve biomedical and social scientific HIV/AIDS research for African women? *Human Rights Review* (Jan–Mar) 7 (2), 130–136.

Stromquist, N.P. (1990) Women and illiteracy: The interplay of gender subordination and poverty. [Electronic version]. *Comparative Education Review (Special Issue on Adult Literacy)* 34 (1), 95–111. Retrieved on 10 October 2005, from http:// links.jstor.org/sici?sici=0010-4086(199002)34%3A1%3C95%3AWAITIO% 3E2.0.CO%3B2-G.

Vavrus, F. (2005) Adjusting inequality: Education and structural adjustment policies in Tanzania. *Harvard Educational Review* 75 (2), 174–2001.

Wakabi, W. (2006) Condoms still contentious in Uganda's struggle over AIDS. [Electronic version]. *The Lancet* 367 (9520), 1387–1388. Retrieved on 29 January

2008, from http://www.thelancet.com/journals/lancet/article/PIIS014067360
6685978/abstract.

Weedon, C. (1987) *Feminist Practice and Poststructuralist Theory.* London: Blackwell.

Wilson, D. (2004) Partner reduction and the reduction of HIV/AIDS: The most
effective strategies come from within. [Electronic version]. *British Medical
Journal* 328 (7444), 848–849. Retrieved on 19 January 2008, from http://www.
pubmedcentral.nih.gov/articlerender.fcgi?artid=387465.

Chapter 8

Learning about AIDS Online: Identity and Expertise on a Gay Internet Forum

RODNEY H. JONES

Introduction

Gay men learn about AIDS from other gay men. They learn about it through informal conversations in bars and chat rooms, and in bedrooms as they negotiate safer sex practices. They learn about it in the context of gossip, insults, jokes, arguments, acts of seduction and a whole range of other 'speech genres' (Bakhtin, 1986) which we do not normally associate with health education. They also learn about it through the media and through more formal educational channels. But the real learning about AIDS, I will argue in this chapter, takes place when they engage in concrete social practices with other gay men, for it is there that they learn not just what to think about AIDS, but what to do about it: how to talk about it, how to position themselves in relation to it and those it affects and how to negotiate the risk that it initials. Such learning involves not just mastering a body of knowledge but also constructing a social identity for oneself within one's peer group. Lave and Wenger (1991) refer to this kind of learning as 'legitimate peripheral participation', arguing that learning is not just a matter of individual cognition, but also a matter of *participation* in 'communities of practice'. From this perspective, learning about AIDS is not just a health issue. It is part of the larger process of learning to 'be gay' within a particular community.

These interactions, of course, do not occur in a vacuum. The images, warnings, exhortations, slogans, narratives and personalities that form our public discourse about AIDS cycle through these informal encounters, and as they do they are appropriated, altered, expanded upon or challenged

(Bakhtin, 1981; Jones, 2002; Wertsch, 1991). In designing AIDS-related messages, therefore, attention must be paid not just to how these messages are constructed, but also to how they are *reconstructed* as people make use of them in their everyday interactions.

AIDS Online

Increasingly, health educators are conducting educational efforts in online environments such as gay websites, chat rooms and message boards (Benotsch *et al.*, 2006; Bolding *et al.*, 2004; Douglas-Brown, 2001; Seeley, 2002), which are increasingly key sites of socialization, community partici- pation and the negotiation of sexual encounters for gay men (Bolding *et al.*, 2002; Jones, 2005; Ross, 2005; Tikkanen & Ross, 2003). There are plenty of good reasons for health educators to venture into these environ- ments: The internet affords a degree of anonymity that makes it easier for people to discuss sex there (Rhodes, 2004); it allows educators to reach men who do not frequent venues typically targeted such as bars and saunas; and it introduces prevention messages into a context where many of the decisions and logistical arrangements leading up to unsafe sex are initiated. Moreover, studies suggest that men who seek sexual partners in these online environments are more likely to engage in unsafe sex (Bentosch *et al.*, 2002; Bull, 2001; Bull *et al.*, 2001; McFarlane *et al.*, 2000).

The most important reason why AIDS educators should pay attention to the internet, though, is because interactions in chat rooms, discussions on message boards and blogs, personal advertisements and online dating sites, IM and webcam sessions, and the host of other ways in which gay men communicate online are precisely the kinds of informal interactions that I was describing above, that is, interactions in which gay men *learn from one another* about the issues affecting them as well as about how to position themselves in relation to these issues in order to be 'a certain kind of gay man'.

However, just as offline interventions in places such as bars, 'beats' and saunas require strategies to be grounded in the culture and perspectives of the different communities using those spaces, online interventions must be informed by an understanding of the cultures, social relationships and interactional norms that exist in these spaces, and the ways in which talk about AIDS is *already part* of these environments. As Brown *et al.* (2005) argue, 'If health promotion initiatives are to maintain (their) effectiveness within cyberspace, they need to engage with participants in ways that are consistent with how the Internet is used and what it means to participants to be part of the environment'.

In this chapter, I will compare the ways in which knowledge about AIDS is discursively constructed in two gay internet forums in Hong Kong, one devoted to informal chats about such issues as dating, celebrities, fashion and sex, and the other devoted exclusively to the topic of HIV/AIDS prevention and moderated by volunteers from a local AIDS service organization. In the comparison, I will focus particularly on how participants use talk about AIDS to claim and impute identities in particular communities of practice, and how these identities amplify or constrain the ways in which they talk about AIDS and the actions they take in response to it.

AIDS Talk and Social Action

The theoretical framework for my analysis is *mediated discourse analysis* (Norris & Jones, 2005; Scollon, 2001), an approach that attempts to understand how people take action with discourse. It focuses, on the one hand, on the larger 'discourses' (Gee, 1996) that circulate through our everyday interactions and, on the other, on the ways in which individuals appropriate and adapt these discursive resources to take concrete social actions in their everyday lives.

From the perspective of mediated discourse analysis, talk about AIDS is seen as a tool for social action – that is, when people talk about AIDS, whether it be in chat rooms or in bedrooms – they are not just appropriating knowledge, attitudes, slogans and concepts from their social environments, they are *using* them to take very specific actions in the world, actions that create their identities and their relationships with other people (Jones, 2002). These actions may be part of social practices as varied as teaching, bragging, seducing, gossiping and insulting. And since cultural tools are inevitably affected by the history of their use, all of these various actions for which AIDS talk is appropriated affect subsequent actions for which it is appropriated, including actions involved in assessing personal risk and managing sexual behavior.

One of the chief ways in which *mediated discourse analysis* tries to understand the role of discourse in social actions is through attention to the ways people use these actions to claim and impute social identities, to 'position' themselves and others, both on the local level of the particular interaction as part of a history of ongoing interactions, and on the social level in relation to the various communities of practice in which they participate.

The concept of 'positioning' was developed by Harré and his colleagues (Davies & Harré, 1990; van Langenhove & Harré, 1999), who describe it as 'the discursive process whereby selves are located in conversations as observably and subjectively coherent participants in jointly produced storylines. By giving people parts in a story, whether it be explicit or implicit, a speaker makes available a subject position which the other speaker in the normal course of events would take up' (Davies & Harré, 1990: 48).

'Storylines' can be looked at in two ways. On the one hand, they are made up of the sequential chains of actions that form the immediate conversational 'performance' in which interactants act out various roles (Goffman, 1959). On the other hand, they are always somehow reproductions of larger cultural storylines, which Gee (1996) refers to as 'metanarratives', stories about the ways people in a culture should act and the ways certain paradigmatic events (like various kinds of sexual encounters) should unfold. Regarding these cultural storylines, van Langenhove and Harré (1999: 18) write, 'neither storylines nor positions are freely constructed; conversations always reflect narrative forms already existing in the culture, which are part of the repertoire of competent members'.

Where mediated discourse analysis is different from the approach of Harré and his colleagues is that it sees positioning within the framework of a theory of social action. People position themselves and others not so much through discourse as through the social actions that they take using discourse and other cultural tools. More importantly, the kinds of positions that people inhabit in these 'chains of action' are determinative of the kinds of subsequent actions they are able to take (Jones, 2008). The main focus of mediated discourse analysis, then, is not so much on positioning as on the relationship of positioning to social action: what kinds of actions make particular positions available and what kinds of positions make particular actions possible.

This perspective provides a practical way of linking the two kinds of 'storylines' Harré and his colleagues identify, the local storyline and larger 'cultural storylines'. All actions and the positions they make possible are mediated through the cultural tools made available in the broader social environment, tools that actors appropriate and adapt to local circumstances. These tools, which include larger cultural narratives and identities, impose upon local actions and the positions they make possible certain affordances and constraints. At the same time, as social actors appropriate these tools and adapt them to specific purposes, they *transform* them. By focusing on the 'mediated action' as the unit of analysis, mediated discourse analysis highlights the 'tension' (Wertsch, 1991) between cultural storylines and the situated storylines of local interactions, and the *transformations* that take place at this point of tension. Understanding this tension and the mechanics of these transformations is especially important for AIDS educators who often see their advice, slogans and 'master narratives' about AIDS transformed (some might say 'distorted') by individuals as they appropriate them to take everyday actions (Jones, 2002).

Finally, this focus on mediation also allows a closer consideration of the role of such mediational means as computer interfaces on the kinds of actions that people can take and the kinds of positions that they can create with these actions. This is also important for AIDS educators planning interventions in online environments, environments in which the affordances and constraints on communication and participation are very different from those in the one-way communication of printed educational materials and the face-to-face interactions of HIV counseling.

Talking about AIDS Online

The online forums I will be analyzing are part of a popular gay portal in Hong Kong, which also has links to a chat room, a gay guide to Hong Kong and an online personal advertisement page. Other forums available include more specialized ones for middle-aged gay men, for 'bears' (larger, hairier men) and for those interested in S and M (sado-masochism). The forums can be read by any visitor to the website, but only members can post. At the time of writing, 24,765 members were registered with the website. As with most forums and newsgroups, participants construct conversations about particular topics, referred to as 'threads'. While each thread may include a single topic, the conversational structure can be complex, with members being able to specifically respond to particular messages within the thread, potentially creating what Marcocia (2004) refers to as 'polylogues', multiple inter-twining interactions among multiple users with complex and dynamic participation frameworks.

This general interest forum that I will be analyzing is the most popular forum on the site with a history of over 2 million messages. It is used by a broad cross-section of the community and includes a broad cross-section of topics including sex, pornography, gay venues like bars and saunas, fashion and grooming, and gossip about local pop stars. The more specialized forum that I will be comparing it with is operated by a local AIDS service organization and is devoted almost exclusively to the discussion of issues of HIV transmission and prevention.

The most striking difference between the general interest forum and the more specialized AIDS prevention forum is the amount of participation they get from users. At the time of writing, there were 107,296 threads available on the general interest forum. Each of these threads had generated an average of 123 responses and each thread had been viewed an average of 9300 times. Threads typically involved multiple participants and sparked debates and discussions that could span weeks – even years. In contrast, the forum devoted to advice about AIDS contained only 256 threads with an average of only 2.25 responses and 300 views per thread.

These statistics reveal not just a difference in the relative popularity of the two forums but also the kinds of conversations that occur on them. Most of the discussions on the specialized AIDS prevention forum involved only two people and were mostly limited to two or three turns, whereas the discussions on the more general forum were more likely to take the form of the complex 'polylogues' discussed above, with multiple users carrying on multiple conversations within a thread.

HIV and AIDS are discussed in both of the forums. The specialized AIDS prevention forum, of course, is almost exclusively devoted to this topic, but it is also prominent in the general interest forum. A search for the acronym AIDS in this forum identified 260 threads containing it, more, in fact, than the total number of threads in the specialized AIDS forum. The main difference between how users talk about AIDS in this forum and how it is discussed in the specialized AIDS forum is the range of conversational contexts in which it occurs. Figure 8.1 shows the range of topics in the specialized AIDS prevention forum and the percentage of threads devoted to them.

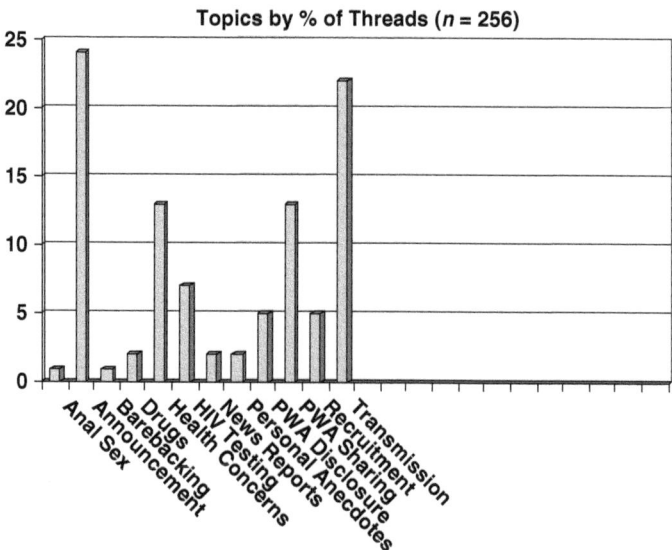

Figure 8.1 Topics in the specialized AIDS forum

Perhaps not surprisingly, most of the discussion on this forum has to do with HIV transmission and other health concerns. Much of the discussion space is also devoted to making announcements about and promoting the activities of the AIDS service organization that operates the forum. Many of the topics involve abstract, decontextualized discussions (e.g. about which sexual acts involve a higher risk of HIV transmission), whereas others involve more interpersonal interaction: people with HIV disclosing their serostatus and sharing their experiences, and participants talking about their health concerns and sharing anecdotes about their AIDS-related experiences. Significantly, although the most frequently occurring threads were those dealing with more abstract discussions on HIV transmission and announcements about AIDS prevention programs and activities, the threads that received the greatest number of 'views' from users were those involving more interpersonal discussion, with the sharing of personal anecdotes being the most frequently viewed topic.

Talk about AIDS in the more general forum is less dominated by didactic, informational discussions and more characterized by interpersonal interaction such as engaging in arguments and disputes, soliciting sexual partners and sharing anecdotes of sexual experiences. Figure 8.2

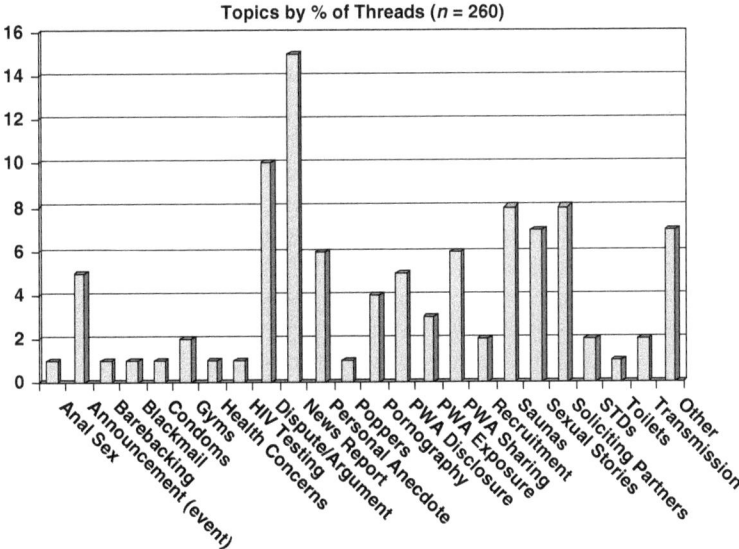

Figure 8.2 Topics in the general interest forum

shows the topics associated with AIDS by the percentage of threads devoted to them.

In this forum, the threads that received the most 'views' were those involving users sharing sexual stories; such threads received an average of more than 800,000 views.

Positioning and Action

These topics do not just represent the content of these conversations, but also implicate different 'activity types' (teaching and learning, soliciting partners, gossiping, and talking about the news) and different 'storylines' within which talk about AIDS is imbedded and is used to take specific social actions and position actors in specific ways.

Discussions in the AIDS prevention forum are generally dialogues between two individuals: a questioner and an AIDS prevention worker. Appendix 1 contains an example of a typical thread with the title 'Do we need a condom for oral sex?' (口交其實係咪應該帶套?). This thread begins, as do an overwhelming majority of those on this forum, with a question. In asking the question, the poster positions himself in contradictory ways. On the one hand, his preface to the question ('I have read in some papers ...') positions him as knowledgeable, while on the other hand, the act of asking the question undermines this position. Similarly, the 'safe identity' constructed through asking the question and being seemingly willing to comply with the answer is undermined by the 'risk taker identity' constructed by the suggestion that one might be able to 'bargain' when it comes to the risk of HIV transmission. The use of the English word 'bargin' (*sic*) code mixed into the Chinese question further positions the poster as well educated. Such multiple and ambiguous positioning is in fact quite common in these forums. As I will argue below, they provide AIDS educators with the opportunity to interpret the question not just as a request for information, but also as an invitation explore with the questioner how to negotiate these contradictory positions between knowledge and ignorance, safety and risk, an opportunity which, in this particular thread and in most of those on this forum, is missed.

Although other participants in the forum may respond to the question, in this particular forum, almost all of the questions are answered by the moderator, an AIDS prevention volunteer, and, as in this example, the answers tend to be lengthy and 'comprehensive' renderings of facts, often with little or no interpersonal content. These answers rarely contain follow-up questions for the initial poster or invitations to other participants to share their opinions or experiences. Rather, they constitute what

Bakhtin (1981) calls 'authoritative discourse', discourse that demands unqualified acknowledgment and does not open up the possibilities of questioning or alternation. By constructing such discourse, the volunteer vigorously takes up the position of 'expert' (a position already imputed on him by the initial poster's action of asking the question).

As with the questioner, the position of expertise taken up by the volunteer is complex and paradoxical, as it is simultaneously claimed and abrogated when the volunteer urges the questioner to 'decide for yourself'. The questioner's ability to do this, however, is dependent on the various ways in which he is positioned by the answerer in the interaction.

On the one hand, the questioner is positioned as someone who is (rightfully) worried about sexual contact (we worry whenever we 'do' it), and as someone who participates in activities such as 'sucking' and 'being sucked' Bull *et al.* (2001). Most importantly, he is positioned as someone who lacks the requisite knowledge to negotiate between these positions, to 'evaluate' his risk behavior.

But the primary position imputed to the questioner is that of an autonomous rational decision maker, and underlying this position is an influential cultural storyline about risk itself: one in which risk behavior is seen as a matter of rational decision making by individuals based on 'facts'. Preventing HIV infection, in this storyline, is a process of first 'accepting facts' ('If you can accept such a fact') and then applying them to a rational evaluation of the situation ('the next step is to evaluate the sexual risk by yourself').

Along with this position of 'rational decision maker', however, a separate and contradictory position is also made available, the position of one who cannot 'accept scientific facts', who, in fact, 'challenges' the expert position of the volunteers, and who 'cannot be persuaded'. This position of the 'willfully irrational self', of course, is made available less as a realistic alternative and more as a foil for the position of the 'rational self' which dominates the discourse.

And so, although the answerer urges the poster to take responsibility for his own decision making, the range of positions from which this decision making can take place is rather limited. The recipient of the discourse can either 'accept the facts' and take up the position of 'individual rational decision maker' or 'ignore the facts' and place himself in danger. Excluded are a host of other positions from which such decisions are often made in real life – positions, for example, in which risk is not a matter of individual decision making but rather negotiated between sexual partners, or positions based on various social identities or interpersonal relationships of intimacy or power. Furthermore, the closed, authoritative discourse structure of the exchange, while placing the burden of decision making on the questioner, does not open up opportunities for him to talk out the decision-making process and explore the various options.

The conversation concludes with a final exchange in which the questioner suddenly switches to English, thanking the prevention worker and judging his response to be 'very professional'. This sudden switch to English, in the context of Hong Kong, helps to further ratify the 'authoritative' status of the reply. English in Hong Kong is usually limited to the formal workplace, governmental or educational contexts, and so in many instances signals 'knowledge' and 'expertise' and marks the exchange as 'professional' rather than 'personal' (Chan, 2002; Lin, 2008; Luke & Richards, 1982). In fact, both the discourse and the participation structure of this forum very much resemble those of more traditional educational activities such as lectures.

This is not to deny the value of information transmission or to suggest that 'facts' are not an important resource in decision making. There is an undisputable role for authoritative discourse in health promotion. In the context of an internet forum, however, such discourse misses the opportunity to exploit the interactive nature of the medium. The problem with authoritative discourse is not that it is not valuable. The problem is that it is a 'conversation stopper'.

In contrast, the thread from the general interest forum I have chosen to analyze, which is typical of threads from this forum, exhibits a much more complex, polylogic participation structure in which multiple participants weave multiple conversations around the issue of risk and claim and impute multiple positions from which it can be evaluated . This thread, entitled 'Not using condoms ... >< ', is reproduced in Appendix 2, represented schematically in a chart in which the numbers next to the posters' names indicate the order in which the post appeared in the thread and the arrows indicate the particular post (or chain of posts) each post was in response to.

The thread begins with a poster named 'tamama10' recounting a sexual experience between him and his boyfriend in which they did not use condoms (Excerpt 8.1).

One of the most striking differences between this thread and the one analyzed above is the way in which posters use language, with posters to this forum using a more informal register characterized by frequent unorthodox punctuation, emoticons and code mixing. In contrast to the *code switching* observed in the thread analyzed above, which signaled formality, here the mixing of English words like 'safe sex', 'check' and 'feel' signals the opposite: informality and involvement (Lin, 2008).

> **tamama10**
>
> 2007-03-27, 5:11 pm
>
> 一直都有safe sex, 點知尋晚同BF.....................><
>
> 如果要去check咪要等3個月 =.="""""
>
> 雖然真係好正feel~
>
> (I always have safe sex, but last night with my boyfriend ......><
>
> If I want to check, then I need to wait for 3 months
>
> But the feeling was great~)

Excerpt 8.1 The opening

In this initial post, the poster recounts the basic storyline that will form the background of all the conversations in this thread, a story of a single action occurring in relation to previous actions ('I always have safe sex') and making necessary certain future actions ('If I want to check, then I need to wait for 3 months'), along with an evaluation of this chain of events ('the feeling was great~'). In the subsequent discussion, this basic storyline is interpreted in various contradictory ways – as a story of irresponsibility, as a story of pleasure and as a story of love and trust – as other members of the forum respond to the initial post and to one another.

These contradictory interpretations in many ways arise from the contradictory positions the original poster himself takes up toward the events and the contradictory storylines he constructs with them. Indeed, he is like a character in two separate stories. First, there is the story of *prevention* in which the poster is portrayed as a responsible individual who habitually acted responsibly before the incident and is acting responsibly in response to it (making plans for HIV testing), and who is able to display sufficient knowledge about HIV ('I have to wait 3 months') in order to deal rationally with the potential danger. In this story, the act of unsafe sex is downplayed – in fact, explicit reference to the act is totally absent, reduced to an extended chain of ellipsis ending with an emoticon (><) (squinting eyes). The 'official absence' of an explicit mention of the main event of the story and the emoticon, which portrays an attitude of consternation toward the unmentioned event, act to distance the poster from it. The naming of the boyfriend further mitigates the poster's guilt by putting the implied action in a context that is (rightly or wrongly) viewed

as 'safer' by members of this community (Jones *et al.*, 2000). In this interpretation of events, unsafe sex is constructed as a temporary excusable
lapse, which will likely not be repeated.

But along with this story of risk there is also the story of *pleasure*,
expressed chiefly in the poster's evaluation ('it felt great~~~'), an evaluation that, in many ways, alters all that has come before it. In this interpretation, the poster is positioned as an emotional individual driven by the
desire for pleasure, especially in the form of intimacy and love. Unsafe sex
in this story is seen as an act of pleasure arising from natural and irresist-
ible drives, one that will likely re-occur as long as these drives persist.
Within this storyline, the various elements in the post take on different
meanings. The 'boyfriend', for example, becomes less a symbol of responsibility and more a symbol of love (with the act of unsafe sex seen as a
consummation of this love).

These contradictory narratives are also reflected in the contradictory
positions that the poster takes up in relation to his readers and the contradictory positions he constructs for them. The act of telling this story is at
once a confession, positioning others as judges, a boast, positioning others
as conspirators in the quest for pleasure, a request for advice, positioning
others as counselors, and an elicitation of sympathy, positioning others as
friends. In the subsequent interaction, other posters develop and elaborate
upon the competing storylines introduced in the first post, and in so doing
take up or challenge the various positions that the poster has made available to them.

The first strand of conversation arising from this thread (Excerpt 8.2)
replays these two themes. The first response comes from 'xxholic', who
repeats the section of the story about the three-month waiting period,
adding to it the more technical term 'window period' (空窗期). In doing
so he both ratifies the original poster's expertise and asserts his own.
Then 'yinge' again repeats the previous sentence about the waiting
period and further adds to it by appropriating another element of the
original story ('it seems that you enjoyed it'). It is in this line that the
narrative of this strand of conversation shifts from the prevention story
to the pleasure story, for the next poster, '404', picks up not on the three-
month waiting period but on the enjoyment associated with the act,
portraying that enjoyment as addictive ('it seems that you can't stop it').
The storyline turns from one of safety and expertise to one of risk and
sexual compulsion.

Meanwhile, another short conversation begins with 'handsome' asking,
'Will you be able to turn back after trying it once?' (會唔會試過一次之後返
唔到轉頭), and a poster named 'snoopy love' adding, 'Please love your

2007-3-27, 5:13 pm
xxholic
要等3個月空窗期
(have to wait 3 months for the window period)

2007-3-27, 5:15 pm
yinge
要等3個月空窗期
不過睇黎你好 Enjoy 咁
(You have to wait for the 3-month window period, but it seems that you enjoyed it very much)

2007-3-27, 5:32pm
404
睇黎會欲罷不能
最終三個月之後又三個月..
(It seems that you can't stop it.
In the end, this 3 months will be followed by another 3 months)

Excerpt 8.2 A turning point

lover and yourself, safe sex please~' (請愛你的愛人同愛自己, safe sex please~). Whereas in the first strand, a narrative of prevention was transformed into a narrative of risk, in this strand, the pleasure narrative is transformed into a prevention narrative, chiefly by 'snoopy love' appropriating the 'love' aspect of the pleasure discourse and turning it to the service of the prevention storyline – 'real love' should result in safe sex, not risk taking.

What is particularly interesting in these strands of conversation is how contributors cooperatively construct these storylines by adding onto (and often repeating verbatim) what previous posters wrote (Figure 8.3).

Tannen (1989) notes that this kind of repetition is actually quite common in casual conversation, helping to create 'involvement' and conversational coherence. It also contributes to the building up of conversational topics

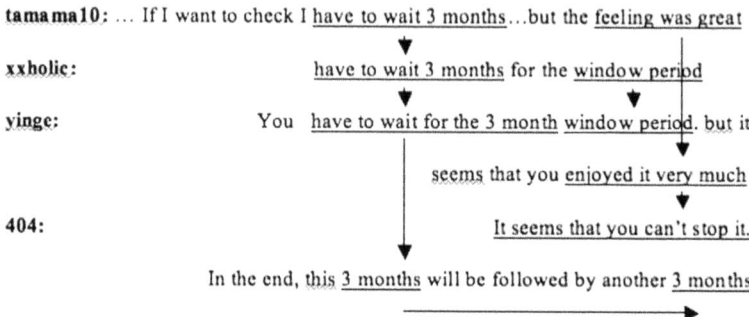

Figure 8.3 Repetition in the thread

and the establishment of common ground'. As participants take up the lines of previous posters, they cooperate in constructing the local storyline of the conversation. These words, however, are not just repetitions of previous posters; they are also often repetitions of words and concepts from larger cultural narratives of AIDS and sex. It is in this incremental co-construction of local talk about AIDS over time, then, that people build up group knowledge schema about AIDS and cultural storylines of safe and unsafe sex, drawing from and adapting the resources available in public discourse.

After these initial exchanges, two longer conversations develop, which reflect and elaborate on the themes the poster established in his first post – the theme of pleasure and the theme of prevention. In each of these conversations, the meaning of the original story is appropriated and negotiated differently by other posters, positioning the original poster as a certain kind of character in this story and resulting in the original poster positioning himself differently in response.

The pleasure conversation begins, with a poster named 'donald duck' taking up the theme of compulsion begun in the first two strands and admitting, 'The feeling is quite good not using condoms I can't turn back after trying it once' (咁唔用 個feel 又真係幾好咁.試過一次就冇得返轉頭家la). Once again, the poster appropriates the words of previous posters, in this case the original poster's admission that 'it felt great' and the accusations of '404' and 'handsome' that he will not be able to stop. Whereas the first few messages distanced the users from the original poster, this poster aligns himself with him, partially by hypothetically taking on the identity of a compulsive pleasure seeker himself. This positioning is immediately responded to by a poster named 'sea son' who uses it to impute on 'donald duck' the negative identity of a 'risk taker': 'It seems that you are quite familiar with it, wow' (睇黎你好有心得wow), to which 'donald duck' replies facetiously with 'It's a good way to save money', on the one hand accepting the 'damaged identity' that is imputed, and on the other hand distancing himself from the original rationale of pleasure and making it more of a rational economic decision. What is most interesting about this short side exchange is the introduction of the theme of 'expertise' as a matter of personal experience (and as an emblem of a 'damaged identity'), a theme that will be taken up again later in the thread.

Finally, the original poster himself replies to 'donald duck' (Excerpt 8.3), elaborating on the relationship between pleasure and romantic intimacy, and, after some time, 'enzo' chimes in, re-entextualizing the original poster's characterization of his partner's semen as 'warm stuff' into 'hot sperm!!!', taking it out of its romantic context and giving it a purely erotic connotation, to which 'bibikun' replies with the exhortation 'be careful~~~', ending this strand of conversation.

2007-3-27, 7:20 pm
tamama10
我覺得係,,,,覺得真係好分別, 仲幾大tim!
覺得同bf親密好多, 同埋feel到佢d好暖既野.....
(I think that … I think it's quite different, really different!
I feel closer to my boyfriend, and I feel his warm stuff …)
2007-3-27, 11:18 pm
enzo
熱精!!!!!!!!!!
(Hot sperm !!!!)
2007-3-28, 12:02 am
bibikun
小心小心ar~~~
(Be careful~~~~)

Excerpt 8.3 The pleasure conversation

Although I have characterized this strand as the 'pleasure conversation', it is clearly made up of a number of 'competing discourses' (Lee, 1992), as posters negotiate together the social meanings of pleasure and its consequences. Pleasure is constructed at different points in the conversation as a matter of compulsion, a creator of intimacy, an emblem of a 'damaged identity', a raw physical drive and a danger, as the discourse of pleasure and the discourse of prevention intertwine, with the conversation ending with what is essentially a prevention message ('be careful'). In this way, as Gee (1996) points out, localized ('small c') conversations become the sites of 'large C conversations' between or among contradictory metanarratives. As posters position themselves as interactants in the 'small c conversation', they also position themselves in relation to the larger discourses and cultural models they invoke in their talk, and so carve out for themselves particular social identities within their particular communities of practice. By invoking a storyline that equates risk with love (rather than with irresponsibility), for example, the poster justifies his action by constructing for himself a recognizable and respectable identity within this community: the identity of a 'passionate lover'.

A similar phenomenon of competing storylines can be seen in what I have dubbed the 'prevention conversation', which begins with a poster named 'fengshen' asking, 'Why didn't you use a condom?'(做乜唔用呢), constructing in his question the underlying presupposition of the prevention storyline, the notion that condom use should be the normal course of events and not using them requires explanation. The original poster replies, 'because ... used up ... and he wanted it. In fact I don't know why they were used up ... When I woke up I thought ... shit <lit.die>'

(因為......冇晒, 咁佢又要 。其實我都唔知點解最終會冇, 醒返先諗....死喇).

This assessment stands in sharp contrast to his reply to 'donald duck' above. Rather than being a passionate lover, the poster is a victim of circumstances and of his boyfriend's insistence, and the act itself, rather than a matter of celebration within a committed relationship, is portrayed as a matter of regret and anxiety. This results in a response from 'fengshen' who begins a three-way debate about the relationship between safe sex, trust and pleasure (Excerpt 8.4) involving the original poster, 'fengshen' and a third user named 'pasukar'.

In this excerpt, 'fengshen' takes up the 'boyfriend' element of the storyline, constructing a monogamous relationship as an effective prevention strategy. 'Pasukar' reiterates this strategy, but frames it as a matter of 'trust', and uses this framing to challenge the original poster ('do you

---

fengshen

2007-3-27, 7:39 pm

不過既然佢係你男友

大家又冇出去偷食

理論上係冇問題架

(However, he is your boyfriend.

If you and he haven't played around with others It should be no problem theoretically)

---

pasukar

2007-3-27, 7:57 pm

其實

如果大家信任對方

唔用都冇問題既

只不過係，你信佢嗎？

(In fact, if you and he trust each other, then not using condoms is okay. However, do you really trust him?)

---

tamama10

2007-3-27, 8:56 pm

唔信都唔會比佢直入喇......hehe

(If I didn't trust him, I wouldn't let him enter me ... hehe)

Excerpt 8.4 The prevention conversation

really trust him?'), to which the original poster replies saying that if he did not trust his boyfriend, he would not have engaged in unsafe sex. Two important transformations have occurred here. The first is the transformation of prevention from a matter of individual judgment to a matter of trust between two people. The second and even more dramatic transformation is the transformation of 'trust' from a *condition* of safe sex (if you and he trust each other …) to a *reason* for unsafe sex. This particular transformation is especially important in understanding HIV risk behavior. Numerous studies have shown that forgoing condom use often functions in romantic relationships as an emblem of 'trust' or 'love' and, conversely, suggesting condom use is sometimes interpreted as an expression of distrust or lack of love (see e.g. Adam *et al.*, 2000). Such associations make prevention efforts even more complex as decisions about personal safety are subsumed within the dynamics of romance. Embedded in this conversation, in fact, is a brief side sequence that parodies this transformation. First, '404' writes: 'Don't employ people you don't trust' (疑人不用), which is the second half of a Chinese proverb:

用人不疑, 疑人不用

Don't suspect those you employ; don't employ those you don't trust.

Then 'pasukar' replies by relexicalizing the first half of the proverb as 'don't suspect those who enter you' (入人不疑), framing trust not as a precondition for unprotected sex but as a result of it: it is in the act of unsafe sex that 'trust' is conferred and communicated.

In the remainder of the conversation (Excerpt 8.5), the original poster and 'pasukar' continue this debate about the relationship between romance and personal responsibility.

Here 'tamama10' again positions himself as a victim of his boyfriend's desires, a move that is challenged by 'pasukar', who re-positions him as an active seeker of illicit pleasure, a positioning that 'tamama10' tacitly accepts with the reply, 'um…'. 'Pasukar' then points out the contradiction in his two positions (being 'for safe sex' and 'trusting his boyfriend'). What is perhaps most interesting about this excerpt is the strategy 'tamama10' uses to counter this move by questioning 'pasukar's' expertise ('have you tried it before?'). Here, the notion of expertise has undergone a profound transformation from being a matter of knowledge and responsible behavior in the beginning of the thread ('I have to wait three months') to being a matter of lived experience. Expertise about unsafe sex comes from having it, and the 'risk taker' identity that was initially portrayed as negative becomes legitimized, a kind of credential within the community. The move opens for 'pasukar' only two possible positions – the position of 'safety' from which he must admit ignorance, and the position of 'risk' from which he can claim status as a legitimate participant in the debate. He answers with the same tacit acceptance of the 'risk taker' position that 'tamama10' issued just a few lines before ('um …'), to which 'tamama10' replies, 'good for you!', thereby completing the imputation of 'risk taker' identity. So, a conversation that begins with unsafe sex being portrayed as

2007-3-27, 8:57 pm
tamama10
我怕佢下次又係咁乍=.= 佢話好正lor
(I'm afraid he'll want it next time. He said the feeling was great.)

2007-3-27, 8:58 pm
karllau
咁咪得LAW~~ 😄
(It's okay~~)

2007-3-27, 8:58 pm
pasukar
咁你覺得正唔正先?
(Then do you think it's good feeling?)

2007-3-27, 9:07 pm
tamama10
嗯..........
(umm. ....)

2007-3-27, 9:10 pm
pasukar
話就話要safe sex
但如果相信佢既
都可以既
(So to say we need safe sex
But if I trust him
It's okay)

(Continued)

2007-3-27, 9:14 pm   **tamama10**   你有冇試過 ☺   (Have you tried it before?)
2007-3-27, 9:16 pm   **pasukar**   嗯~   (umm~)
2007-3-27, 9:52 pm   **tamama10**   你又好喇   (Good for you!)

Excerpt 8.5 Debate

dangerous and irresponsible ends with it becoming an emblem of expertise and status within the community.

Engineering the Heterogeneous

There is much in this second thread that would undoubtedly make health promoters uncomfortable, not least being the fact that participants seem to be encouraging one another in risky behavior more than supporting and promoting safer sex. What is important for educators to understand is the *process* through which this occurs. Storylines of HIV risk and safety in everyday conversations are not just a matter of scientific knowledge and individualistic decision making; they are a matter of social identity, formulated cooperatively through a complex process of positioning and re-positioning of social actors in real-time interactions.

Within this process, AIDS prevention discourse is reframed and transformed through interaction with other discourses, in particular the discourse of pleasure, a discourse which, while conspicuously absent from most health promotion texts, including the example from the AIDS prevention forum included here, is central to how people make decisions about sexual risk. The important thing about pleasure seeking, which is missed by individualistic perspectives on health communication, is that it is not merely a matter of the individual but also an important part of social identity, particularly in many communities of gay men. The identity of the 'risk taker' in such contexts is often ambiguous, contingent and not necessarily negative or stigmatized – suggesting that someone engaging in unsafe sex is simultaneously an accusation and a compliment, a marker of 'ignorance' and a marker of 'expertise'.

What we see in conversations on the general interest forum is a process of learning dependent less on the 'authoritative discourse' of traditional health promotion and more on the negotiation of the meanings of risk and pleasure that involves the interaction and tension among multiple competing discourses. Part of the complexity and dynamism of this negotiation is a result of the unique set of affordances and constraints offered by the medium itself. The interactivity of the internet, the tools it provides for managing identity, the egalitarian relationships it seems to foster (Sproull & Kiesler, 1986; Walther, 1992) and the potential it has for facilitating polylogic interaction all help to create opportunities for posters to take up multiple (sometimes contradictory) positions within complex participation frameworks, and thus to shift the 'economies of knowledge' around AIDS talk from traditional hierarchical forms of discourse to forms that involve more lateral processes of knowledge exchange (Richardson, 2001: 58) . In fact, what is most striking about the interaction on the more formal AIDS education forum is that posters *do not* avail themselves of these opportunities, reconstructing more traditional participation frameworks in this new medium.

In order to participate meaningfully in such contexts, health educators need to focus not so much on 'delivering messages', but on what Gherardi and Nicolini (2000), in their work on organizational safety, refer to as 'engineering the heterogeneous': working within this complex negotiation of multiple storylines and acknowledging how, in this negotiation, the meaning and functions of discourse can undergo profound and sometimes unpredictable transformations.

The first step in being able to effectively 'engineer the heterogeneous' is understanding how it works, understanding how knowledge about AIDS is received, rejected, redefined, resisted and accepted within communities through complex social processes of negotiation, transformation, reinterpretation, distortion and rediscovery.

References

Adam, B.D., Sears, A. and Schellenberg, E.G. (2000) Accounting for unsafe sex: Interviews with men who have sex with men. *Journal of Sex Research* 37 (1), 24–36.

Bakhtin, M.M. (1981) *The Dialogic Imagination: Four Essays by M.M. Bakhtin* (M. Holquist, ed.; C. Emerson and M. Holquist, trans.) Austin: University of Texas Press.

Bakhtin, M.M. (1986) *Speech Genres and Other Late Essays* (C. Emerson and M. Holquist, eds; V.W. McGee, trans.) Minneapolis: University of Minnesota Press.

Benotsch, E., Kalichman, S. and Cage, M. (2002) Men who have met sex partners via the internet: Prevalence, predictors and implications for HIV prevention. *Archives of Sexual Behavior* 31, 177–183.

Benotsch, E., Wright, V.J., deRoon Cassini, T.A., Pinkerton, S.D., Weinhardt, L. and Kelly, J.A. (2006) Use of the internet for HIV prevention by AIDS service organizations in the United States. *Journal of Technology in Human Services* 24 (1), 19–35.

Bolding, G., Elford, J. and Sherr, L. (2002) *Gay Men's Survey in London Gyms 2002*. London: City University London. On WWW at http://www.city.ac.uk/barts/gymsurvey.

Bolding, G., Davis, M., Sherr, L., Hart, G. and Elford, J. (2004) Use of gay internet sites and views about online health promotion among men who have sex with men. *AIDS Care* 16 (8), 993–1001.

Brown, G., Maycock, B. and Burnes, S. (2005) Your picture is your bait: Use and meaning of cyberspace among gay men. *The Journal of Sex Research* 42 (1), 63–73.

Bull, S.S. (2001) HIV and sexually transmitted infection risk behaviors among men seeking sex with men on-line. *American Journal of Public Health* 91 (6), 988–989.

Bull, S.S., McFarlane, M. and King, D. (2001) Barriers to STD/HIV prevention on the Internet. *Health Education Research* 16 (6), 661–670.

Chan, E. (2002) Beyond pedagogy: Language and identity in post-colonial Hong Kong. *British Journal of Sociology of Education* 23 (2), 271–285.

Davies, B. and Harré, R. (1990) Positioning: The discursive production of selves. *Journal for the Theory of Social Behavior* 20 (1), 43–63.

Douglas-Brown, L. (2001) Prevention efforts are going online. *The Washington Blade.*, October 12.

Gee, J.P. (1996) *Social Linguistics and Literacies* (2nd edn). London: Taylor & Francis.

Gherardi, S. and Nicolini, D. (2000) The organizational learning of safety in communities of practice. *Journal of Management Inquiry* 9 (1), 7–18.

Goffman, E. (1959) *The Presentation of Self in Everyday Life*. New York: Doubleday.

Jones, R. (2002) Mediated action and sexual risk: Discourses of sexuality and AIDS in the People's Republic of China. Unpublished PhD dissertation, MacQuarie University, Sydney.

Jones, R. (2005) The internet and gay men. In J.T. Sears (ed.) *Youth, Education and Sexualities* (pp. 433–437). Westport, CT: Greenwood/Oryx Press.

Jones, R. (2008) Good sex and bad karma: Discourse and the historical body. In V.K. Bhatia, J. Flowerdew and R. Jones (eds) *Advances in Discourse Studies*. London: Routledge.

Jones, R., Yu, K.K. and Candlin, C. (2000) *A Preliminary Study of Risk Behavior and HIV Vulnerability of MSM in Hong Kong* (A Report to the Council for the AIDS Trust Fund). Hong Kong: Council for the AIDS Trust Fund, HK Department of

Health. On WWW at http://personal.cityu.edu.hk/~enrodney/Research/ MSM/MSMindex.html.

van Langenhove, L. and Harré, R. (1999) Introduction to positioning theory. In R. Harré and L. van Langenhove (eds) *Positioning Theory: Moral Contexts of Intentional Action* (pp. 14–31). London: Blackwell.

Lave, J. and Wenger, E. (1991) *Situated Learning: Legitimate Peripheral Participation.* Cambridge: Cambridge University Press.

Lee, D. (1992) *Competing Discourses: Perspective and Ideology in Language.* London: Longman.

Lin, A.M.Y. (2008) The ecology of literacy in Hong Kong. In N.H. Hornberger (ed.) *Encyclopedia of Language and Education* (pp. 3170–3182). New York: Springer.

Luke, K.K. and Richards, J.C. (1982) English in Hong Kong: Functions and status. *English World-wide* 3 (1), 47–64.

Marcocia, M. (2004) Online polylogues: Conversation structure and participation framework in internet newsgroups. *Journal of Pragmatics* 36, 115–145.

McFarlane, M., Bull, S.S. and Rietmeijer, C.A. (2000). The internet as a newly emerging risk environment for sexually transmitted diseases. *JAMA* 284, 443–446.

Norris, S. and Jones, R. (eds) (2005) *Discourse in Action: Introducing Mediated Discourse Analysis.* London: Routledge.

Rhodes, S.D. (2004) Hookups or health promotion? An exploratory study of chat room-based HIV prevention intervention for men who have sex with men. *AIDS Education and Prevention* 16 (3), 315–327.

Richardson, K. (2001) Risk news in the world of internet news groups. *Journal of Sociolinguistics* 5 (1), 50–72.

Ross, M.W. (2005) Typing, doing and being: Sexuality and the internet. *Journal of Sex Research* 42 (4), 342–352.

Scollon, R. (2001) *Mediated Discourse: The Nexus of Practice.* London: Routledge.

Seeley, S. (2002) CAMP Safe: Launches Internet based prevention program. *Letters from CAMP Rehoboth,* 12 (1). On WWW at http://issue02_01_02/campsefe.htm. Accessed 30.7.03.

Sproull, F. and Kiesler, S. (1986) Reducing social context cues: Electronic mail in organizational communication. *Management Science* 32, 1492–1512.

Tannen, D. (1989) *Talking Voices: Repetition, Dialogue and Imagery in Conversational Discourse.* Cambridge: Cambridge University Press.

Tikkanen, R. and Ross, M.W. (2000) Looking for sexual compatibility: Experiences among Swedish men in visiting gay chatrooms. *Cyber-psychology and Behavior* 3 (4), 605–616.

Walther, J. (1992) Interpersonal effects in computer-mediated interactions: A relational perspective. *Communication Research* 19 (1), 52–90.

Wertsch, J.V. (1991) *Voices of the Mind: A Sociocultural Approach to Mediated Action.* Cambridge, MA: Harvard University Press.

Appendix 1

我睇過一d paper, 話其實口交雖然風險底, 但係都有機會傳染愛滋, 或其他性病如梅毒等. 咁到底口交時 (比人含、含人)帶唔帶套, 到底係可以 bargain, 定係無得傾, 一定要帶?	I have read in some papers that although oral sex is low risk, there is still a chance of getting Aids or other STDs like syphilis, etc. So do we need to wear condoms for oral sex (suck by others, suck others). Can we bargain on that or it is a must to use?
gymtogether 你好啊 近排 member 圈內·愛滋感染數字持續上升, 真係會令人「做」親都提心弔膽。 不過, 事實上, 除·自瀆之外, 冇 種性行為係完全冇風險既。 如果你係性活躍既話, 就要承受某 程度既風險, 呢樣係難以避免。 若能·接受呢個事實, 下一·就係幫自己衡量自己既性風險 同埋懂得點樣去預防感染愛滋病病毒／性病。 講到口交, 透過口交而感染愛滋病病毒既機會確實係有既, 不過冇戴套口交既風險 (正如你 d paper 所講) 比冇戴套肛交既風險就低好多。之所以好少人透過口交而感染愛滋病病毒既原因, 係因為口水本身有抑壓愛滋病病毒既作用 (但係唔係百分百)。 只要能夠保持口腔健康, 口交既時候口裏面冇明顯既傷口, 咁感染 HIV 既機會就會比較細。 含人會遠遠比俾人含既風險高好多。俾人含只會接觸到對方既口水, 而口水係唔會傳播到愛滋病病既。除非對方口裏面係流緊血, 而血係含有大量既病毒, 咁俾人含既一位就肯定有風驗。但係如果對方口係流緊血既話, 都唔會「血淋淋」咁俾佢含啦, 所以透過俾人含而感染 HIV 既機會確實好微。	Hello gymtogether Recently the number of Aids infections keeps growing among members to the point that we worry whenever we "do" it. However, in fact, other than masturbation, there is no sexual behavior that is free of risk. If you are active in sex, you need to bear a certain degree of risk and this is unavoidable. If you can accept such fact, then the next step is to evaluate the sexual risk by yourself and know how to prevent the infection of Aids or STD. Talking about oral sex, while there is a chance of Aids infection through oral sex, the risk is much lower for oral sex without condom than anal sex without condom (as your papers have said). The reason why not many people get Aids through oral sex is because saliva can inhibit the Aids virus. If you can keep the oral cavity healthy and there is no obvious wound inside the mouth, then the chance for HIV infection is comparatively small. The risk for sucking others is much higher than being sucked. Being sucked only results in contact with saliva and saliva does not transmit the Aids virus unless the oral cavity is bleeding, and the blood contains a large amount of virus. Then certainly there is a risk for the one being sucked. If the oral cavity of the other is bleeding, you would not let him suck you with his bleeding mouth. So getting HIV through being sucked is rare.

含人既風險就有 d 唔同啦, 因為咁樣會接觸到對方既射前分泌物(透明 o 個 d) 同埋精液, 而精液係會含有大量 HIV 既。不過, 正如以上所講, 如果能夠保持自己口腔健康, 就算唔好採對方係你口裏面射精, 只要你能夠即時吐左佢, 唔好俾愛滋病病毒留係你身體裏面, 咁絕對可以減低感染呢個病毒既機會	The risk for sucking others is different because one will have contact with the secretions and semen of the partner. Semen can contain a large amount of HIV. However, as mentioned above, if you can keep the mouth in a healthy condition, even if the partner ejaculates in your mouth, you just need to spit it out to reduce the chances for infection.
不過話時話, 雖然透過口交而感染愛滋病病毒唔係咁容易既事, 感染其他性病就容易好多啦。例如淋病/非淋病性尿道炎、梅毒、性病疣 (椰菜花) 都可以透過口交傳染。所以, 回答你第一個問題 : 「口交時 (比人含、含人)帶唔帶套, 到底係可以 bargain, 定係無得傾, 一定要帶?」, 理性 d 講,好明顯係戴好過唔戴。但係一咁樣講就好多人都會開 : 「咁咪乜都唔做得？重有乜野樂趣？」講到呢度, 情願冇乜樂趣, 還是有機會感染性病, 就要自己決定啦, 幾多科學證據都未必說服到一個人！	However, although it is not easy to get the Aids virus through oral sex, it is easy to get other STDs. For example, gonorrhea/non-gonorrhea inflammation of the urine duct, syphilis, and warts can be transmitted through oral sex. So, to answer your question "Whether to wear condom for oral sex (suck by others, suck others). Can we bargain on that or it is a must to use?" Theoretically speaking, obviously it is better to use rather than not to use. But when we say that, many people might challenge us and say 'Then you cannot do anything fun?' Regardless of the fun, or chances for STDs, **you have to decide yourself**. No matter how many scientific facts you give, you cannot really persuade a person!
thanks, i think your answer is really professional and good!!	
Dear gymtogether You are most welcome. Hope the information helps! Take care.	

Appendix 2

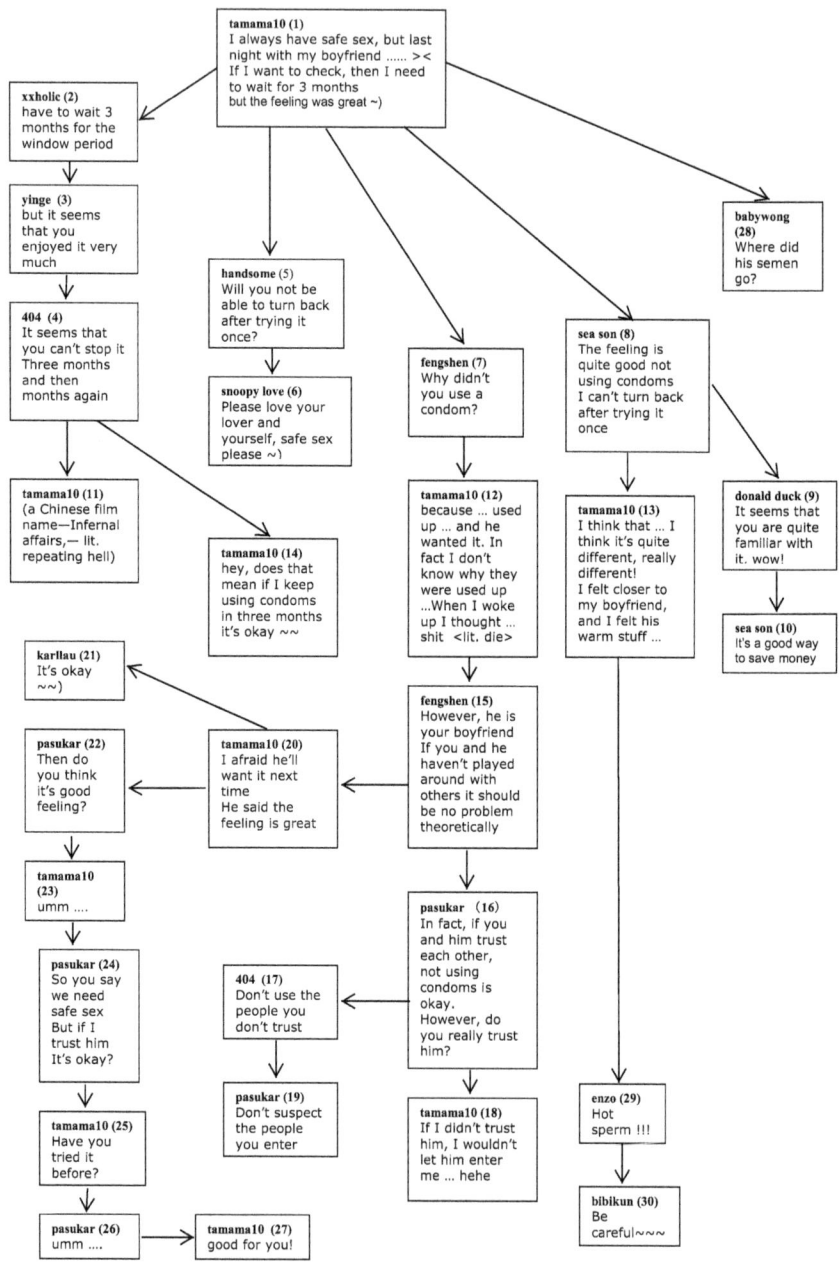

tamama10 (1)
I always have safe sex, but last night with my boyfriend ...... >< If I want to check, then I need to wait for 3 months but the feeling was great ~)

xxholic (2)
have to wait 3 months for the window period

yinge (3)
but it seems that you enjoyed it very much

babywong (28)
Where did his semen go?

404 (4)
It seems that you can't stop it Three months and then months again

handsome (5)
Will you not be able to turn back after trying it once?

fengshen (7)
Why didn't you use a condom?

sea son (8)
The feeling is quite good not using condoms I can't turn back after trying it once

snoopy love (6)
Please love your lover and yourself, safe sex please ~)

tamama10 (11)
(a Chinese film name—Infernal affairs,— lit. repeating hell)

tamama10 (12)
because ... used up ... and he wanted it. In fact I don't know why they were used up ...When I woke up I thought ... shit <lit. die>

tamama10 (13)
I think that ... I think it's quite different, really different! I felt closer to my boyfriend, and I felt his warm stuff ...

donald duck (9)
It seems that you are quite familiar with it. wow!

tamama10 (14)
hey, does that mean if I keep using condoms in three months it's okay ~~

sea son (10)
It's a good way to save money

karllau (21)
It's okay ~~)

fengshen (15)
However, he is your boyfriend If you and he haven't played around with others it should be no problem theoretically

pasukar (22)
Then do you think it's good feeling?

tamama10 (20)
I afraid he'll want it next time He said the feeling is great

tamama10 (23)
umm ....

pasukar (16)
In fact, if you and him trust each other, not using condoms is okay.
However, do you really trust him?

pasukar (24)
So you say we need safe sex But if I trust him It's okay?

404 (17)
Don't use the people you don't trust

enzo (29)
Hot sperm !!!

tamama10 (25)
Have you tried it before?

pasukar (19)
Don't suspect the people you enter

tamama10 (18)
If I didn't trust him, I wouldn't let him enter me ... hehe

bibikun (30)
Be careful~~~

pasukar (26)
umm ....

tamama10 (27)
good for you!

Chapter 9
Contextualizing Local Knowledge: Reformulations in HIV/AIDS Prevention in Burkina Faso

MARTINA DRESCHER

Introduction

In comparison to South Africa, HIV/AIDS prevalence rates in West-African Burkina Faso are quite low. According to UNAIDS (2007), approximately 2% of the estimated 13 million Burkinians are living with AIDS. Knowledge about the pandemic is less disseminated than in the high prevalence regions of Austral Africa. Thus, informing people about the disease and the ways to avoid an infection are still the most urgent goals of HIV/AIDS awareness campaigns in the Sahel region. This chapter investigates the place of local and global knowledge in HIV/AIDS education from a linguistic point of view (Drescher, 2004, 2006, 2007). The data consist of video-taped training sessions for young adults intending to work as *peer educators* in HIV/AIDS campaigns in Burkina Faso. Drawing on interactional sociolinguistics and Bakhtinian discourse analysis, the focus of the analysis is on the interaction of different knowledge systems on HIV/AIDS as they become manifest in the corresponding discourses. I am particularly interested in the linguistic devices and interactive strategies the participants use to refer to local knowledge. Among these strategies, a specific type of reformulation, which I will call *intertextual reformulation*, is very prominent. The purpose of this chapter is to provide a detailed and empirically grounded description of both the structural and the functional aspects of intertextual reformulations as prototypical means of the 'multi-voiced' character of HIV/AIDS education.

Theoretical and Methodological Background

Health education relies on media (radio, television, movies, billboards, etc.) and on direct personal communication (discussion groups, individual counseling, etc.). Since Burkina Faso is among the poorest countries in the world, both media use and literacy rates are very low. HIV/AIDS education thus relies strongly on personal communication where professional social workers, together with *peer educators*, that is, specially trained members of the target group, aim at creating awareness about the pandemic in direct interactions.

Most health education programs are based on the premise of a knowledge gap. They presume that risky behavior is due to an absence of knowledge, and that in return the availability of this knowledge will trigger the appropriate behavior changes. According to one of the most popular prevention messages this means in the case of HIV/AIDS either abstinence, faithfulness or the avoidance of sexual intercourse without a condom. Health education focuses primarily on knowledge communication. Even if this take on prevention has largely been criticized, especially for overlooking emotional and cultural aspects, it still characterizes most health education programs (Hurrelmann & Leppin, 2001). This is also true for the training sessions where my data come from. Here, the emphasis is exclusively on the successful transmission of knowledge.

However, in developmental contexts, knowledge communication looks frequently like a one-way street, that is, knowledge and practices rooted in Western traditions are exported to developing nations and intended to supplant, at least partially, local knowledge. In HIV/AIDS awareness campaigns, it is the biomedical knowledge on the disease, conveyed in a now global discourse, that is disseminated. Prevention has become a prototypical mediator of global messages and influences (Barnett & Whiteside, 2002). Yet the global biomedical discourse on HIV/AIDS does not take place in a vacuum. It rather has to face local conceptions and beliefs on sexuality, illness and so on, which are conveyed in local discourses. With Foucault (1969) I argue that discourses organize and structure knowledge, which means in return that knowledge has a discursive facet. The result is *discursive heteroglossia* (Bakhtin, 1990), that is, a plurality of generally competing knowledge systems, each of them establishing a different discourse. Although the local discourse on HIV/AIDS is assumed to be part of the shared knowledge of all participants, the dissemination of its global counterpart constitutes the genuine topic of the trainings. Consequently, local conceptions and beliefs remain in general implicit. In the data, references to the local knowledge are scarce, and they always seem to appear in specific contexts where the legitimacy of the local discourse is challenged. With regard to the place of local and global knowledge, it is thus interesting to investigate the interactional sequences where local discourse emerges and to examine the strategies and linguistic devices the participants use to make it interactionally relevant, and finally to have a closer look at its functions in the context of discursive heteroglossia.

Again, I do not aim at a reconstruction of the underlying knowledge system – this belongs to the realm of medical anthropology (Charmillot, 1997; Vidal, 2004). The focus here is rather on the linguistic surface, that is, the manner in which the local discourse is indicated and framed in order to become relevant for the ongoing interaction. In Gumperz's (1992) words, the purpose is to gain an understanding of the *contextualization cues* that allow for a shared, yet implicit knowledge to become part of the current and active context of interaction. I thus share Goodwin & Duranti's (1992: 31) dynamic view, where context and talk 'stand in a mutually reflexive relationship to each other, with talk, and the interpretative work it generates, shaping context as much as context shapes talk'. This means that context is the outcome of participants' joint efforts to make it available. In my data, reformulations are a particularly prominent contextualization cue when it comes to turn elements of the local discourse on HIV/AIDS from interactionally irrelevant to relevant.

I undertake a closer examination of the reformulations occurring in the data by using tools from discourse analysis and interactional linguistics where more strictly linguistic interests are combined with conversation analytic methodology. In accordance with Couper-Kuhlen and Selting (2001), linguistic forms and structures are seen as resources for the organization of interaction, and their description goes hand in hand with an investigation of their interactional tasks. The focus of the analysis is on the relationship between a specific form or structure and their function(s) in interaction. Here two different, yet complementary perspectives are possible, which address the following two concerns: (1) 'what linguistic resources are used to articulate particular conversational structures and fulfill interactional functions? and (2) what interactional function or conversational structure is furthered by particular linguistic forms and ways of using them?' (Couper-Kuhlen & Selting, 2001: 3). In both cases, the embedding in a particular context and the ethnographic background of the data become crucial.

Since, from a structural point of view, reformulations are a very heterogeneous phenomenon with various interactive tasks, I start by differentiating two types of reformulation that both occur in the data. Very frequent are the so-called *paraphrastic* reformulations where a speaker comes back to a first expression and replaces it by a second expression presented as an equivalent of the former. The relation between the two components may

be made explicit by a marker such as *that is* in English. Paraphrastic reformulations play an important role in the mediation of biomedical knowledge. In the data, especially technical terms like *vaginal secretion, antibody*
or *ovule* trigger paraphrastic reformulations, but there are also colloquial
expressions like *problem of hygiene* that is rephrased by *it is not clean.*
Together with metaphors, word explanations, examples and so on this
technique supports the successful transfer of the biomedical knowledge
about HIV/AIDS.

In contrast to paraphrastic reformulations, there is a second, structur-
ally different and less frequent type of reformulation that seems to be
limited to specific sequential environments. These reformulations activate
the *intertext* of the communication, that is, knowledge that speakers
assume to be shared by their interlocutors. I therefore call them *intertextual
reformulations.* Unlike paraphrastic reformulations, intertextual reformulations do not have a three-part structure. Rather, they consist of more or
less fixed meta-communicative expressions like *it seems that (il paraît que),
people say that (les gens disent que),* which convey to what follows the status
of a quotation or reported speech. In general, the origin of the citation
remains vague or is not indicated at all. Intertextual reformulations allow
the speaker to introduce a different 'voice' or point of view without assuming the responsibility for what has been said. At the same time, a speaker
may insinuate that what is said was already known by the interlocutors.
Intertextual reformulations are thus good examples for the fundamentally
dialogic character of speech as observed by Bakhtin (1990).

In the trainings, intertextual reformulations frequently appear when the
asymmetric turn-taking mechanism typical of classroom interaction is
temporarily abandoned in favor of more egalitarian formats with a higher
participation and involvement of the class. Sometimes such sequences are
initiated by the teacher, who invites his students explicitly to ask *other
questions about AIDS the things you have heard perhaps in your areas between the
young people well things to discuss and that you would like to debate today* (quote
from the data, my translation). These requests generally open question
periods where the future peer educators reveal ideas about HIV/AIDS,
sexuality and so on, which diverge clearly from the biomedical discourse
put forward in the trainings, a discourse that embraces not only scientific
results, but also moral values. The sequences give place to the local
discourse and they are also rich in intertextual reformulations. In the training sessions, it is almost exclusively the students who resort to intertextual
reformulations. Generally, they use this technique to turn elements of the
local knowledge on HIV/AIDS from interactionally irrelevant to relevant.

Data

As mentioned before, my data come from HIV/AIDS education in Burkina Faso. I work with video-taped training sessions for future community workers guided by the principles of peer education. The dominant interaction type is classroom interaction. The trainings take place in French, the official language of multilingual Burkina Faso. However, with the exception of the trainer who speaks an acrolectal French close to the standard, the participants who belong to different ethnic groups and thus have different African mother tongues (Moore, Jula, Fulfulde) speak a heavily indigenized meso- or even basilectal variety of French (Lafage, 1990). Hence language choice is an important issue for HIV/AIDS awareness campaigns in multilingual countries.

In Burkina Faso, for instance, there are about 60 different local languages, and only a small, urban and generally well-educated percentage of Burkinians – an estimated 20% – knows French. On the one side, most of the manuals and kits for HIV/AIDS education provided by international nongovernment organizations are in French. On the other side, the community workers sometimes only have a reduced command of the official language. Consequently, the transfer of complex biomedical knowledge may be hindered or even threatened. And what is more, most of the peer educators will have to work in their own African language, since members of their community – especially in rural regions – will not understand French. Aside from diverging levels of competence in French, another challenge for the future peer educators is the task of translating information and recommendations for HIV/AIDS prevention in local languages without any assistance. This translation task becomes even more challenging when one considers that not only the words, but also the ideas and moral values they convey might be ignored in the local context, and that there is no equivalent in the African languages. A good example is the word *faithfulness*, one of the key concepts of HIV/AIDS education, which has no direct equivalent in traditionally polygamic societies (cf. Drescher, 2007).

Analysis

I now turn to a closer investigation of some pieces of data. The focus lies on the contribution of intertextual reformulations to the contextualization of the local discourse on HIV/AIDS. The analysis will show that intertextual reformulations can have different sequential positions depending on the context and especially on the evaluation of the quoted source. Although in the first three examples, intertextual reformulations appear at the beginning of a turn and are used in relation with the introduction of a new topic, extracts (4) to (6) exemplify an argumentative function where the reformulation helps to support a previous statement. In both cases the speaker declines the responsibility for what has been said. This allows him either to avoid direct critique by presenting a point of view as a mere quote and thus distancing himself from the get-go, or to back challenged claims by reference to a presumed authority.

The following two examples stem from one of the question periods initiated by the trainer. The topical coherence inside these sequences is rather weak. Every student addresses a new topic. The intertextual reformulation comes at the very beginning of the turn and introduces a new topic. Here the technique denotes a speaker's immediate distancing from the contents he or she evokes. As we will see, the contextualization of elements of the local discourse by one of the peer educators is regularly followed by a refutation or depreciation from the part of the trainer. Referring to the local discourse thus can be a face-threatening activity that necessitates particular interactive care. Intertextual reformulations seem to be an appropriate answer to this problem because they allow the speaker to mention a questionable issue without really saying it.

In example (1), Davidson (Da), one of the peer educators, comes onto the issue of different types of viruses. He establishes a link between an infection with HIV 2 and putting on weight that might thus be interpreted as a symptom of an infection[1].

(1) *That fattens up man/ça engrossit l'homme*

01 E   là, (.) c'est ça tu prends, (?bon),
        that is what you catch (?well)
02 Da   mais il paraît que le vé i ach deux-là, que:
        but it seems that this HIV 2 that
03 E   oui'
        yes
04 Da   bon, (..) en partant de ceci:, (.) le commencement
        well starting from this the beginning
05   euh ça engrossit l'hOmme,
        uhm that fattens up man
06 E   NON, (.) <vite> non non non non,+ NON, (.) je vous ai
        no <fast> no no no no no I told you
07   dit que tous les vé i ach, (.) okay' <lent> il vaut
        that all the HIVs okay <slowly> it is
08   mieux ne pas, les prendre point,+ (.) grossir l'homme'
        better not to catch them at all to fatten up man

```
09      pourquoi' c'est pas possIBle,
        why that's not possible
10  Da  <riant> okay,+
        <laughing> okay
11  E   <vite> non non non non,+ ça peut pas être possible,
        <fast> no no no no that cannot be possible
```

Using the meta-communicative formula *it seems that* (line 02) Davidson presents such a link as an established fact, without specifying the source of his knowledge. It is also clear that he does not assume the responsibility for this assertion. As the teacher had suggested, he presents his talk as something one knows by hearsay without necessarily agreeing with it. Hence the contents are submitted to the judgment of the audience, especially of the trainer (E) who, for his part, contests emphatically the existence of such a link (line 06) and thus contradicts the assumption put forward by Davidson. The student ratifies the answer without insisting (line 10), and the floor goes to another participant.

In example (2), one can observe the same technique. Davidson (Da) takes the floor and discusses the – very delicate – issue of a conscious and voluntary transmission of the virus by people infected with AIDS. He alludes to a quite widespread belief in Burkina Faso where people assume that the 'gift' of the disease in the literal sense of the word, that is the infection of another person who takes over the illness, may help the infected person to recover from AIDS.

(2) *Bissap*

```
01  Da  <lent> mais il paraît aussi qu'il y avait une femme
        <slowly> but it seems also that there was a woman
02      qui était atteinte du sida, (.) mais elle a enlevé son
        who was infected with aids but she removed her
03      sang là pour mettre dans le bissap tout ça (?....)
        blood in order to put it into the bissap and so on (?...)
04  E   <fort> vous'+ (.)/vous devriez savoir, <accentué>
        <loud> you/you should know <emphasized>
05      que sI on met le sang dans le bissap, (.) sI le sang
        that if one puts the blood into the bissap if the blood
06      est contaminé, (.) si le sang contient le virus de
        is contaminated if the blood contains the virus of
07      sida, si vous le mettez dans le bissap, (.) il mEUrt
        aids if you put it into the bissap it dies
08      cinq secondes après,+ (.) c'est pas son milieu de vie,
        five seconds later it's not his natural environment
09      (.) c'est comme si tu prends faroukou aller le jeter
        it's as if you take Faroukou [first name] and go and throw him
```

10   `dans le mE:r, au pôle nord,`
        into the sea at the North Pole
11 XX `<riant>`
        <laughing>

Davidson tells the story of a woman living with AIDS who sells *bissap* – a traditional red-colored beverage, made from dried flowers – spoiled with her infected blood. Again the meta-communicative formula *it seems also that* (line 01) signals that Davidson refers to shared knowledge while he is only the spokesman who does not assume the responsibility for the contents. The expression *there was* (line 01) also contributes to his strategy of depersonalization as it asserts merely the existence of a fact. The trainer (E) prompts by contesting vigorously the possibility of a viral transmission with an infected beverage. In his answer, he emphasizes mainly the conditions the virus needs to survive and thus relies on scientific arguments belonging to the biomedical discourse (*if one puts the blood into the bissap if the blood is contaminated if the blood contains the virus of aids if you put it into the bissap it dies five seconds later it's not his natural environment*; lines 05–08). Then the scientific reasoning is taken up in an analogy where the virus is compared to Faroukou, one of the members of the group, and the blood to the sea at the North Pole, implying that a virus cannot survive in a beverage like a human cannot survive in the icy water (lines 09–10).

The next example is different from the previous inasmuch as it is the trainer (E) who refers to elements of the local knowledge. Here, intertextual reformulations obviously serve a didactic strategy that aims to point out 'wrong' beliefs and assumptions in order to dismantle them subsequently. In correlation with the already discussed understanding of the disease as something one can get rid of by contaminating somebody else, the trainer mentions another traditional explanation that is particularly strong in the African context: HIV/AIDS is caused by 'bad spirits', and – this would be the consequence – beyond the influence of humans.

(3) *Bad spirits/mauvais esprits*

01 E   `<accentué> si vous voulez+ <vite> contaminer tout`
        <emphasized> if you want <fast> contaminate everybody
02   `le monde,+ vous serez peut-être la première personne`
        you will perhaps be the first person
03   `à partir, (.) c'est des mauvais esprits,`
        to leave it is bad spirits
04   `(.) okay' c'est sûr que vous avez entendu des`
        okay sure that you have heard
05   `choses comme ça, (.) dans vos quartiers, (.) mais'`
        things like that in your area but

```
06    c'est peut-être parce qu'ils ne savent pAs,↑(.)
```
it's perhaps because they don't know
```
07    et s'ils ne font pas attention, (.) ils peuvent
```
and if they don't pay attention they can
```
08    prendre une autre (?...) et ainsi augmenter (.)
```
catch another (?...) and in this way increase
```
09    leur charge virale, et précipiter le <vite>
```
their viral charge and speed up the <fast>
```
10    processus vers la mort,+ . okay' (.) donc, s'ils
```
process towards death okay so perhaps if they
```
11    avaient peut être cette information, (.)
```
had this information
```
12    ils ne: diraient pAs' qu'ils vont (.) contaminer
```
they wouldn't say that they will contaminate
```
13    (.)le maximum de personnes, (.) okay'
```
the maximum of people okay

The assertion *it is bad spirits* (line 03) is introduced quite abruptly. Only retroactively is it framed as a quote by an elaborated meta-communicative sequence. The trainer presents this belief as an element of the shared knowledge of the group, presuming that the peer educators have heard similar explanations in their community (lines 04–05). The whole sequence forms the first part of a concessive movement, keyed by the markers *okay sure* (line 04). The second part is opened by the adversative marker *but* (line 05), that introduces an opposition. The following sequence consists of a series of suppositions why people stick to the traditional beliefs: *it's perhaps because they don't know and if they don't pay attention they can catch another* (lines 06–08) that leads up into a description of the consequences, that is the infection with a second type of HIV and a yet increased decline of the person living with AIDS. The whole sequence ends up with a plead for health education since it will put an end to this kind of behavior: *if they had this information they wouldn't say that they will contaminate the maximum of people* (lines 10–13). The example thus illustrates the reference to local discourse in a didactic perspective. Elements of the local knowledge are brought to light in order to combat them and to replace them subsequently by elements of the biomedical knowledge. They also allow the trainer to provide the peer educators with arguments for their future work in the community.

In the next examples, the sequential position of the intertextual refor-mulations is different: They are now used in the course of an argument where they support previously challenged claims. References to the local knowledge thus function as argumentative backings. They are part of longer exchanges, characterized by recursive structures of claims and refutations, that oppose the trainer (E) and generally one of the peer educators. In example (4), Evariste (Ev) asserts that the absence of a woman's menstrual period could be compensated for by other bleedings such as nosebleeds, and then she makes use of an intertextual reformulation to respond to a refutation of this assertion.

(4) *Bleedings/saignements*

01 E   oui´
             yes

02 Ev   il y a certaines qui ne voient pas leurs règles mais
             there are some who don't see their periods but it

03   ça se manifeste d'une autre façon
             shows up in another way

04 E   ça se manifeste où´
             where does it show up

05 Ev   par exemple, (.) les saignements´ (.)
             for instance bleedings

06 E   où´
             where

07 Ev   et voilà´ (.) par le nez
             well through the nose

08 E   ça n'a pAs de liEn, je pense pas que ça ait un lien,
             there is no such connection I don't think that there is a connection

09 Ev   MOI j'ai entendu comme ça,
             I heard it that way

10 E   <fort> les rè:gles,+ les règles (.) c'est un autre
             <loud> the period the period that's another

11   système, (.) les saignemENTs au <vite> niveau du nez
             system the bleedings on <fast> the level of the nose

12   non, +
             no

13 Ev   oui oui,
             yes yes

14 E   nOn, ça/ce n'est pas la même chose, (.) ce n'est pA::s
             no that this is not the same thing this is not

15   le: même chemin, (.) ce n'est pA:s les mêmes organes
             the same way it's not the same organs

16   qui sont en cause, (.) okay´ (.) les règles,
             that are concerned okay the period

17 Fk   c'est pas la même chose,
             it's not the same thing

18 E   c'est quAnd´ l'Ovule, (.) est pondue,
             it's when the ovum is laid

19 Xf   hein´
             what

20 E   l'Ovule descend <vite> au niveau+ de l'utérus, (..)
             the ovum goes down <fast> at the level of the uterus

Evariste first presents her claim without epistemic modalization or any other mitigation. However, the teacher categorically denies the existence of a connection between the two types of bleedings (*there is no such connection*; line 08) and then reformulates his assertion with a slight epistemic modalization that emphasizes the subjective character of his judgment (*I don't think that there is a connection*; line 08). Evariste does not accept the objection and prompts by indicating the source of her information (*I heard it that way*; line 09). By doing so, she retroactively frames her statement as an intertextual reformulation. The intertextual reference thus occurs in a situation of 'argumentative distress'. The re-labeling of questioned previous talk as hearsay reduces the responsibility of the speaker, because it allows him or her both to 'hide' behind the different voice and to strengthen his or her own position by referring to an authority. This contrasts with the foregoing examples where the speaker presents the statement from the beginning as a quote, rather than taking on any personal responsibility for the claim.

In example (5), the intertextual reformulation is again part of an argument between the trainer (E) and Maximilien (Max), one of the peer educators.

(5) *Certain relatives/certains parents*

```
01  E     okay' (.) oui' euh: toé,
          okay yes uhm toé [first name]
02  Max   mais moi je voulais leur dire aussi:, je connais
          but I also wanted to tell them I know
03        certains parents <bas> (?. . .), +
          certain relatives <low> (?...)
04  E     bOn:, je pense que c'est un peu exagéré, (?ils vont)
          well I think that it is a bit exaggerated (?they don't) go
05        pas jusqu' à tuER, (.) mais on SAIT qu' (?il y en a)
          as far as to kill but one knows that (?there are people) who
06        qui cAchent, (.) <vite> y en a+ qui veulent pas qu'on
          hide <fast> and there are people who don't want that you talk
07        pArle, y en a qui cachent, <plus bas> mais, aller
          and there are people who hide <lower> but to go as far
08        jusqu'à tuER' je pense que ça c'est un peu trop fort, +
          as to kill I think that this is a bit too strong
09  Max   (?. . .) c'est ce qu'on dIt,
          (?...) it's what people say
10  E     <vite> non non non non non, les docteurs ne vont
          <fast> no no no no no the doctors will
11        jamais faire ça, (.) quoi,
          never do that right
12  Max   à force de trop de dépenses
          forced by too much expenses
```

```
13  XX    <rient>
          <laughing>
14  E     non non, faut pas payer
          no no don't have to pay
15  Max   (?...)
16  E     aucun médecin, ne va accepter faire ça
          no doctor will accept doing that
```

According to Maximilien, some people living with AIDS are killed by their own relatives who are no longer able to pay the expenses caused by the disease. The teacher first judges this claim as exaggerated (line 04), then he replaces *kill the sick persons* (lines 04–05) by *hiding the sick persons* (lines 05–06). Finally, he fleshes out his argument with some paraphrastic reformulations and concludes with a subjective statement: *I think that this is a bit too strong* (line 08). The epistemic modalization *I think* mitigates his objection which remains – given the topic – surprisingly moderate. Maximilien prompts with a partially unintelligible statement that concludes with the meta-communicative expression *this is what people say* (line 09). Here again, the previous utterances are framed retroactively as intertextual reformulation. The trainer contradicts emphatically with a series of *no* and points out that *doctors will never do that* (lines 10–11). Maximilien still insists by putting forward as another argument in favor of his position the costs caused by the illness of a parent (*forced by too much expenses;* line 12). The trainer denies again by rephrasing his previous statement in a more categorical way (*no doctor will accept doing that;* line 16) and the argumentation still continues for a few turns.

The last example I will discuss here shows how an intertextual reformulation is used to contest an explanation given by the trainer (E). Abdou (Ab), one of the peer educators, takes the floor by asking whether animals can carry HIV (line 01).

(6) *Animals/des animaux*

```
01  Ab   est-ce que (.) les animaux, ont le vé i ach,
          do animals have hiv
02  E     qui peut répondre à ça, (.) oui, Faroukou,
          who can answer to this yes faroukou [first name]
03  Fk    les animaux ne sont:/portent pas (.) le vé i ach,
          animals are not/don't carry the hiv
04  E     <fort, accentue chaque mot> le virus de
          <loud, emphasizing each word> the virus of human
05        l'immunodéficience humaine, +
          immuno-deficiency
06  Ab    NON,(?...) certains disent que,/que ça
          no (?...) some people say that/ that this
```

07   (?vient) des animaux, parce qu'il y a des situations
        (?comes) from animals because there are situations
08   vous êtes/(?...) de/de faire l'amour avec les animaux,
        you are (?...) to to make love with the animals
09 E   bOn, je vous ai co/bon c'est comment' (?ce que
        well I had you/well how is it (?what
10   vous dites), ça veut dire que, au début, (.)
        you say) this means that at the beginning
11   on cherchait l'o:rigine du virus, (.) les
        one was searching for the origin of the virus
12   gens ont raconté n'importe quoi, (.) y en a qui
        people talked nonsense there are some that
13   disent que c'est les sin:ges, y en a qui disent
        say that it is the apes there are some that say
14   c'est: (.)/je sais pas moi, (.) okay' mais je te
        it is/I don't know okay but I
15   dis que, (.) euh en tout cas, on a/on a/on a pu
        tell you that uhm anyway it has/it has/it has been
16   démontrer, (.) quE' le vé i ach:, tel quE on le
        demonstrated that the HIV as we
17   connaît, ne peut pAs se retrouver chez les animaux,
        know it cannot be found in animals

The trainer delegates the answer to Faroukou (Fk), another student, who denies that animals can carry the virus (line 03). He then takes up by spelling out the acronym HIV while detaching and emphasizing each word with a staccato prosody (line 04). In this way he highlights the adjective *human* contained in the acronym and thus ratifies the answer given by Faroukou. At this point Abdou, apparently not satisfied by the previous answers, takes up the floor again (line 06). He opens his turn by an emphatic *no* and – after an unintelligible passage – brings up the idea of a possible human infection through sexual intercourse with animals. This explanation of the transmission of the disease is framed as a reference to local knowledge and introduced by the expression *some people say*. Indeed, the belief that the epidemic may have its origin in sexual intercourse with infected animals, especially apes, is very popular among the future peer educators and – perhaps because of its taboo infringing, spicy character – a topic that the students seem to relish. The subject is brought back several times during the training sessions.

At first, the trainer obviously displays the difficulty in responding to this delicate issue. After he has taken up the floor, one can observe self-repairs and re-starts (line 09). He then continues by reformulating Abdou's question (lines 09–10) and giving it a new focus. He reframes it as a request for information about the scientific research on HIV/AIDS in earlier years and especially about the different hypotheses regarding the origin of the virus. By turning the question in this way, the trainer evades the tricky topic of zoophilic relationships and comes back on safer scientific grounds. He argues that there were various different explanations and that some people just talked nonsense (line 12). This statement is immediately followed by an allusion to apes, yet now without the sexual connotation, that may count as an illustration of absurd hypotheses. The whole sequence is framed as a quote (*people talked, there are some that say*; lines 12–14), but it is not clear whether the trainer refers here only to the local discourse or gives his claim a more general scope. He then cuts short to the list of possible origins of the virus, keys this issue as one that is not really to the point (*anyway*; line 15) and concludes with a statement that is presented as a scientific truth and thus makes explicit reference to the biomedical discourse: *anyway it has been demonstrated that the HIV as we know it can not be found in animals* (lines 15–17).

Conclusion

The previous analysis has shown that more or less fixed meta-communicative expressions – utterances like *it seems that*, *people say that* or *I have heard that* – are fundamental for the identification of intertextual reformulations as they make a reference to shared knowledge explicit. Shared knowledge belongs to the context of the communication. The intertextual reformulations refer to this source and make it available for the ongoing interaction. They may be considered as traces of the underlying discursive heteroglossia, as they bring in different points of view. Such reformulations are always framed as 'it is not me, it is somebody else who is saying it'. The resulting principal communicative function is distantiation. According to Nølke (1994), the expression *il paraît que* ('it seems that'), a prototypical marker of intertextual reformulations, serves to dilute the 'enunciative responsibility' (*reponsbilité énonciative*) inherent to the act of assertion.

This distancing effect of language such as *il paraît que* holds for intertextual reformulations in general. Speakers always present themselves as mere spokespersons and thus reduce or even cancel their own involvement. Intertextual reformulations share this feature with other patterns of evidential and/or epistemic modalization (cf. Chafe & Nichols, 1986; Dendale & Tasmowski, 2001; Palmer, 1986). Yet, such a distantiation of the speaker has repercussions on the interaction, because his withdrawal signifies 'for the co-enunciator the possibility to question, or even to refute the content of the received message' (Guentchéva, 1996: 11, my translation).

If an utterance already displays a low commitment of the speaker, it is easier for the interlocutor to take issue with its contents since the face-threatening act that all refutation entails is mitigated. This explains also why, in the pieces of data presented here, a majority of intertextual reformulations appears in disagreement sequences with a fairly stable distribution of the interactional roles: Generally, it is the peer educators who resort to intertextual reformulations, whereas the trainer usually questions information framed in such a way. It seems that intertextual reformulations already hint to the contentious character of the contents they introduce. So the mere format of distantiation might be an incentive to refutation.

With regard to the functions of intertextual reformulations in the data, we also have to take into account the sequential position of the intertextual reformulation. As we have seen, the technique appears in at least two different environments: On the one hand, it marks the beginning of a turn and accompanies the introduction of a new topic. Here the fixed modal and evidential expressions are used as 'disclaimers'. Given the asymmetric situation of the trainings, this strategy reduces the speaker's risk to be blamed for a deviant opinion and offers nevertheless the possibility to put forward potentially controversial positions. On the other hand, intertextual reformulations are quite common in argumentative contexts where they support previous assertions. In this case, the speaker appeals to another voice that is supposed to be more cogent or to have greater authority, in order to defend his claim. It becomes evident that, while the common denominator of either the 'disclaiming' and the 'backing' use of intertextual reformulations lies in the decrease of the speaker's responsibility through the recourse to another voice, the prestige one assigns to this voice plays an important role too. If the source of information is considered reliable, the reformulation can be used to support the argumentation. But if the quoted voice has only a low prestige in the given context, the information has little value as well.

This aspect is crucial for the training sessions, because the intertextual reformulations contextualize almost exclusively the local discourse on HIV/AIDS and related subjects as sexuality or death. Yet, this discourse is opposed to the biomedical discourse, and both struggle for hegemony. In other words, they intend to eradicate any knowledge incompatible with their own logic. As the data show, in HIV/AIDS education in Burkina Faso, the local knowledge is in a weak position. It lacks legitimacy and is supposed to be supplanted or at least completed by biomedical knowledge. Therefore it is not surprising that intertextual reformulations that do not fully commit the speaker are used to frame references to the local discourse. Since intertextual reformulations participate in the contextualization of competing knowledge systems, that is biomedical or global knowledge and traditional or local knowledge, they are particularly interesting with regard to the discursive heteroglossia that characterizes the HIV/AIDS education. Inasmuch as they belong to the linguistic traces of the struggle for hegemony that opposes the concurrent discourses and surfaces in these processes of negotiation, they can also provide interesting insights into the place of local and global knowledge in HIV/AIDS education (cf. Chilisa's, 2005, critique of HIV/AIDS campaigns in Botswana). Finally, intertextual reformulations and the strips of talk they frame may to some extent contest the biomedical explanations of the pandemic and therefore be understood as acts of resistance to the predominant global discourse on HIV/AIDS. Hence research on reformulations and similar linguistic devices can give insight into the dissemination, valorization or depreciation of different knowledge forms and the power relations inscribed in HIV/AIDS education.

Appendix: Transcription Conventions

/	word fragments without a pause
(.)	very short pause
..	short pause
...	mid-length pause
haut'	rising intonation
malade,	falling intonation
↑	high peak
MALIN ROsé bAr	emphasis of a word/of a syllable/of a sound
oui: et::: no:n	prolongation of a syllable/of a sound
(? toi aussi)	uncertain transcription
(? ...)	(passage of an) unintelligible utterance
<bas> . . . +	comment by the transcriber; precedes the utterance
<souriant> . . . +	and stays valid until the +-sign

Note

1. Cf. Appendix for the transcription system that follows the conventions developed at the University of Bielefeld (Germany). In the discussion of the data, I will quote the translated gloss rather than the original text for the sake of easier reading.

References

Bakhtin, M. (1990) *The Dialogic Imagination*. Austin: University of Texas Print.

Barnett, T. and Whiteside, A. (2002) *AIDS in the Twenty-First Century. Disease and Globalization*. Houndmills and New York: Palgrave Macmillan.

Chafe, W.L. and Nichols, J. (eds) (1986) *Evidentiality: The Linguistic Coding of Epistemology in Language*. Norwood, NJ: Ablex.

Charmillot, M. (1997) *Les savoirs de la maladie. De l'éducation à la santé en contexte africain*. Genève: Faculté de psychologie et des sciences de l'éducation [Cahiers de la section des sciences de l'éducation 81].

Chilisa, B. (2005) Educational research within postcolonial Africa: A critique of HIV/AIDS research in Botswana. *International Journal of Qualitative Studies in Education* 18 (6), 659–684.

Couper-Kuhlen, E. and Selting, M. (2001) Introducing interactional linguistics. In M. Selting and E. Couper-Kuhlen (eds) *Studies in Interactional Linguistics* (pp. 1–22). Amsterdam and Philadelphia: John Benjamins.

Dendale, P. and Tasmowski, L. (2001) Introduction: Evidentiality and related notions. *Journal of Pragmatics* 33, 339–348.

Drescher, M. (2004) Zur Interkulturalität der Wissenskommunikation. Das Beispiel der HIV/AIDS-Prävention in Burkina Faso. *Gesprächsforschung. Online-Zeitschrift zur verbalen Interaktion* 5, 118–147.

Drescher, M. (2006) Sprachliche Markierungen alltagsweltlicher Diskurse in der HIV/Aids-Prävention Burkina Fasos. In M. Drescher and S. Klaeger (eds) *Kommunikation über HIV/Aids. Interdisziplinäre Beiträge zur Prävention im subsaharischen Afrika* (pp. 15–47). Münster: LIT Verlag.

Drescher, M. (2007) Global and local alignments in HIV/AIDS prevention trainings. A case study from Burkina Faso. *Communication & Medicine* 4 (1), 3–14.

Foucault, M. (1969) *L'archéologie du savoir*. Paris: Gallimard.

Goodwin, C. and Duranti, A. (1992) Rethinking context: An introduction. In A. Duranti and C. Goodwin (eds) *Rethinking context* (pp. 1–42). Cambridge: Cambridge University Press (CUP).

Guentchéva, Z. (1996) Introduction. In: Z. Guentchéva (ed.) *L'énonciation médiatisée* (pp. 11–18). Louvain and Paris: Editions Peeters.

Gumperz, J.J. (1992) Contextualization revisited. In P. Auer and A. di Luzio (eds) *The Contextualization of Language* (pp. 39–53). Amsterdam and Philadelphia: John Benjamins.

Hurrelmann, K. and Leppin, A. (2001) Moderne Gesundheitskommunikation – eine Einführung. In K. Hurrelmann and A. Leppin (eds) *Moderne Gesundheitskommunikation* (pp. 9–21). Bern: Huber.

Lafage, S. (1990) Regionale Varianten des Französischen außerhalb Frankreichs. In G. Holtus, M. Metzeltin and C. Schmitt (eds) *Lexikon der romanistischen Linguistik* (Vol. V/1) (pp. 767–787). Tübingen: Niemeyer.

Nølke, H. (1994) La dilution linguistique des responsabilités. *Langue Française* 102, 84–94.

Palmer, F. (1986) *Mood and Modality*. Cambridge: Cambridge University Press.

UNAIDS (2007) On WWW at http://www.unaids.org/en/Regions_Countries/Countries/burkinafaso.asp. Accessed 12.12.2007.

Vidal, L. (2004) *Ritualités, santé et sida en Afrique. Pour une anthropologie du singulier*. Paris: IRD-Karthala.

Chapter 10

What Difference Does This Make? Studying Southern African Youth as Knowledge Producers within a New Literacy of HIV and AIDS

CLAUDIA MITCHELL, JEAN STUART, NAYDENE DE LANGE, RELEBOHILE MOLETSANE, THABISILE BUTHELEZI, JUNE LARKIN and SARAH FLICKER

Introduction

'Can the visual arts make a difference in South Africa in addressing HIV and AIDS'? asks Marilyn Martin (2003). To Martin's provocative question one might also add, if so, 'how', 'under what circumstances', 'when', 'what kind of evidence is useful' – and critically, to whom? Specifically, what difference can visual and arts-based participatory HIV and AIDS interventions make in the lives of young people in South Africa? How can a study of the 'the afterlife' of participatory youth-focused arts-based projects help to deepen an understanding of the impact of this kind of work?

Nowhere is Martin's question more relevant than in relation to young people in Southern Africa. Globally, sub-Saharan Africa remains the worst affected region in the world with almost one in three people who are infected with the virus living in the region (UNAIDS, 2006). In particular, South Africa has been hit hard, with HIV and AIDS emerging as the first cause of mortality among youth (United Nations, 2005). For example, evidence from epidemiological studies shows that the peak incidence of HIV and AIDS occurs in young people aged 15–24 years. A survey of HIV and sexual behavior among young South Africans conducted by the Reproductive Health Research Unit (RHRU) in 2007 found that young women were at higher risk of infection than young men. Furthermore, the survey highlights that more than two thirds of youth report changing their sexual behavior because of awareness about HIV and AIDS, and substantial increase in reported condom usage at last sex. The concern however is the high percentage of young people, including those already infected, who underestimate their risk for HIV.

KwaZulu-Natal province is at the epicenter of the HIV pandemic in South Africa, where, in some rural areas more than 25% of young people between the ages of 15 and 24 are HIV positive. This chapter addresses two main facts of life in this province: (1) death and dying as a result of HIV and AIDS, and (2) a paucity of solutions that recognize the pivotal leadership role that young people can play in addressing health-related issues. For the past three years, our research team has been testing a variety of visual methods with young people and their teachers which have centered on the idea of engagement through participation. We have regarded approaches such as photo-voice[1] and participatory and collaborative video[2] as critical to both understanding how young people frame issues of stigma, voluntary counseling and testing, gender violence and safe sex practices and learning more about how to 'get the message out' in culturally relevant ways to peer audiences. In this chapter, we explore ways of framing this type of engagement (both for producers and consumers) in the context of knowledge production. How do young people 'give voice' to their concerns, and how might we read their visual images within a framework of social change? How can arts-based methodologies be used with young people in rural schools to create a more youth-focused and learner-centered approach to knowledge production and behavior change in the context of HIV and AIDS?

When these questions were posed several years after the completion of a CIDA-funded study called the *Soft Cover* project, an intensive peer education and arts intervention project with a group of 15 young people in schools in two townships in the Western Cape, we were struck by the difficult transitions young people must make in going from high school and out into the world, and the challenges of maintaining an activist agenda. Over the course of the project, a partnership between the Centre for the Book in Cape Town and the Faculty of Education, McGill University, young people from Khayelitsha and Atlantis participated in a number of workshops organized around various arts-based approaches to 'getting the message out' about HIV and AIDS (including hip-hop, graffiti and book-making/creative writing). As published authors in *In My Life* (see Mitchell, 2006a), a small collection of poems and stories written about AIDS in their lives, they also spoke out in their schools and communities.

Unfortunately the end of funding for the project coincided with the time when the group was completing secondary school. We regard it as unfortunate because the transition in the face of poverty, drug abuse, gangs, illness as a result of HIV and AIDS and high levels of unemployment in townships like Khayelitsha has been far from smooth. At the same time, as our preliminary 'two-years later' individual and small group interviews revealed, the spark that had been lit in their work as peer educators in local schools had not been extinguished. One young man had participated in an international forum on youth and HIV and AIDS in Germany and he, along with several of the others from Khayelitsha talk about forming a performance group to continue their work on HIV and AIDS education. And one young woman, while struggling to find any work other than a part-time 'internship' in a Checkers Food Market, nonetheless looks back at some of the writing she did as part of the *Soft Cover* project and wonders how she could get back into writing. Understanding the 'afterlife' of their participation (and the involvement of the young people in local schools) in a project that took up so much of their lives several years earlier is exactly the type of 'what difference' that we see as contributing to responding to Martin's provocative question.

Youth as Knowledge Producers within a New Literacy of AIDS

Our question, 'what difference does this make'?' is framed within our broader project of what we have termed elsewhere, a new literacy of AIDS (Mitchell, 2006a). In an article called 'Sick of AIDS: Life, literacy and South African youth' (Mitchell & Smith, 2003), we first argued for a re-examination of the meanings of literacy in the age of AIDS. The point of that article was to draw attention to the importance of youth engagement and youth participation as a way to counter what was clearly a type of 'AIDS fatigue'. Now several years later these issues remain, and there is still relatively little 'up close' research on youth-focused projects and the meanings that young people themselves are making of the pandemic. In the meantime, many more young people are becoming infected, many more young people are dying and many more young people have had to assume new responsibilities such as heading up households. Thus, we look to the emerging challenges within literacy itself. Language, for example, itself is critical. There are 11 official languages in South Africa. How do language policies relate to emerging 'new literacy' issues? Life-Skills teachers that we interviewed a few years ago in a township school noted that they always conduct classes on HIV and AIDS in the learner's first language regardless of school policy (Mitchell & Smith, 2003). The information, they said, is too 'life-and-death' (their words) to be lost as a result of only partial comprehension. Another issue relates to obtaining appropriate identity documents and death certificates (of parents) in order to apply for the Social Grants that are available to eligible children who have lost parents. A third issue, as a result of the increased number of orphans and vulnerable children, relates to financial literacy and managing a household. Now that antiretrovirals are increasingly available, there are also new literacy issues in relation to compliance and adherence. These concerns appear to be remarkably similar to the kinds of issues that fit within work around multiliteracies (Kress, 2003) and situated literacies more broadly (see e.g. Barton *et al.*, 2000).

But beyond these situated literacies, we have been interested in the emergence (and reinforcement) of community literacy practices that speak to voice and to the role of participation within a context that acknowledges the particularities of the pandemic. One that we explore elsewhere relates to role of Memory Boxes and Memory Books – and the practice of parents who are ill 'leaving something behind' for their children (Mankell, 2004; Mitchell, 2006a, 2006b). Pertinent to young people is the idea of peer publishing. The *In My Life* book noted above demonstrated that there are new stories to be told *for* and *by* young people in South Africa today, ones that are almost *beyond the imagination* of many adults who did not themselves grow up in the age of AIDS but are currently writing fiction for young adults. This youth voice is critical and not just in South Africa, as Michael Hoechsmann and Bronwen Low observe in their analysis of reading youth writing (Hoechsmann & Low, 2008). Contained within a cultural materialist reading of *In My Life* (Mitchell & Moletsane, 2007) is a recognition of the place and cultural currency of a local text like this 'on the streets'. Not only were many copies of the book in circulation when it first came out, but its authors were also in circulation as public figures. Shortly after the book was published, some of the authors took on celebrity status in Khayelitsha and Atlantis and were given opportunities to speak at AIDS events and looked for advice from neighbors and friends. In follow-up evaluations to the project, the majority of the young authors said that this experience had been very empowering and was one of the critical aspects they took away from writing their stories. Status became a kind of social commodity. This work speaks to the significance of ordinary citizens (in this case young people) taking action as cultural producers (Buckingham & Sefton-Green, 1994).

Both within and beyond the classroom, our work embraces the possibilities that result from a recognition of the importance of working beyond the confines of verbal language, which is why we have given so much attention to visual and arts-based participatory methodologies such as photo-voice and participatory and collaborative video. In relation to classroom pedagogies, Stein and Newfield (2006: 10) have noted:

> Multimodal pedagogies acknowledge learners as agentive, resourceful and creative meaning-makers who communicate using the communicative potential and multiple resources of their bodies and of their environment to interconnect. Learners engage with different modes differently: they have different relationships, histories and competencies in relation to modes. In multimodal pedagogies there is a conscious awareness of the relationship between modes, learning and identity.

Responding to the socially and culturally embedded aspects of HIV and AIDS and its multifaceted nature is complex, and as individuals and communities struggle to do so, the value of multimodalities and multiliteracies is evident. For instance, performative and visual modes communicate more easily across language barriers, and provide a different 'grammar' to articulate ideas and experiences.

Within a new literacy of AIDS, we are drawing on the term 'youth as knowledge producers' (Lankshear & Knobel, 2003) to describe the body of work that explicitly involves youth themselves as producers of both traditional and new media (e.g. drumming, hip-hop graffiti, photography, video documentary, radio, writing, and so on) in the context of HIV and AIDS education. As with the work of Kendrick *et al.* (2006), Stein and Newfield (2006) and Newfield and Maundegzo (2006), these approaches speak to the significance of multimodalities in cultural expression. While the work is also located within the broader study of arts-based research (Cole *et al.*, 2004; Knowles & Cole, 2007) and more specifically in relation to the use of the arts in health education, work with youth and HIV and AIDS has become its own research area as the vast range of youth-focused artistic participatory initiatives mapped out in a recent study for UNESCO of several hundred organizations around the world attest (Mitchell, Low & Hoechsmann, 2006). As organizations such as UNICEF and UNESCO have cautioned, unless youth are given a more significant role in producing locally relevant messages, prevention programs are doomed to failure (Ford *et al.*, 2003). Such a position recognizes that although young people are sometimes victims of an invincible attitude that says 'it can never happen to me', simultaneously they are more likely to believe that they can make change. And while there may be a 'sick of AIDS' phenomenon among youth (Mitchell & Smith, 2003), they are also more likely to want to do something! As with the work of

Pattman (2006) in studying with young people their sexual identities, the idea of youth as knowledge producers also positions youth as assets to each other. The studies our research team has conducted form a body of work that has been organized around empowering youth in school-based programs, community-based programs and in programs involving pre-service teachers as an often under-studied 'youth-based' population (Stuart & Mitchell, 2007). Within these studies focusing on youth and HIV, we have tested out photo-voice (Mitchell *et al.*, 2005; Moletsane *et al.*, 2007), participatory video (Mak, 2006; Mitchell *et al.*, 2009), collage (Norris *et al.*, 2007), drawing (Mitchell, Walsh & Moletsane, 2006; Stuart, 2006a, 2006b) and hip-hop and forum theatre (Stuart & Mitchell, 2007). In one project, beginning teachers participated in a series of arts-based HIV and AIDS workshops as part of a guidance and counseling module (Stuart, 2004, 2007). In another, a group of beginning teachers as peer educators on the campus of the University of KwaZulu-Natal have been involved in a series of 'youth as knowledge producers' workshops on video, photo-voice, forum theatre and hip-hop to address HIV and AIDS. Based on their own participation in these workshops, the beginning teachers have been working in rural schools with grades 9 and 10 learners (Stuart *et al.*, 2007). The studies span both rural and urban settings and offer the possibility for examining both short-term impact as well as impact over several years beyond the life of a project. These include the *Soft Cover* project noted above (Mitchell, 2006a, 2006b; Walsh & Mitchell, 2006), as well as a series of interventions in Swaziland and in the Vulindlela district of KwaZulu-Natal. We have also embarked upon projects that link South African youth and Canadian youth such as the TIGXpress HIV and Aids project, a photo-voice project involving young people in Toronto and in the Mariannhill district of KwaZulu-Natal (Larkin *et al.*, 2007).

These projects can also be viewed in the context of a Media Education orientation where there is growing recognition of the value of positioning learners (young people) as producers (Buckingham, 2003; Buckingham & Sefton-Green, 1994). Early on in the emergence of media education, much of the focus was on arming youth against what was seen as the corruptive influence of media and 'common' culture, but as the discipline matured, this focus was balanced by a recognition that critical awareness and (arguably) empowerment could result when media production was encouraged. By producing their own media texts, whether through the medium of traditional print media such as newspapers, visual media such as photographs, audio media such as radio or in line with global communication development, new media – websites, chat rooms, SMS and blogging, young people could give voice to their own ideas and interact with those of people in ever widening social and cultural circles.

Evaluating What and for What Purposes?

An emerging agenda for this work is one of fine-tuning analytic frameworks and tools of evaluation within arts-based research and within development studies more broadly. This is a critical area for assisting arts-based youth groups who are committed to social change and who depend on donors for financial support. How can what we are doing as academics and researchers spill over into their community-based projects that, among other things, need to be funded? There is much written already about the failure of traditional, didactic HIV and AIDS programming with youth and the need to shift towards more participatory approaches (Campbell, 2003) and it is within this context that the burgeoning body of work on visual and arts-based participatory approaches has flourished. However, while the field of arts-based participatory work is rapidly growing, it seems that ways of evaluating or studying this work are less developed. While this gap is to be expected in such a new field of study, it poses serious problems in the context of the urgency of AIDS, particularly in South Africa. Indeed, the relative absence of documenting the effectiveness of these approaches means the programs and many small-scale interventions in place could have fatal consequences if, in fact, the approaches are found to be ineffective or require serious revision. At the same time, policy makers who are in a position to advocate for such approaches will fail to be convinced of their usefulness in the absence of evidence. Too often, for example, evaluations rely solely on quantitative measures which may not be sufficiently nuanced to respond to such critical areas as engagement or empathy.

The need for strengthening work in this area was made evident at a recent conference on evaluating the impact of the arts held in Paris in January 2007 (Centre Pompidou, 2007) and it is also a point taken up by Gould (2007). Concomitantly, school-based, community-based organizations and national programs such as loveLife need to be able to show evidence of the overall effectiveness of their programs. This point took on national proportions several years ago when loveLife lost a substantial amount of its funding when it was not able to demonstrate through evidence-based evaluation techniques its overall impact on reducing the spread of AIDS among young people (see also Epstein, 2007). This led to more recent external studies that have incorporated a range of evaluative techniques (Pettifors *et al.*, 2005) and analyses of the potential benefits of this work (Lesko, 2007), although as Jewkes (2006) points out in her critique of the evaluative studies, defining 'youth participation' in the context of HIV and AIDS is itself a complex issue.

Obviously there are many different aspects of this work that need to be studied, critiqued and evaluated. As Gould (2007) in her report on culture and HIV and AIDS points out, it is not necessarily the messages *per se*, or even what has traditionally been regarded as behavior change that is the point, so much as the actual engagement and reflexivity process that is critical. In essence, this kind of approach might be regarded as a necessary precursor to behavior change. And while in single issue interventions it may be easier to determine indicators of success (e.g. a number of young people between the ages of 15–24 reporting using condoms; or a number of young people who report knowing their status), the indicators themselves (and means of testing) may not speak to the complexity of the issues. The afterlife is broader than just 'during' and immediately 'at the end of the project' types of evaluations and it is vital that we find ways of expanding the 'what difference does this make?' questions towards studies that extend into young adulthood.

In working to deepen an understanding of the long-range impact of this work, we are interested in identifying critical features of youth-focused visual and arts-based participatory work that need to be replicated or improved. It has been suggested, for example, that involving youth in the creation of new media (e.g. using the internet, photography, video and music production software) can promote community development, critical literacy, artistic expression, civic engagement and social activism (Flicker *et al.*, in press; Goodman, 2003; Mitchell, 2006b; Ross, 2001; Tyner, 2003; Tyner & Mokund, 2004). By encouraging creativity and personal expression, youth media projects may promote self-awareness, empathy and critical dialogue (UNESCO, 2005). By taking successful concrete actions towards improving their communities, youth, it is argued, can build their self-respect and confidence to cope with other life situations (Carroll *et al.*, 1999) while becoming better connected with their communities and cohorts (Bradley & Selby, 2004). Furthermore, engaging in community action projects has been found to foster positive relationships with caring adults (Camino, 2005; Mercier *et al.*, 2002) and allow marginalized youth who have few positive outlets to feel like they can make a positive difference (Harper & Carver, 1999). In projects with peer educators, an additional dimension is related to the nature of social activism and 'taking action' (Allen, 2004, 2005; Ebreo *et al.*, 2002). And in some of the recent interventions on masculinities, gender violence and HIV and AIDS, the significance of critical reflection is highlighted (Morrell & Makhaye, 2006). This is a feature of the *Soft Cover* project noted above and is also central to several projects underway by team members involving hip-hop, forum theatre, photo-voice and video production (Stuart & Mitchell, 2007). The extent to which it is the post-reflection process and the extent to which it is during the actual production (of the photographs or videos), which makes a difference, is an example of what could be explored through youth-focused self-study (see e.g. Childs, 2005; Stuart, 2006a). We are also interested in what kind of follow-up action takes place, particularly in the context of policy change? Finally, as we have found in our work on the gendering of HIV and AIDS, this work requires a careful gender and age lens which in and of itself opens up further questions about the differing impact of various interventions on girls and young women and boys and young men (Larkin *et al.*, 2007; Walsh & Mitchell, 2006). The various features point to the importance of a participatory and iterative process that offers young people themselves the opportunity to contribute to mapping out 'what makes a difference'.

The challenge is to develop systematic approaches to studying the long-term impact of our visual and arts-based participatory work with youth. Five domains that we have identified as starting points to this work include critical reflection, empathy, engagement, social activism and policy change. Critical reflection, one might argue, is a precursor to behavior change. Empathy we have seen is important particularly because of the impact of stigma on communities. And elsewhere we have begun to look at ways of studying engagement, using as a starting point the photographs taken of participants involved in activist projects by the research team itself (Pithouse & Mitchell, 2007). Social activism is key, so that the works in which young people are involved extend into their larger communities. Finally, policy change is the ultimate marker for larger project impact.

Towards a Framework for Evaluation: Studies of Policy Change

Here we focus on two of the projects that come out of photo-voice initiatives: the 'Feeling safe/not so safe' Project in Swaziland and the 'Friday Absenteeim' Project in an informal settlement north of Durban. While we are interested in the actual literacy skills of the children, we focus in particular on the ways in which the visual texts they produce might be examined within policy change.

'Feeling safe/not so safe' project: 'You can be raped in the toilets'

In the 'Feeling safe/feeling not so safe' project, 7th grade students in a school just outside of Mbabane in Swaziland participated in a photo-voice project where they were given disposable cameras and asked to photo-graph where they felt safe and not so safe. The one-day project, part of a larger study on participatory methodologies with youth for addressing issues of sexual abuse was carried out in three short stages: In stage 1, the 30 or so young people gathered in groups and were given a short explana-tion of the point of the project, which was to find out where they felt safe and not so safe in school – particularly in the context of sexual abuse. They were also given a short demonstration on the use of disposable cameras and were grouped with three or four others of the same sex. In stage 2, which lasted for approximately 40 minutes, they were free to go anywhere on the school premises to take photographs. Stage 3 was the 'looking at photographs' stage. The students gathered in small groups on the play-ground and were each given their envelopes of photographs to look at and to choose several that they wanted to write about on the back of the photographs.

In the process of the children viewing their photographs and developing captions for them, their teachers also had an opportunity to see what the children photographed. Many were surprised – not at the conditions of the toilets since obviously they knew that the doors were broken (Figure 10.1), but at the danger experienced and expressed so directly by the girls.

In relation to literacy skills, the children were engaging in meaning-making around the production of photo images. Because they were

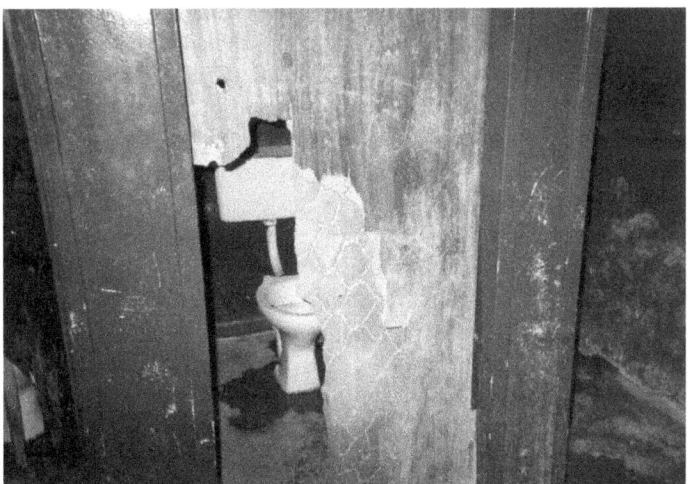

Figure 10.1 Broken doors on girls' toilets

working in small groups, they needed to collaborate and engage in dialogue, and because they were taking pictures at the school, they also had to negotiate with teachers and other students and obtain informed consent. After their photographs had been developed at the local one-hour photo shop in Mbabane, they worked directly with the photographs, selecting the ones they thought best addressed the issues of 'feeling strong' and 'feeling not so strong' and writing captions. In relation to policy, we learned that as a follow-up to this exercise, the school actually embarked upon the practice of monitoring the toilets. The pictures were critical to this. At a later point when these same photographs were shown to a Child Protection committee of UNICEF in New York, several people who were involved in developing policies on water and sanitation noted the importance developing programs and policies to monitor toilets in the context of gender-based violence and HIV and AIDS.

Friday Absenteeism Project

In this project, children from an informal settlement became involved in a photo-voice project which led to several policy changes in relation to food security and gender violence – both critically linked to HIV and AIDS (see also Mitchell *et al.*, 2005, 2006; Moletsane & Mitchell, 2007). A critical issue in the school was the fact that many of the children missed school on Fridays. The school is located in the Ilembe district, about 160 km inland and north of Durban and it serves a large number of children who live in informal settlements surrounding, but not adequately served by, a cluster of small factories and light industries (since these do not offer adequate employment opportunities to the majority of adults in the area). Instead, the usual problems of poverty, unemployment and high rates of HIV infection and illness abound in the community, and these contribute to the many interruptions to schooling as children miss classes for a variety of reasons related to these causes.

The principal and staff at the primary school and others in the area already knew why the children missed school: Friday was market day and many of the children in the senior primary grades, all 11, 12 or 13 year olds, were often called on to work in the market to earn money to at least provide for the basic nutritional needs of the families over the weekend. This is an important point since although there was a school feeding-scheme from Monday to Friday; no provision existed for help with food over the weekends. The principal was concerned because the learners could not afford to miss a day a week of school, and this behaviour sent a message to other learners, as well, that school was not important. However, finding effective strategies to address the problem remained a challenge. While there were a variety of approaches the principal and staff might have taken to address the problem (including doing nothing, given the range of curricular, administrative and social issues that confront school staff), the participation of the principal in a university module on cinematic and documentary texts was instrumental to his belief that working with the visual would yield transformative results among the learners, and possibly in the community as well (Mitchell *et al.*, 2006). From this understanding, he saw the potential for the young people to use photography not only to document the problems they faced, but also to identify and/or influence the development of strategies, within the school, the community, as well as in the government departments responsible for their well-being. So, through a photo-voice project, he involved his grade 6 class in analysing the problems and identifying possible solutions to this and others affecting the community.

The children's narratives in the photographs, posters and writing revealed a variety of issues. These included alcoholism among adults in the community, as captured in a caption to a photograph: 'If we look at these people who are living in this shack, they are drinking alcohol. They are not working. The schoolchild cannot survive in this condition'. Other issues they identified included high levels of unemployment, the need for housing, the lack of clean water and sanitation and the danger to children of even coming to school because they have to cross a wide highway that has no bridge over it. Most importantly, the photographs draw attention to the effects of poverty, and they provide visual evidence of why children as young as 11 or 12 must supplement the family income. Poverty also led to some of them having to miss school to take care of younger siblings. As a caption to one of the photographs, the students note: 'This photo shows us the rate of children who are absent from schools. These children are absent because they have to look after their baby sister or brother while their parents are working'. The photographs taken in the market not only showed images of the adults who run the market trying to make a living, but also showed the children's peers at work, so, very obviously, not at school. The children also took pictures of learners from nearby schools, demonstrating that Friday absenteeism was a widespread problem in the district. One particular photograph was of a boy who was working in the market to raise money for a school trip to Durban, which he could not otherwise afford: 'He absented himself from school because they had a trip to Durban. He decided to look for a part-time job because he needs the money. He has no parents'. The photographs and captions also reflected upon the conditions of the school itself. For example, one of the girls who was working in the market spoke about issues of safety and security in her classroom. Her teacher, she indicated, had been making sexual advances towards her. Being away from school on Fridays was an escape from this unwanted attention.

As with the Friday Absenteeism Project, the children were engaging in meaning-making as community photographers. Going beyond the scope of the 'one-day' project in Swaziland, their work extended from the preliminary discussions about school attendance, through to two photography fieldtrips during school hours, one to their own community in the informal settlement and the other to the market. When they returned to the classroom, they worked in small groups to create posters of their work, and it was these posters that were eventually presented to stakeholders in the community. Because the children were involved in every step of the process, the links between producing the visual images and taking action in the community contribute to the idea of the new literacy of AIDS noted above.

The rich insider data produced by the children in the project had major implications for policy development at school and community level. For example, from the data, the principal instituted disciplinary action against the teacher who allegedly was sexually harassing a female learner. He also raised the issue of absenteeism with other principals in the district, and planned for a community-based stakeholders' forum where the children were to present their posters. From this work, and because the school was registered as a not-for-profit company, he was able to approach donors and corporate funders and attract financial support for a feeding scheme for the weekends as well as during the week.

Discussion

Clearly, this work with the visual is not without its challenges, ranging from the costs of photo equipment and film development, the ethical issues of working with photo and video images, the limited access many of the young people in rural areas have to on-line sexual health information (Mitchell *et al.*, 2004; Mitchell & Reid-Walsh, 2007) and challenges in distributing their own images. However, as we write elsewhere (Weber & Mitchell, 2007), the widespread use of mobile phones has meant that young people are often very creative in how they are able to use the technology available. In a video-making project with young people, for example, in rural KwaZulu-Natal (Mitchell *et al.*, 2009; Weber & Mitchell, 2007), participants imported their own soundtrack into the production using their mobile phone. And, in other work with young people in

Nigeria (Mitchell & Sokoya, 2007), we saw the ways in which internet cafes are transforming digital access. Even in rural areas of South Africa a 'Spaza' shop (local convenience store) or a petrol station may have a set of terminals.

What was important in both projects was the involvement of the children, often the invisible stakeholders in schools and communities, as influential participants in social and political action. While we acknowledge that in the Friday Absenteeism Project the children's photographs and photo-stories enabled the principal, as the adult, to speak at a district meeting about the problems and issues, the fact that the children themselves produced documentary evidence made the stories authentic and, we argue, more useful for conceptualizing, developing and implementing interventions that work. As the various essays in *Putting People in the Picture* (De Lange *et al.*, 2007) document, critical engagement of young people and their teachers in addressing HIV and AIDS may be a way to combat AIDS fatigue.

The visual itself is important. We have ample evidence from journalism – from, for example the famous photograph of the Hector Pieterson from Soweto, 16 June 1976 – of the power of photographs to move people to action. This is an area that warrants further study but is clearly central to arts-based research more broadly as we see in the work of Knowles and Cole (2007) and many others. What is it about the girls' photograph of the empty and broken down toilet that moves the policy makers of the United Nation to add safety and security of toilets to their strategic plans?

Finally, we are interested in the ways in which visual arts-based tools such as photo-voice capture a 'through the eyes' of children and young people. As adults we may not see the world quite the same way. We were fascinated for example when the teachers and community health care workers took photographs of the challenges and solutions in addressing HIV and AIDS how many of their photographs 'demonized' young people, positioning them as being not very responsible in their 'jolling' [having a good time] and engaging in unprotected sex (Mitchell *et al.*, 2005). Interestingly, when we asked young people in the same schools to document through photo-voice some of the challenges and solutions in addressing stigma, in particular, in relation to HIV and AIDS it was clear that there is a lot of despair. One photograph even shows a group who stage a scene of a young boy hanging himself. We are not dismissing the comments of the teachers. Rather, we see that there is a need for more dialogue between these two scenarios – promiscuity and despair. It is worth noting that when the same group of young people were involved in making video documentaries – which could be on any topic they wanted – they chose to highlight gender-based violence (Mitchell *et al.*, 2009). In the scenarios they acted out, it was clear that a lot that goes on under the banner of 'jolling' and 'unprotected sex' is not necessarily consensual. It does appear, however, to be normalized – and perhaps that is the place to start in terms of policy issues around sexual health.

Why is sexual violence and coercive sex normalized? How do young people participate in the normalization of sexual violence, and how are the adults (teachers, parents and community health care workers) complicit? In other words, how could these images become the starting point for new policy dialogue? Beyond documenting policy change though even within these two projects, broader questions related to the participants themselves would be interesting to follow up: How for example did the children in the Friday Absenteeism Project regard the follow-up actions of the principal? How aware were they of their own participation in bringing about policy change? What difference might that awareness make to their own sense of efficacy, agency or future interest in political work? And, what difference might these shifts have in challenging the fatalism that make so many youth so vulnerable to HIV? While these are questions that run beyond more conventional notions of literacy, if the project is about saving lives, we regard them as ones that suggest critical alliances between those working within participatory methodologies and those working with the visual within multimodalities and multiliteracies frameworks.

Acknowledgments

We gratefully acknowledge the financial support of the Social Sciences and Humanities Research Council of Canada and the National Research Foundation (South Africa).

Notes

1. The term 'PhotoVoice' was patented by Caroline Wang (1999). Using a simple point shoot camera, participants themselves produce their own photo images, making visible their 'voice' around a particular social issue. A carefully considered prompt is provided to encourage participants to explore, through the lens of a camera, issues of concern. The created images themselves contain elements of social critique, which is further interrogated by eliciting responses about the photographs. Weber (2008) refers to such images as making visible the often difficult to access 'emic' points of view as well as lending credibility to it. The photographs created by the youthful participants are powerfully raising issues around safety, food security and attendance of school.
2. Participatory and collaborative video refers to a set of community-based film-making practices. In some cases participants, working alongside a filmmaker, are responsible for all aspects of the film-making process. In others, there are

various levels of participation (ranging from story-boarding through to the production of a rough cut, to participating as a member of a team led by the filmmaker to produce the film). Mak (2006) also refers to the participation of audiences as a type of participatory video.

References

Allen, L. (2004) 'Say everything': Exploring young people's suggestions for improving sexuality education. *Sex Education* 5, 389–404.

Allen, L. (2005) *Sexual Subjects: Young People, Sexuality and Education*. New York: Palgrave Macmillan.

Barton, D., Hamilton, M. and Ivancic, R. (2000) *Situated Literacies: Reading and Writing in Context*. Routledge: London and New York.

Bradley, B.S. and Selby, J. (2004) The 'Voices' project: Capacity building in community development for youth at risk. *Journal of Health Psychology* 9 (2), 197–212.

Buckingham, D. (2003) *Media Education: Literacy, Learning and Contemporary Culture*. London: Polity Press.

Buckingham, D. and Sefton-Green, J. (1994) *Cultural Studies Goes to School*. London and New York: Routledge.

Camino, L. (2005) Pitfalls and promising practices of youth–adult partnerships: An evaluator's reflections. *Journal of Community Psychology* 33 (1), 75–85.

Campbell, C. (2003) *'Letting Them Die': Why HIV/AIDS Prevention Programmes Fail*. Bloomington: Indiana University Press.

Carroll, G.B., Hébert, D.M.C. and Roy, J.M. (1999) Youth strategies in violence prevention. *Journal of Adolescent Health* 25, 7–13.

Centre Pompidou (2007) Evaluating the impact of the arts and culture education on children and young people. A European and International Research Symposium, 10–12 January. On WWW at http://www.centrepompidou.fr/Pompidou/Pedagogie.nsf/Docs/IDD9E5FCOE.

Childs, K. (2005) Self-study in working with youth. In C. Mitchell and S. Weber (eds) *Just Who Do We Think We Are? Methodologies for Autobiography and Self Study in Education*. London and New York: Routledge Falmer.

Cole, A., Knowles, G. and Luciano, T. (eds) (2004) *Provoked by Art: Theorizing Arts-informed Research*. Halifax, NS: Backalong Books.

De Lange, N., Mitchell, C. and Stuart, J. (eds) (2007) *Putting People in the Picture*. Amsterdram: Sense.

Ebreo, A., Feist-Price, S., Siewe, Y. and Zimmerman, R.S. (2002) Effects of peer education on the peer educators in a school-based HIV prevention program: Where should peer education research go from here? *Health Education and Behavior* 29 (4), 411–423.

Epstein, H. (2007) *The Invisible Cure: Africa, the West and the Fight against AIDS*. New York: Viking.

Flicker, S., Maley, O., Ridgeley, A., Biscope, S., Lombardo, C. and Skinner, H. (in press) e-PAR: A model for engaging youth in health promotion. *Journal of Action Research*.

Ford, N., Oddalo, D. and Chorlton, R. (2003) Communication from a human rights perspective. Responding to the HIV/AIDS pandemic in Eastern and Southern Africa. *Journal of Health Communication* 8, 519–612.

Goodman, S. (2003) *Teaching Youth Media: A Critical Guide to Literacy, Video Production and Social Change*. New York: Teachers College Press.

Gould, H. (2007) What's culture got to do with HIV/AIDS? *Findings, Health World Links*, 7, February. On WWW at www.healthlinks.org.uk

Harper, G. and Carver, L. (1999) 'Out-of-the-mainstream' youth as partners in collaborative research: Exploring the benefits and challenges. *Health Education and Behavior* 26 (2), 250–265.

Hoechsmann, M. and Low, B. (2008) *Reading Youth Writing: New Literacies, Cultural Studies and Education*: New York: Peter Lang.

Jewkes, R. (2006) Response to Pettifors *et al. AIDS* 20 (6), 952–953.

Kendrick, M., Jones, S., Mutonyi, H. and Norton, B. (2006) Multimodality and English education in Ugandan schools. *English Studies in Africa*, 49 (1), 94–114.

Knowles, G. and Cole, A. (2007) *Handbook of the Arts in Qualitative Research: Perspectives, Methodologies, Examples and Issues*. London: Sage.

Kress, G. (2003) *Literacy in New Media*. London and New York: Routledge.

Lankshear, C. and Knobel, M. (2003) *New Literacies*. London: Open University Press.

Larkin, J., Lombardo, C., Walker, L., Bahreini, R., Tharao, W., Mitchell, C. and Dubazane, N. (2007) Taking IT Global Xpress: Youth, Photovoice and HIV/AIDS. In N. de Lange, C. Mitchell and J. Stuart (eds) *Putting People in the Picture: Visual Methodologies for Social Change* (pp. 31–43). The Netherlands: Sense.

Lesko, N. (2007) Talking about sex: The discourse of loveLife peer educators in South Africa. *International Journal of Inclusive Education* 11 (4), 519–530.

Mak, M. (2006) Unwanted Images: Tackling Gender-Based Violence in South African Schools through Youth Artwork. In F. Leach and C. Mitchell (eds) *Combating Gender Violence in and Around Schools* (pp. 113–123). London: Trentham Books.

Mankell, H. (2004) *I Die, But the Memory Lives on: The World AIDS Crisis and the Memory Book Project*. London: The Harvill Press.

Martin, M. (2003) HIV/AIDS in South Africa: Can the visual arts make a difference? In K. Kauffman and D. Lindauer (eds) *AIDS and South Africa: The Social Expression of a Pandemic* (pp. 120–135). New York: Palgrave Macmillan.

Mercier, C., Piat, M., Peladeau, N. and Dagenais, C. (2002) An application of theory-driven evaluation to a drop-in youth centre. *Evaluation Review* 24 (1), 73–91.

Mitchell, C. (2006a) In My Life: Youth Stories and Poems on HIV/AIDS: Towards a new literacy in the age of AIDS. *Changing English* 13 (3), 355–368.

Mitchell, C. (2006b) Visual arts-based methodologies in research as social change. In T. Marcus (ed.) *Shifting the Boundaries of Knowledge*. Pietermaritzburg: UKZN Press.

Mitchell, C. (2009) Geographies of danger: School toilets in sub-saharan Africa. In O. Gershoern and B. Penner (eds) *Ladies and Gents* (pp. 62–24). Philadelphia: Temple University Press.

Mitchell, C., De Lange, N., Moletsane, L., Stuart, J. and Buthelezi, T. (2005) The face of HIV and AIDS in rural South Africa: A case for photo-voice. *Qualitative Research in Psycholog* 3 (2), 257–270.

Mitchell, C., De Lange, N., Moletsane, R., Stuart, J., Taylor, M., Buthelezi, T. and Walsh, S. (in press) Addressing gender violence in and around South African schools through participatory video. In F. Ogunleye (ed.) *The Video Book Project*. Swaziland: Academic Publishers.

Mitchell, C., Low, B. and Hoechsmann, M. (2006) Developing a webtool on arts-based and other participatory approaches to HIV and AIDS education. Report to Culture and HIV, UNESCO, Paris.

Mitchell, C., Moletsane, R., Stuart, J., Buthelezi, T. and De Lange, N. (2005) Taking pictures/taking action! Using Photo-voice Techniques with Children. *ChildrenFIRST* 9 (60), 27–31.

Mitchell, C., Moletsane, R., Stuart, J. and Nywanyana, C.B. (2006) Why we don't go to school onFridays: Youth participation and HIV and AIDS. *McGill Journal of Education* 41 (3), 267–82.

Mitchell, C. and Reid-Walsh, J. (2007) Culture and digital technologies in the age of AIDS. In S. Weber and S. Dixon (eds) *Growing up on Line* (pp. 195–210). New York: Palgrave Macmillan.

Mitchell, C., Reid-Walsh, J. and Pithouse, K. (2004) 'And what are you reading, Miss? Oh, it is only a website'. Digital technology as a South African teen's guide to HIV/AIDS. *Convergence* 10 (1), 191–202.

Mitchell, C. and Smith, A. (2003) Sick of AIDS: Literacy and the meaning of life for South African youth. *Culture, Health & Sexuality* 5 (6), 513–522.

Mitchell, C. and Sokoya, G. (2007) New girl (and boy) at the internet café: Digital divides, digital futures. In S. Weber and S. Dixon (eds) *Growing up on Line* (pp. 211–225). New York: Palgrave Macmillan.

Mitchell, C., Walsh, S. and Moletsane, R. (2006) 'Speaking for ourselves: A case for visual arts-based and other participatory methodologies in working with young people to address sexual violence'. In F. Leach and C. Mitchell (eds) *Combating Gender Violence in and Around Schools*. London: Trentham Books.

Moletsane, R., De Lange, N., Mitchell, C., Stuart, J., Buthelezi, T. and Taylor, M. (2007) Photo-voice as a tool for analysis and activism in response to HIV and AIDS stigmatization in a rural KwaZulu-Natal school. *Journal of Child and Adolescent Mental Health* 19 (1), 19–28.

Moletsane, R. and Mitchell, C. (2007) On working with a single photograph. In N. De Lange, C. Mitchell, and J. Stuart (eds) *Putting People in the Picture: Visual Methodologies for Social Change* (pp. 131–140). Amsterdam: Sense.

Morrell, R. and Makhaye, G. (2006) Working not blaming: Masculinity work with young African men in KwaZulu-Natal. In F. Leach and C. Mitchell (eds) *Combating Gender Violence in and Around Schools* (pp. 153–162). London: Trentham.

Newfield, D. and Maundegzo, R. (2006) Mobilizing and modalising poetry in a Soweto classroom. *English Studies in Africa* 49 (1), 48–71.

Norris, G., Mbokasi, T., Rorke, F., Goba, S. and Mitchell, C. (2007) Where do we start? Using collage to explore very young adolescents' knowledge about HIV and AIDS in 4 senior primary classrooms in KwaZulu-Natal. *International Journal of Inclusive Education* 11 (4), 481–499.

Pattman, R. (2006) Making pupils the resources and promoting gender equality in HIV/AIDS. *Journal of Education* 38, 89–116.

Pettifors, A., Rees, H., Kleinschmidt, I. and Steffenson, A. (2005) Young people's sexual health in South Africa HIV prevalence and sexual behaviour. *AIDS* 19, 1523–1534.

Pithouse, K. and Mitchell, C. (2007) Looking at looking. In N. de Lange, C. Mitchell and J. Stuart (eds) *Putting People in the Picture*. Amsterdam: Sense.

Reproductive Health Research Unit (2007) *Reproductive Health and HIV Research Unit National Youth Survey*. RHRU: Johannesbug.

Ross, J. (2001) *Youth Making Media, Making Movies: A Report from NAMAC's Online Salon.* San Francisco, CA: National Alliance for Media Arts and Culture.

Stein, P. and Newfield, D. (2006) Multiliteracies and multimodality in English in education in Africa: Mapping the Terrain. *English Studies in Africa* 49 (1), 1–22.

Stuart, J. (2004) Media matters – producing a culture of compassion in the age of AIDS. *English Quarterly* 36 (2), 3–5.

Stuart, J. (2006a) From our frames: Exploring with teachers the pedagogic possibilities of a visual arts-based approach to HIV and AIDS. Unpublished doctoral dissertation, University of KwaZulu-Natal.

Stuart, J. (2006b) From our frames: Exploring with teachers the pedagogic possibilities of a visual arts-based approach to HIV and AIDS. *Journal of Education* 38 (3), 67–88.

Stuart, J. and Mitchell, C. (2007) Where are the youth in faculties of education? Preservice teachers as cultural producers in addressing HIV and AIDS. *Fourteenth International Teaching and Learning Conference*, Wits University, Johannesburg, 26–29 June.

Stuart, J., Mitchell, C., De Lange, N., Moletsane, R., Buthelezi, T. and Taylor, M. (2007) Participatory video in addressing HIV and AIDS in a rural community: A methodology for dialogue? *Third South African AIDS Conference* Durban, 5–8 June.

Tyner, K. (2003) *Mapping the Field: Knowledge Network Focuses on Youth Media.* San Francisco, CA: National Alliance for Media Arts and Culture.

Tyner, K. and Mokund, R. (2004) Mapping the field: A survey of youth media organizations in the United States. In K. Tyner (ed.) *A Closer Look: Media Arts 2003 Case Studies from NAMAC's Youth Media Initiative.* San Francisco, CA: National Alliance for Media Arts and Culture.

UNAIDS (2006) Report on the global HIV/AIDS epidemic: Executive Summary. On WWW at http: data.unaids.org/pub/Global Report/2006.

UNESCO (2005) *Learning to Live, Living to Learn: Perspectives on Arts Education in Canada* (Preliminary Report on Consultations conducted by the Canadian Commission for UNESCO) (p. 50). Ottawa, ON: UNESCO.

Walsh, S. and Mitchell, C. (2006) 'I'm too young to die' Danger, desire and masculinity in the neighbourhood. *Gender and Development* 14 (1), 57–68.

Wang, C. (1999) Photovoice: A participatory action research strategy applied to women's health. *Journal of Women's Health* 8 (2), 185–192.

Weber, S. (2008) Visual images in research. In J.G. Knowles and A.L. Cole (eds) *Handbook of the Arts in Qualitative Research* (pp. 41–53). Thousand Oaks, CA: Sage.

Weber, S. and Mitchell, C. (2007) Imaging, keyboarding and posting identities: Young people and new media technologies. In D. Buckingham (ed.) *Youth, Identity and Digital Media* (pp. 25–48). Cambridge, MA: MIT Press.

Chapter 11
Articulations of Knowing: NGOs and HIV-Positive Health in India

MARK FINN and SRIKANT SARANGI

Introduction

Health promotion practices in the so-called new public health of the late 20th and early 21st centuries have different dimensions, couched as they are in discourses of prevention, risk management, quality of life and healthy lifestyles, for example. In the development of a concern for public health and its social determinants, the emergent central figure and target of various health promotion efforts is the responsible and self-managing 'knowing' individual. Mainly, health promotion and prevention measures are targeted at the 'healthy' individual, with non-government organiza-tions (NGOs) around the globe coming to play a significant role in the promotion of health and health prevention agendas. Some NGOs have taken up the position to address these issues from the perspective of the disadvantaged and the 'unhealthy'; that is, those who are suffering from a chronic and incurable condition such as HIV. Our overall interest in this chapter lies with how HIV-related NGOs in India can frame the experi-ence of HIV-positive people in 'positive' terms and as a demonstration of a regulative 'empowerment' that has become a main aim of global health intervention and health promotion campaigns in low- and middle-income countries. As Petersen (1997: 196) points out, in fulfilment of the World Health Organization's (WHO) goal of 'Health for All', health promoters (and here we include HIV-related NGOs) are 'helping to forge a new conception of the political and see themselves as closely allied with the new social movements in their concern to "empower" citizens'.

In particular, we empirically and critically explore the operations of 'enabling knowledge' and 'empowerment' as inter-related key elements

233

in promotions of (HIV) health and as twin technologies of neoliberal subjectivity and its (self) management. In light of perceived limitations to do with targeting the individual as the mere *object* of information, an 'empowerment' approach to HIV prevention and the promotion of a 'positive' quality of life for people living with HIV and AIDS (PLHA) can be seen as being favoured in Indian HIV-NGO accounts as a more productive way of assembling the individual as the *subject* of knowledge and effecting behaviour. These accounts are accomplished through a privileging of certain types of language of discourse. As we illustrate, an important aspect of health promotion among the NGOs participating in our study is one that we suggest involves the apparent distinction between an 'information-based choice' that may not always lead to changed and preferred behaviour, and a 'knowledge-based decision' upon which the subject of neoliberally fashioned notions of 'health' and health promotion is more likely to act and self-manage.

We move on to provide a brief background to neoliberal political ideology and the governance of the 'healthy' subject. We situate the particular technologies of 'enabling knowledge' and 'empowerment' as elements of a transnational, neoliberal discourse of knowledge about health and as covert but powerful forms of rule in the global promotion of public health. In the analysis section that follows the methodological and theoretical framing, we illustrate ways in which HIV-related NGOs in India can deploy the discourse of empowerment and discuss the implications of associated ways of 'knowing' in relation to the HIV-'positive' subject in India.

Theoretical Framings

The 'healthy' and the 'knowing' neoliberal subject

Along with the medico-ethical privileging of patient perspectives and 'patient-centred' outcomes from the late 1940s, Sullivan (2003) notes that patients moved from being simply understood as unknowing bodies to be healed to being regarded as people with autonomy, values, self-awareness and the capacity for choice in relation to their health and well-being (cf. Armstrong *et al.*, 2007; Petersen & Bunton, 1997). Propped up by humanist psychological sciences that were at the same time prescribing the ideals of psychological health and a worthy life as involving autonomy, self-actualization, self-fulfilment and a sense of freedom (Rose, 1985), the 'knowing' and rational subject of the health professions became increasingly individualized in the years following World War II and was credited with significant responsibility for health outcomes (Sullivan, 2003). People in general were encouraged to maximize themselves through a complete-ness of physical and mental 'health' that was thought to be discoverable through acts of choice and result in an overall quality of life (cf. Rapley, 2003; Rose, 1990). As such, medical culture and the psychological sciences have been theorized as having a vital role in the forging of identity in the name of health (Crawford, 1994; Lupton, 1994).

Having (re)endowed the individual with liberal-humanist capacities for self-awareness, independence and free choice, however, particular political problems came to the fore in terms of how the 'healthy' and self-knowing subject is to be effectively, but covertly, governed in a liberal age of ostensible autonomy and freedom. In being ascribed the ability to know and effect one's own health, and choose from available health options, self-knowledge and a capacity for choice were themselves to become principles of rule (Osborne, 1997; Rose, 1990, 1999), even though power to choose and access to choice are unevenly distributed in a given societal context.

Drawing on Foucault's (1978) thesis of the relationship between knowl-edge and power (his theory of 'governmentality'), critical theorists (e.g. Osborne, 1997; Rose & Miller, 1992) argue that the solution to the problem of liberal governance lies with a 'neoliberal' style of governing that 'advances' liberal principles of rule. According to Foucault (1978), since the 18th century liberal governance involved techniques and procedures for directing individual conduct that presupposed the 'freedom' of the governed. In effect, exploiting a presupposed 'freedom' as a form of rule, subtle forms of discipline were mobilized so that individuals would responsibly 'know' themselves in prescribed ways and thus self-regulate through making suitable choices for health (among other things) with government agencies (and in our case, non-governmental agencies) being seen to operate from a distance.

In developing a liberal form of rule that exploits assumed freedom so as to be seen to govern from a distance, from the 1970s in Europe and America *neo*liberalism as a politico-economic philosophy began to operationalize a 'politics of lifestyle' wherein various programmes, procedures and tech-nologies of the self are assembled as the means by which we routinely understand and manage ourselves (Rose, 1999; Rose & Miller, 1992). From this time, governing 'from a distance' began to explicitly involve the creation of a demand for holistic forms of 'health' and 'quality of life' that people would 'freely' enact on themselves while effectively self-managing with the help of experts. This was (and remains) a notion of health and well-being not predicated exclusively on the absence of disease and illness but on correct conduct, healthy lifestyles and individual 'rights' and 'freedoms'. By creating a demand for an all-inclusive health, which equates with well-being, the individual is fashioned and regulated according to ways in which one is obliged to act on oneself and improve their lives in the name of health. As Osborne (1997) suggests, a neoliberal rationality for global socio-economic reform recognizes the indeterminacy and abstractness of the 'absolute health' ideal and instead opts for determinant strategies, targets and specifics that are cost-effective in having the 'responsible' and 'knowing' individual take control of one's health and thus reduce dependency on state health and welfare services.

In being mutually constructed by government and the 'psy-complex' (Rose, 1985), 'empowerment' can be understood as one determining strategy and target for an otherwise indeterminate health. By the 1980s, 'empowerment' came to stand as a measure and display of comprehensive health and warrant its responsible pursuit (Finn & Sarangi, 2008; Powers, 2003). Aligned with the advent of advanced liberalism and the global discourse of empowerment that accompanies it, was the ascendancy and active involvement of NGOs in international moves to improve international health standards and inequalities (alongside other concerns such as human rights and world poverty).

NGOs and empowerment

In a 21st-century 'bottom-up' approach to neoliberal socio-economic development, NGOs have been theorized, and critiqued, as principal agents of change in acting as mediators between government bodies, health agencies and local communities (Kamat, 2004; Mercer, 2002; Sharma, 2006; Townsend *et al.*, 2004). As agents of change in a mediatory role, NGOs the world over remain crucial arms of small government in their provision of various empowerment programmes. In this they can be seen as being pivotal to a neoliberal order wherein the interests of society are thought to be ideally served through the self-regulation and empowerment of 'knowing' individuals, particularly those deemed to be 'at risk' or 'risky' (Kamat, 2004). NGOs are in this way an act of empowerment, so to speak, with governments 'empowering' NGOs through various means (e.g. via capacity building, training and supervision), and NGOs, in turn, are working at ground level to 'empower' targeted individuals and communities to overcome risk and move towards health and prescribed forms of well-being.

In the global fight against HIV and AIDS, the various health care and advocacy services provided by NGOs have become particularly prominent from the 1990s (see Finn & Sarangi, 2008). Targeting 'risky' health behaviour and aiming to provide solutions to health and wider socio-economic problems, from the late 1990s in particular, Indian HIV-related NGOs have been working to increase awareness of HIV issues and disseminate information in a widespread promotion of responsible conduct and healthy lifestyle. As Sharma (2006) notes in her account of a state-initiated empowerment programme for rural women in India, empowerment agendas that are being framed and articulated by Indian NGOs resemble the neoliberal agenda of self-rule and self-care against the downsizing of state responsibility. By virtue of the policies laid out by international health and aid organizations such as WHO and UNAIDS, a transnational discourse of health, along with the knowledge, practice and decisions that accompany it, filters into the policies and practices of NGOs the world over. In the Asia-Pacific region, for example, the United Nations global development network actively works with affiliated NGOs to empower and support PLHA to take a more active role in fighting HIV/AIDS and associated stigma. This includes the provision of online and consultancy support for the establishment and running of positive speakers' bureaus as one such empowering strategy (see Finn & Sarangi, 2009). Alongside Sharma (2006), who theorizes empowerment projects in India as tying disenfranchised populations into western neoliberal aspirations and ways of living, other scholars have argued that moves to fashion the responsibilized 'empowered' individual serve to produce and regulate compliant subject positions and forms of health (Holt & Stephenson, 2006; Lupton, 1994) while glossing over cultural diversity (Finn & Sarangi, 2008; Powers, 2003).

What we focus on in our analysis of Indian NGO talk is the ways in which NGOs, as the 'knowers' of good health and the techniques necessary to procure it, can construe 'enabling knowledge' and its 'empowering' properties as not so much emanating from information-based choice but a knowledge that is based on personal decision and more likely to change behaviour. In doing so, we attend to how a 'knowledge-based decision' approach to health and empowerment can be seen to intensify the regulative effects of neoliberal ideology by summoning the knowing, decision-making subject to know itself, and be known, as one who thoroughly consumes politically conducive notions of 'empowered' health and life.

Methodology and Analytical Perspective

Our analysis draws on data consisting of 19 one-to-one interviews with male and female workers from HIV/AIDS-related NGOs that have been operating in metropolitan and/or rural areas in India generally from the late 1990s. Participants were recruited from internet sites (e.g. the Indian AIDS Forum) and through networking in India. The client bases of the NGOs, and thus the people spoken of in the extracts presented, are working and middle-class people living with HIV in rural and city areas. This includes 'high-risk' groups such as women, truckers, commercial sex workers, migrant labourers and 'men who have sex with men'. Services offered by the NGOs included primary health care, education, advocacy, counselling, HIV testing, home-based care, and the training of HIV health and medical professionals. All participating NGOs shared the common goals of promoting awareness of HIV/AIDS and related issues such as stigma and discrimination, and developing access to services that aim to ensure the well-being and 'empowerment' of PLHA.

Interviews were conducted between 2003 and 2005 by a researcher based in a British university. With the one exception of an American ex-patriot who was permanently residing in India, all interviewees were Indian. English was chosen as the language to conduct the interviews in because the interviewer did not speak any Indian language. Given that English is the lingua franca, all participants spoke English with confidence and to a good standard. In no interview was communication or understanding between interviewer and interviewee impeded from either's point of view. Interviews were generally one hour in duration and were loosely structured as far as interviewer-initiated questions were concerned. This allowed the interviews to proceed according to what was important for participants without imposing pre-conceived areas of significance.

Discussion usually centred on the aims and work practices of the NGO in relation to HIV prevention. This was in particular relation to their HIV and community health care and support programmes, health promotion and risk management strategies, HIV-related policy and legislation, capacity building, HIV-related stigma and discrimination, and human rights. Specific questions were typically about the effectiveness of local programmes and initiatives; governmental/state and global efforts in relation to HIV prevention and care; the challenges of working with particular groups and communities; medical treatment and practices; the involvement of PLHA in support initiatives and policy recommendations; women's issues; funding issues; the socio-cultural conditions of stigma and discrimination in India; HIV-related quality of life and media representations of HIV/AIDS in India.

The analytical premise we adopt is that discourses as sets of systematic statements for making objects, 'realities' and experiences known do more than simply describe 'realities' but actively produce various forms of knowledge, subject positions and power relations (Foucault, 1972, 1977; Henriques *et al.*, 1998). The term 'discourse analysis' covers a broad spectrum of language-oriented approaches that, generally speaking, are concerned with the analysis of talk, text and other signifying practices. Our focus in what follows is not on the linguistic, rhetorical or micro specificities of the accounts but on the global or 'macro' aspects underlying such accounts. In this, we seek to ascertain ways in which emergent discursive constructions and patterns and variation of meaning in the data worked to constitute certain kinds of knowledge (or 'regimes of truth'; Foucault, 1977) and subjectivities (ways of being), particularly in relation to health prevention, HIV-positive health, empowerment and associated quality of life.

Thus, in our discourse analytic approach, we take discourses as not operating independently from their social, cultural or historical conditions of emergence or from wider ideologies. Within this theoretical framing, we understand the 'self' as non-unitary, discursively constituted and deeply enmeshed in contemporary political practices and moral values (Henriques *et al.*, 1998). In our analysis, we are also concerned with the 'power relations' (or capillaries of power) that are evoked and played out in the deployment of various discourses and the various knowledges and identities they generate. By 'power relations' we are referring not merely to domination and repression, but to the productions of ostensible 'truth' in configurations of knowledge and the normalizing and disciplinary effects that underpin such knowledge. In this, we are drawing on Foucault's (1977) understanding of the 'knowledge–power' axis wherein 'power' refers to any 'reality' and 'truth' that is supporting (and supported by) types of knowledge and where knowledge and power thus both directly imply one another. In other words, knowledge linked to productive power and the generation of 'reality' comes to assume the guise and authority of 'truth'.

As Fairclough (2000) points out, the ongoing project of neoliberalism is primarily one of language and discourse where discursive and power-inducing narratives of progress, labour flexibility, risk and empowerment, for example, work to actualize new forms of knowledge, production, social relations, identities and values. The discursive structuring of the diversified neoliberal order, he suggests, produces a particular knowledge–power that configures social problems as problems for individuals. Thus in a 'truth-making' system of inter-lacing knowledge and power that is worked up and legitimized by neoliberal discourses, 'welfare dependency' is re-framed as individual deficiency, 'flexibility' is construed as individual virtue and 'risk' is made 'real' as individual choice and responsibility.

Behaviour Change and the Inadequacy of Information

In the following sections that explore NGO talk of enhancing a thorough-going knowledge of health among the people they work with, our central concern is for ways in which the HIV-positive individual is made responsible for themselves within a neoliberal fashioning of productive and 'positive' health, as commonly constructed across the interviews. We begin our analysis by exemplifying the way in which the NGO workers interviewed can commonly articulate the perceived inadequacy of health promotional information that aims to merely promote awareness of HIV and risk.

As a response to HIV and AIDS, participating NGO workers commonly spoke of, and relied on, prevention programmes that aim to promote behaviour change among PLHA and so-called vulnerable populations such as sex workers, truckers, drug users, youths in slums and 'men who have sex with men', for example. This kind of approach, fixated on notions of risk and behaviour change, is the driving force of many international programmes for HIV prevention (Aggleton, 2005). One of the ways in which the NGO workers accounted for their attempt to effect behaviour change was by promoting general awareness of HIV/AIDS and associated 'truths' and risks through the provision of information. Consider the following two extracts where workers from two NGOs talk about health intervention and promotion among 'vulnerable' groups and the wider communities being worked with. These two extracts come from the lengthy opening phase of the interviews where the interviewees are talking about the work of the NGOs they are involved with.

Extract 1[1]

I think, see as far as HIV is concerned you can say now that the awareness level is okay. It's good actually, at least everyone knows what is HIV and AIDS. They know there is no cure, they know, ah, okay, at least this information everyone knows, whether they are rural or city at least they know this.

Extract 2

[I]ntervention is creating awareness among the vulnerable and marginalized population groups, make them to perceive the risk perception. Promote safer sex initiatives and provide STD treatment and referrals, main thing, condom promotion, counselling [...] Our task is to see that we have a change to take place in Andhra Pradesh (name of state) among these vulnerable and marginalized populations. That is our overall goal, how to bring behaviour change.

In these extracts, disseminating information about the existence and facts of HIV, and how to prevent it, is framed as one basis for intervention. In Extract 1, the success of intervention efforts is measured by the level of community awareness of HIV and AIDS. By providing information and promoting general awareness, the condition for behaviour change is thought to be created or at least aimed for (Extract 2). Merely heightening the awareness is presumed to serve the primary goal of behaviour change among vulnerable groups, that is, those deemed to be 'backward', ignorant and therefore most in need of intervention by way of information (Nettleton, 1997). As talked up in these examples, the information-induced behaviour change approach can be seen to involve the implicit assumption that the association between information as input and attitudinal and/or behaviour change as output is straightforward (Aggleton, 2005). In the following extracts, however, this presumption is problematized by other HIV-NGO workers where a perceived gap between information (Extract 3), or information-based knowledge (Extract 4), and behaviour change is identified. Respondents are here talking about how they perceive the effectiveness of their (across social class) health intervention programmes. Again, Extracts 3 and 4 are taken from general and non-directed introductory talk about an NGO which in both cases involves the discussion of behaviour change strategies.

Extract 3

The thing is, when people have a lot of information they are able to make choices about what they do. But you would be surprised at how many people know what HIV is and they still go out and are risky [...] These are educated people and they say I didn't think it was a serious thing.

Extract 4

Knowledge is very high, but why in behaviour is there no change? Why then the knowledge is so high we expected that they may not at least go, or even among those that were involved in multi-partner sexual behaviour, at least they will be using condoms, but it was a surprise that knowledge did not match with behaviour [...] So we thought 'Fine, we got the message', so we transferred to behaviour.

Extract 5

There's a lot of social change that has to happen, a lot of attitudinal change has to happen because I really believe that unless a person changes in his or her heart nothing else will happen. You can have a lot of laws and reforms and lecturing but nothing is going to happen unless the person decides for himself that this is what I'm going to do and I'm going to change the way I think about this issue.

Here the limits of NGO efforts to raise awareness of HIV and AIDS are acknowledged as individuals can still indulge in risky behaviour despite their access to a rich information base. That information-based knowledge (or factual knowledge) does not 'match with behaviour change' is in Extract 4 framed as a surprise finding. For these NGO workers, mere information (or information-based, factual knowledge) is perceived to be ineffective in bringing about HIV prevention and behaviour change inasmuch as informed individuals can 'surprisingly' maintain risky behaviour contrary to the information they are given and the knowing this is assumed to impart. In other words, information is seen to present people with a range of choices but not necessarily to ensure the preferred one. In Extract 3, the mere provision of choice is perceived as superficial and likely to fuel irrational risk-taking even among the allegedly educated. For this reason, the speakers of Extracts 4 and 5 deploy a health promotion discourse in which focus is transferred from providing factual knowledge (e.g. about risk and condom use) to targeting, and changing, actual behaviour. It is behaviour itself that is to be targeted if health and HIV prevention are to be guaranteed, with behaviour change made conditional on personal decision rather than the mere provision of choice.

As illustrated by these extracts, beyond mere information that does not necessarily bring about behaviour change, an individual's capacity to correctly decide and act on the information provided is held up as being crucial. Indeed, central to behaviour change models and health promotion discourse is the self-managing individual who is exhorted to take responsibility for his or her own life satisfaction and well-being through making healthy lifestyle decisions and maintaining them (see Jones, 1997, and Lupton, 1999, in relation to HIV/AIDS). It is 'empowerment' as one such motivation and technology for the making of healthy lifestyle decisions and the self-management of these decisions that we go on to explore.

Enabling Knowledge as Empowering

In the following extracts, health promotion and behaviour change are described as operating not along the problematic 'information-choice' axis, as we have highlighted it, but rather along the lines of enabling knowledge and decision. The extracts are taken from the same interview as that of Extract 3 above (Extract 6) and from a further interview with another NGO worker (Extract 7). Both speakers are talking about NGO programmes of behaviour intervention in terms of an 'empowerment' approach that is geared towards enabling PLHA and vulnerable groups to make and sustain 'right' and personally owned decisions.

Extract 6

Interviewer: It (peer education programmes) must be quite a difficult thing to monitor.

Interviewee: Very very difficult but no, it's very nice also. What has happened now is it has become a people's movement […] It's an empowerment model […] We thought we should give them right knowledge. So we should work on the right knowledge, give them as much as possible. Give them knowledge on disease, give them knowledge on sex and sexuality, give them knowledge on legal issues, give them knowledge on rights so all these groups (such as commercial sex workers, truckers and youths in slums) are empowered with knowledge […] So when the knowledge on health came they started perceiving how it's important to have quality of life. How quality of life is important for their future. Then you see behaviour change […] See it should not stop with the test result getting into the hands of the user. It should be more than that. He or she should be able to make decisions in their life to decide on the quality of life in future. So all these things will be focused on (their) future.

Extract 7

Interviewer: What are the things that impact most on quality of life?

Interviewee: Quality of life? What I understand is a person who gets first diagnosed with HIV getting information then and there will definitely have a good quality of life because he has got better information (for) changing behaviour. Like if he's smoking or drinking. Like a lot of things, eating in time, taking medication in time […] So simple just to explain. It all helps quality of life as well as

always enforcing them how they can have safe sex so
they can enjoy the sexual life and don't transmit the
infection to others and don't get re-infection so they
can have a healthy life and a healthy sex life and liberty
[…] So you have to explain to people what is right,
what is wrong. Everybody will do the right one,
nobody will choose the bad one […] They get more
hope, their life changes […] Then they get empowered,
self-esteem (is) developed so quality of life is improved
[…] So I feel these are the things initially we can give
them so they can start monitoring themselves.

On the one hand, the speaker of Extract 6 presents herself as the provider
of straightforward health information but she also positions herself as the
benevolent provider of a 'better' information, which means information
beyond the narrow confines of HIV/AIDS to include life circumstances
more generally. What also contributes to a 'better' information is the moral
distinction between what is ostensibly 'right' and 'wrong'. There is also an
implicit sense here that in making information 'better' by assigning it clear
moral weight, information is transformed into an enabling *knowledge* that
induces the (across social class) psychologized subject to subscribe to techniques of self-empowerment wherein 'bad' choices will potentially not be
made. In this, an enabling knowledge is made the province of the rational,
moral and self-monitoring decision-maker, as is clear from Extract 6.

In both extracts, an all-inclusive 'right' knowledge is constructed as
that which is stocked up and not free floating, as something that 'empowers' people by bringing the importance of having a 'quality of life' into
view and as that which ideally leads to the making of positive decisions
that supports this vision. As opposed to being purely information-based
choice (although this is also an element of empowerment as described
here), the particular 'knowing' articulated in the above extracts is infused
with the power of enablement. As such, the conduct of vulnerable groups
and HIV-positive individuals is held up to be more thoroughly directed by
the affordance of a maximally grounded knowledge that does more than
present options and guarantee little (as in 'information-based choice')
but as that which effectively directs behaviour through the process of a
decision-making that can enhance self-esteem, change lives and alter
perception. In Extract 6, in particular, decision-making amounts to being a
kind of future-oriented responsible act. In this process of making decisions –
the 'more than' just providing people with information about their health
status – the 'empowered' individual is constituted as a rational and

responsible agent who can properly (or at least potentially) act on information and 'monitor' themselves. As Aggleton (2005) notes, empowerment models of health promotion focus on an individual's ability to see clearly and take control through developing skills of communication and negotiation, and by exploring possibilities for self-growth and change (cf. Holt & Stephenson, 2006; Lupton, 1994; Powers, 2003).

Importantly, the invocation of a 'quality of life' in these extracts serves to prop up an enticing 'empowerment' and can be seen as legitimizing a decision to change behaviour and opt for health. Submission to moralized and enabling knowledge is talked up as bringing into focus a vision of a quality of life that both reinforces and potentially sustains the very knowledge and decision that reveals it. Here the productive power of 'enabling knowledge' is associated with a certain transparency, one that brings a 'quality' future and a particular perception of life and 'self' into view as opposed to the opaqueness of mere information that is disassociated from the production of the knowing and visionary, and thus pliable, subject. In these excerpts, an empowering knowledge can be seen to serve a disciplinary function in that it enjoins the self-determining, knowing subject to a 'right' and moralized knowledge and a particular regime of health while justifying this enjoinment as being essential for one's freedom and future. A 'quality of life' that is made to invoke and confirm a knowledge of health can be seen to weigh health as non-ambiguous, positive and alluring, and thus lend it added force as a technology for self-management (see Finn & Sarangi, 2008). As Crawford (1994) understands it, 'health' operates as a key organizing technology for the good, moral and responsible self, and a 'knowledge-based-decision' approach to the promotion of health, as illustrated here, can be seen as a crucial aspect of this.

In the following section, we further explore what kind of subjectivity is being produced and promoted through the uptake of the power infusing 'knowledge-based-decision' strategy for health promotion and behavioural change.

Configurations of Empowered Subjectivity

In the next extract taken from an interview with another NGO worker who is himself HIV-positive and a self-professed 'empowered' individual, the theme of empowerment is elaborated on. The people specifically spoken of in this extract are PLHA from poor socio-economic backgrounds and thus generally under-resourced. As one who sees himself as self-empowered, this speaker is able to position himself as the 'knowing' agent of change by perceiving others as less 'positive' and capacitated and therefore in need of empowerment. The extract comes from a response to the researcher's question about the practice of some support agencies merely giving out rations and money to PLHA in need.

Extract 8

> Let them (PLHA) know what HIV is exactly. Let them know how to speak actually. If you are able to educate yourself and know the issues then you can work and do some like creative income generation. That's the thing, I don't (like seeing) people sitting idle because I'm seeing people who are living five or six years and they are dying. Since they found out they are HIV positive they just go to the NGO, collect something and come back and always they are feeling that they are sick actually and they go to the care centre and there they pass their lives. Two years and then they die. It is not a life actually. I don't want to go into that kind of life [...] I want to empower people, that is important actually. You can give people three thousand (rupees) a month. That is also not going to help, it makes (for) laziness [...] And always there is no positiveness. We have to develop some positiveness. I believe in empowerment, encouragement, (the) possibility of people fighting for their rights [...] We want to encourage them (PLHA) to learn something rather than depend on some support.

Again, correct and affirming knowledge (along with the ability to articulate it) is held up as being crucial for personal empowerment and for directing the lives and conduct of PLHA. Different from the information-based knowledge that is imparted to a more passive subject, here a knowledge that delineates and brings into view an altogether 'positive' quality of life is made the essence of an 'empowered' individual, one who learns how to articulate and act on this embodied knowledge. Overtly contrasted with this enabling knowledge is an ignorance and inactivity that allegedly lead to dependency, sickness and death. As the opposite of an ignorance that is aligned with weakness and a kind of non-life, 'enabling knowledge' is infused with its privilege and productive power. For this NGO worker, a provided for and self-taught 'enabling knowledge' has productive effect in terms of shaping a particular and morally preferred 'positive' subjectivity and lifestyle. The 'knowing' subject of empowerment is in essence constructed and idealized as independently self-sufficient, economically productive, politically aware (if not also active), optimistic and healthy. In this kind of knowing, the informed subject is at the same time being constituted and normalized according to the particular standards and truths that this way of knowing oneself marks out.

As illustrated in the following extract from talk about the importance of 'getting right information' (the same speaker as Extract 7), an empowered approach to life, which is being referred to here, incorporates a complete distancing from 'any sickness', one that relies on antiretroviral treatment and the construction of HIV as 'just a chronic disease'.

Extract 9

So basically what we are trying to do in our treatment of HIV positive people is like this. There are still many people who are not getting right information. People living with HIV are not getting right information ... Yes okay, therapy is not a cure but we can control the virus multiplication by lessening the viral load, improving the CD4 so the patient, people, can have a healthy life without any sickness and have a productive life. They can support their own treatment, they can support their own family [...] HIV is just a chronic disease and you can live a quality life.

A notion of 'quality life' that involves the absence of illness is clearly informed by functionalist conceptualizations of 'health' as the optimum capacity for the effective performance of socially (and politically) valued tasks, and illness as a deviation from social expectations and responsibilities (see Lupton, 1994, for discussion of Talcott Parsons and functionalism). In promoting the entrepreneurial life of income generation, self-sufficiency and activism, the principle of empowerment, as construed in these extracts, can be seen as being clearly linked to advanced liberalism and its privileging of the productive and autonomous subject (Finn & Sarangi, 2008; Powers, 2003; Rose, 1990, 1999). As illustrated in these not isolated examples from our data corpus, a neoliberal subjectivity is significantly configured according to the ways in which one is obliged to know and act on oneself in the name of complete health and its responsible pursuit.

Summary and Implications

The point that we have attempted to draw out from our analysis of the data and want to emphasize is that the strategy of 'information-based choice' as a way of inducing behaviour change can be perceived as being somewhat ineffective for a more thorough subjectification and regulation of the 'informed' risk-taking individual, and especially the newly diagnosed. With a 'knowledge-based-decision' strategy that functions as an alternative conduit for behaviour change, and as that which moreover provides an individual with the capacity to enact and sustain it, productive power can be located at the point at which the transnational neoliberal subject is conjoined to the constitutive and regulative enactments of rationality and responsibility. Tied up with this move away from the individual as being the mere *object* of information and irrational surveyor of choice to being the *subject* of rational decision-making, is not only the lure of good health but also the promise of a 'quality of life' that the empowered decision-maker is able to envisage and is equipped to settle on. This constitutive and disciplinary process can be interpreted as involving the responsibilized individual who, for the sake of health and freedom, is ideally obliged to consume 'right', life-affirming knowledge as a pathway to empowerment and a liberated life of quality. In highlighting ways in which a 'knowledge-based-decision' strategy is absorbed into neoliberal proliferations of 'free choice', we suggest that a form of health governance deploying such a strategy has significant implications for how the subject of health is regulated and compelled to adopt neoliberal norms of a healthy life.

As illustrated, the neoliberal promotion of 'enabling knowledge' as a vital empowerment measure in global health and social programmes can be seen to function as a circuit of knowledge and power, one that HIV-related NGOs in India can have an active role in. In this respect, our interpretation of the data lends support to existing research and commentary that associates NGOs across the world with the ideology and workings of neoliberal governance (Kamat, 2004; Sharma, 2006). We do not claim, however, that our sample is representative of all Indian NGOs working with HIV and AIDS. Nor do we intend to dismiss ways in which NGOs can provide the means for effective political mobilization and resistance, as others have argued (e.g. Sharma, 2006; Townsend *et al.*, 2004). What we can emphasize is that there are clear connections between participating NGOs and the health agendas of international health organizations such as WHO and UNAIDS, with participants supporting their neoliberal premises.

Generally speaking, there is an apparent mismatch between a western-centric neoliberalism and the inability of many PLHA in India – particularly women (Kohli *et al.*, 2005; Sharma, 2006) – to access health services, afford medication, remain economically self-sufficient and overcome stigma (see Elamon, 2005; Sarangi, 2007). For the HIV-positive subject to self-identify and know oneself as 'empowered' must, we contend, present significant difficulty in a country where the unknowability and unpredictability of HIV pathways are particularly acute (Kielmann *et al.*, 2005). Indeed, empowerment and a 'right' knowledge that demonstrates and compels it can be seen as working to downplay and devalue disadvantaged socio-economic circumstances and obscure the limits to what many PLHA in India (and elsewhere) may be capable of (Crossley, 1998; Holt & Stephenson, 2006).

The implications that can be drawn from the analysis presented here are that in thinking of ways of promoting health that do not perpetuate a normalizing and across-culture neoliberal order, it would be necessary to forgo presumptions of a lacking irrational subject who is deemed unable to choose 'healthy' options and to critically attend to the power effects of a 'knowledge-based-decision' approach to health promotion and care. As Fairclough (2000) argues, insofar as the neoliberal project is partly a language project, the challenge is very much a challenge of language. That is to say, struggles against neoliberalism and its relations of power can be significantly pursued in and through language. For Fairclough, attending to how language and discourse can figure in resistances to the neoliberal order and delineate plausible alternatives should be a coordinated effort of critical, and applied, language researchers. As such it would be necessary to address ways in which language, discourse and the communication of health could, on the one hand, work to formulate a resistance to global neoliberal ideology and policy, and on the other, promote culturally sensitive alternatives to ways in which 'health' and its promotion are being universally conceptualized, practiced and regulated.

Acknowledgments

This chapter derives from a Leverhulme Trust funded programme in 'Language and Global Communication' (Grant No. F/00 407/D, 2001–2006). We wish to thank the NGO workers who participated in this study and are grateful to Annabelle Mooney for collecting the data.

Note

1. In the extracts [...] indicates where part of a transcript has been omitted and brackets are used around added information.

References

Aggleton, P. (2005) HIV/AIDS: Lessons for and from health promotion. In A. Scriven and S. Garman (eds) *Promoting Health: Global Perspectives* (pp. 115–124). Hampshire: Palgrave Macmillan.

Armstrong, D., Lilford, R., Ogden, J. and Wessely, S. (2007) 'Health-related quality of life and the transformation of symptoms'. *Sociology of Health & Illness* 29 (4), 570–583.

Crawford, R. (1994) The boundaries of the self and the unhealthy other: Reflections on health, culture and AIDS. *Social Science & Medicine* 38 (10), 1347–1365.

Crossley, M.L. (1998) 'Sick role' or 'empowerment'? The ambiguities of life with an HIV positive diagnosis. *Sociology of Health & Illness* 20 (4), 507–531.

Elamon, J. (2005) A situational analysis of HIV/AIDS-related discrimination in Kerala, India. *AIDS Care* 17 (2), 141–151.

Fairclough, N. (2000) Language and neo-liberalism. *Discourse & Society* 11 (2), 147–148.

Finn, M. and Sarangi, S. (2008) Quality of life as a mode of governance: NGO talk of HIV 'positive' health in India. *Social Science & Medicine* 66, 1568–1578.

Finn, M. and Sarangi, S. (2009) Humanizing HIV/AIDS and its (re)stigmatising effects: Public 'positive' speaking in India. *Health: An Interdisciplinary Journal for the Social Study of Health, Illness and Medicine* 13 (1), 47–65.

Foucault, M. (1972) *The Archaeology of Knowledge and the Discourse on Language*. New York: Pantheon Books.

Foucault, M. (1977) *Discipline and Punish: The Birth of the Prison*. London: Penguin.

Foucault, M. (1978) Governmentality. In J.D. Faubion (ed.) *The Essential Works of Foucault 1954–1984* (Vol. 3, pp. 201–222). London: Penguin.

Henriques, J., Hollway, W., Urwin, C., Venn, C. and Walkerdine, V. (1998) *Changing the Subject: Psychology, Social Regulation and Subjectivity*. London: Routledge.

Holt, M. and Stephenson, N. (2006) Living with HIV and negotiating psychological discourse. *Health: An Interdisciplinary Journal for the Social Study of Health, Illness and Medicine* 10 (2), 211–231.

Jones, R.H. (1997) Marketing the damaged self: The construction of identity in advertisements directed towards people with HIV/AIDS. *Journal of Sociolinguistics* 1 (3), 393–418.

Kamat, S. (2004) The privatization of public interest: Theorizing NGO discourse in a neoliberal era. *Review of International Political Economy* 11 (1), 155–176.

Kielmann, K., Deshmukh, D., Deshpande, S., Datye, V., Porter, J. and Rangan, S. (2005) Managing uncertainty around HIV/AIDS in an urban setting: Private medical providers and their patients in Pune, India. *Social Science & Medicine* 61, 1540–1550.

Kohli, R.M., Sane, S., Kumar, K., Paranjape, R.S. and Mehendale, S.M. (2005) Assessment of quality of life among HIV-infected persons in Pune, India. *Quality of Life Research* 14, 1641–1647.

Lupton, D. (1994) *Medicine as Culture: Illness, Disease and the Body in Western Societies*. London: Sage.

Lupton, D. (1999) Archetypes of infection: People with HIV/AIDS in the Australian Press in the mid 1990s. *Sociology of Health & Illness* 21 (1), 37–53.

Mercer, C. (2002) NGOs, civil society and democratization: A critical review of the literature. *Progress in Developmental Studies* 2 (1), 5–22.

Nettleton, S. (1997) Governing the risky self: How to become healthy, wealthy and wise. In A. Petersen and R. Bunton (eds) *Foucault, Health and Medicine* (pp. 207–222). London: Routledge.

Osborne, T. (1997) Of health and statecraft. In A. Petersen and R. Bunton (eds) *Foucault, Health and Medicine* (pp.173–188). London: Routledge.

Petersen, A. (1997) Risk, governance and the new public health. In A. Petersen and R. Bunton (eds) *Foucault, Health and Medicine* (pp. 189–206). London: Routledge.

Petersen, A. and Bunton, R. (eds) (1997) *Foucault, Health and Medicine*. London: Routledge.

Powers, P. (2003) Empowerment as treatment and the role of health professionals. *Advances in Nursing Science* 26 (3), 227–237.

Rapley, M. (2003) *Quality of Life Research: A Critical Introduction.* London: Sage.

Rose, N. (1985) *The Psychological Complex.* London: Routledge.

Rose, N. (1990) *Governing the Soul: The Shaping of the Private Self.* London: Routledge.

Rose, N. (1999) *Powers of Freedom: Reframing Political Thought.* Cambridge: Cambridge University Press.

Rose, N. and Miller, P. (1992) Political power beyond the state: Problematics of Government. *British Journal of Sociology* 43 (2), 173–205.

Sarangi, S. (2007) The micropolitics of disclosure, stigma and (dis)trust surrounding HIV/AIDS in India. In I. Markova and A. Gillespie (eds) *Trust and Distrust: Sociocultural Perspectives* (pp. 153–177). Greenwich: Information Age Publishing.

Sharma, A. (2006) Crossbreeding institutions, breeding struggle: Womens' empowerment, neoliberal governmentality and state (re)formation in India. *Cultural Anthropology* 21 (1), 60–95.

Sullivan, M. (2003) The new subjective medicine: Taking the patient's point of view on health care and health. *Social Science & Medicine* 56, 1595–1604.

Townsend, J.G., Porter, G. and Mawdsley, E. (2004) Creating spaces of resistance: Development NGOs and their clients in Ghana, India and Mexico. *Antipode* 36, 871–889.

Chapter 12
Signs Show the Way: Reading HIV Prevention on the Andaman Islands

ANNABELLE MOONEY

Introduction

Finding a way of capturing success in HIV prevention appears to be as elusive as it is important. I suggest that close linguistic analysis of what appear to be unremarkable prevention signs, coupled with an understanding of the local context, may be a way of being precise about what is required. In the Port Blair region of Andaman India, we find a realization of what Sarangi and I have elsewhere called an 'ecological intervention' (2005); that is, an HIV intervention that seeks out root causes and manages these rather than managing HIV as such. Seeing prevention efforts in this way means that HIV is always symptomatic of these root causes. Without changing the causal conditions sustainable prevention is impossible. The starting point for the analysis in this chapter is prevention signs found in the Port Blair region. I suggest that a pragmatic and semantic reading of these signs tells us exactly which root causes need to be addressed.

Both signs are in a sense unremarkable. The first urges addressees to 'use condom, avoid HIV'. The second provides information on the three main routes of HIV transmission: unsafe sex, blood transfusions and intravenous drug use (IDU). They were both found in prominent public spaces, though attached to the outside of a hospital and a health clinic. These signs are worth spending time on. A close semantic–pragmatic analysis of the signs provides exactly the conditions that need to be in place for their messages to be understood and taken up. Further, there is evidence from interview and fieldwork data that these conditions are in place. Hence, I argue, the signs can be understood as indexing the resilient and robust social environment present in and around Port Blair.

In this context, I adopt C.S. Peirce's terminology in relation to his tripartite distinction between icon, index and sign. Peirce defines an index 'as a sign determined by its dynamic object by virtue of being in a real relation to it' (Peirce, 1977 [1904]: 33). If a prevention sign is an index, the object is the ecology of the community. It is this real, rather than iconic or arbitrary (symbolic), relationship that I want to draw attention to. The indexical relationship, in this sense, is one of 'real' connection. It seems to me that this connection is traceable in ways other than the strictly semiotic, in that 'An Index is a sign which refers to the Object that it denotes by virtue of being really affected by that Object' (Pierce, 1998 [1903]: 291–2). If the object alters, so in a sense will the index. Further, in the context of prevention signs, if the index (the sign) changes, this may also change the object. This understanding of the indexical relationship foregrounds an organic connection that is particularly appropriate to a discussion of root causes and the ecology of a community.

The argument that the prevention signs index a social situation is in many ways the logical corollary of the concept of ecological interventions. Given that,

> ... ecological interventions take account of issues such as gender empowerment, economic status, language issues and cultural positioning (whether a group is a stigmatized one, for example) ... [and] also work towards solutions that are possible with existing resources. (Mooney & Sarangi, 2005: 277)

It should be possible to find evidence of such an ecological intervention. One would expect to find little evidence of the root causes of HIV vulnerability (such as poverty and gender discrimination). One would also expect to see the 'existing resources' mobilized in ways that are appropriate to local needs. Evidence confirming exactly this is collected during a period of fieldwork in the Port Blair region (November 2004), which included semi-structured interviews with four NGOs working in the field of HIV prevention and sexual health education as well as with the State AIDS Control Organization. Three of the NGOs were identified by virtue of past funding by the National AIDS Control Organization (NACO) through information available on the national website at the time (October 2004). One further organization was identified through contact with the State AIDS Control Organization in Port Blair. The target populations that these groups work with include prisoners, commercial sex workers (CSW), fishermen, children, tribals and migrants. While none were being funded at the time, most continued their work in the field of HIV prevention and awareness education. The interviews sought to elicit information about the kind of work these organizations engaged in, the challenges faced, the methods of outreach and communication used, and their relationship with other stakeholders. The strategy was to start with low-risk information, with the aim of building rapport in the early stages of the interaction, before exploring the more difficult and sensitive areas related to the difficulties and challenges in communication and prevention, as particular to this part of India. The interview questions and probing strategies were designed to be as informal as possible with the particular group, in order to access the discourses and practices of the particular organizations, rather than a performance more suited to familiar yet formal footing often taken with funders and donors.

Because of the relationship between index and object, it is important to understand the field site. Port Blair is the capital of the Andaman Islands, a territory of India lying off the east coast of the mainland in the Bay of Bengal. The islands have a population of about 300,000, with a third of these living in the capital region. In Port Blair one finds the ruins of a cellular jail that was used by the British to incarcerate and punish Indian freedom fighters. In this way, the area is tied closely to concepts of Indian national identity. Indeed, British rule properly represents a second period of colonization for Andaman although it seems to have eclipsed the first, that is, people from the Indian subcontinent coming to occupy an area with existing indigenous populations. (The important issues, health and otherwise, of indigenous people on Andaman are not addressed here [see Kailash, 1997].) However, given the time and expense to travel to the region, as it is accessible only by air or a three-day boat trip, it is not a common destination for people living in India. While there is some tourism, this appears to be largely confined to specific resort areas, including small islands off the main island. There is some backpacking activity; however, this is normally done by those interested in wildlife or in 'roughing it'. All interviewees reported that the majority of the population in the area are employed by the government. This in itself results in high levels of affluence and, less directly, in gender equality, especially when compared to other semi-urban areas of India. This, as well as the cohesiveness of community that comes from living in relative isolation, may also assist in the low levels of HIV.

The levels of HIV in the area are remarkably low. Currently, according to official statistics, there are 37 cases in the region. Monitoring of HIV in India is undertaken at sentinel sites, where specific populations are tested for HIV. Hence, those tested in Andaman as a matter of course are women presenting at ante-natal clinics and patients attending STD clinics. In 2004, there were no cases among women presenting at ante-natal clinics, and only 1.6% of patients treated for STD tested positive. In 2005, the figures were 0.58% and 0.4%, respectively. It is important to see these claims in relation to other Indian states and in their particular context, if only because NGOs in mainland India insist that the levels are higher than government figures suggest.

In Tamil Nadu, a state widely acknowledged as having reacted quickly and well to the issue of HIV, the levels at sentinel sites are much higher. The prima facie reliability of Tamil Nadu figures is suggested by the inclusion of intravenous drug users and men who have sex with men (MSM) as relevant testing populations. Inclusion of the latter signals clearly that the state is aware of new (for the Indian context) vulnerable populations. For 2004, while ante-natal levels were low at 0.5%, 8.4% of patients presenting for STD treatment tested positive, as did 39.9% of people with a history of IDU and 6.8% of MSM. In the case of Andaman, there are other factors which suggest that the low figures are accurate. The presence of sentinel sites in the area is significant; these are by no means a given in the Indian or the global context. Neither is there a culture of denial about the existence of HIV at the state level (as is the case in many parts of the world; see Altman, 2006; Dyer *et al.*, 2004). The number of positive people also needs to be seen in a medical context; that is, Andaman provided antiretroviral therapy (ARVT) even before this was rolled out at a national level in India. Because of this, the number of positive cases is arguably higher than it would have been without ARVT exactly because positive people are living longer.

The official, and I suggest reliable, figures are clear signs of success with respect to HIV prevention. The cause of this success, I argue, can be retrieved from a close reading of the two prevention signs mentioned. That is, I am reading these signs as *symptoms* of success. I see them not so much as causal agents, which they also must be, but rather as indexical of a sound basis for the prevention of HIV, that is, a robust and resilient social environment. I argue that the relevant root causes for success can be isolated by means of a close pragmatic reading of the prevention texts found. This analysis is both textual and semiotic drawing on speech act theory and pragmatic understandings of language. The targeted way of identifying root causes means that rather than proposing an almost impossible social transformation into a near utopia, programs of social change can be constructed around particular, and possible, priorities. In short, this mode of analysis provides a way of replicating success with respect to prevention without ignoring local conditions. If nothing else, the signs suggest a way of mapping the success of Andaman.

First, however, I consider alternative explanations for the low levels of HIV in the region. Such explanations are linked to the absence of 'risk groups' as conceived in the official Indian context. This survey also provides some initial background about the socio-economic context of the area.

By the Book: 'Risk Groups'

One of the dominant discourses in India in relation to HIV prevention is that of risk group and risk behavior. It is possible to explain the low levels of HIV in Andaman in terms of the absence of risk groups, but I suggest that such analysis may not provide enough specific information about what is going well in the Port Blair region. Nevertheless, given the importance given to 'risk groups' in the Indian policy context, it would be remiss not to consider the area in such terms. The three risk groups identified and targeted in India are (1) CSW, (2) long-distance lorry drivers and (3) migrant workers (for a discussion of this, see Mooney & Sarangi, 2005).

If we begin with sex workers, unusually, in Andaman there are no red light areas where sex workers can be found. While none of my informants suggested that sex work did not take place, it was at far lower levels than in, for example, even the Westernized and affluent Bangalore. Ravi, from the NGO working with sex workers and their clients, explained the reasons for engaging in commercial sex work as follows:

> some people work some people just for money some people only for pleasures (.) most people have their jobs and poor peoples are doing for their daily [job] for their family (.) their family background family background is very poor. (Ravi: 17–19)

Working for money is hardly surprising; working for pleasure is. As will be seen later, 'clients' were often lexicalized as 'boyfriends'. While this may be explained in terms of patriarchy, the admission that women derive pleasure from sex was unusual. However, the very absence of any identifiable area where CSW could be found was unprecedented in my experience.

The small size of Andaman means that there are no lorry drivers of the kind included in the second risk group on the mainland. On the subcontinent, lorry drivers are *long-distance* lorry drivers and may be away from their wives and families for weeks at a time. Truck stops along lorry routes routinely serve as brothels and 'lodges' for CSW and clients. In Andaman, there is one trunk road that runs up the middle of the island (see http://www.andaman.org/ for a discussion of this, especially in relation to the indigenous Jarawa). Indeed, during fieldwork, local authorities had finally resolved not to close the road altogether, even though having it open is technically illegal as its closure was ordered in 2002. In relation to lorry drivers, however, as Dr Thulsi, head of the State AIDS Control Organization, explained,

But there is no highways here or anything (.) they close down their vehicle by 6 o'clock or 7 and goes home (.) so that problem is not there (,) now the hotels and that but still I don't find that much type of these things like in Mainland (.) like [there?] they are camping somewhere away from the home (.) so those type of drivers are mostly involved in the casual sex so that doesn't apply here. (Dr Thulsi: 208–212)

In relation to MSM, again, while no one denied that there must be some men who had sex with men, there was certainly no visible community or, what is more usual in India, cruising spots. As with CSW, this is not from a lack of space. While Andaman is small enough not to need long-distance lorry drivers, it is large enough for such cruising spots to be established if there was a sizable community.

The final risk group, migrants, is also minimal and tends to be seasonal. Port Blair does not have the attraction that Bangalore, Mumbai or Delhi have. Moreover, given the difficult journey from the mainland, 'migrants' are poachers from South East Asian countries, most usually Thailand and Myanmar (Burma). As such poaching is illegal, if caught, they are imprisoned. In prison, they are provided with good facilities, a doctor on call, and specific education about STDs and HIV from an NGO working specifically with the prison population.

While not usually recognized as a 'risk group', because of gender roles in relation to sexual activity, women are more vulnerable than men with respect to any STD. Thus gender empowerment and the education of women have often been noted as crucial in any national HIV campaign (Chaterjee, 2003; Go *et al.*, 2003; Laurance, 2007; Shrotri *et al.*, 2003). Again, in Andaman we find, if not paradise, at least something more equitable as regards gender than in many other states. Thus women work, even after marriage, and have some economic and social independence. As suggested above, this may be linked to their employment in prestigious government jobs. Children, boys and girls, attend school unless they do not wish to. Thus while informants admit that there must be child labor, it is not at levels found elsewhere in India. While it is apparent that a sound ecology will limit the emergence of women as a risk group, similar arguments can also be made for the three primary risk groups. At the very least, a sound social ecology will change the way in which CSW, migrants, lorry drivers and MSM live, such that the activities that make them vulnerable to HIV (which make them 'risk groups') will be altered.

Signs: Pointing in Another Direction

While the absence of risk groups as an explanation for low levels of HIV is a straightforward one, it seems to me that it is not wholly satisfying. If one accepts such an explanation, one also accepts at one level some inherent vulnerability connected to occupation, sexuality or displacement: identity profiles that are of a different order than viruses and blood. In short, risk groups, and even risk behavior, are only a partial answer. The microscopic level of the virus invites a microanalysis of the prevention signs in the area.

Because of the low levels of HIV in Andaman, it is possible to argue that preventative measures are being used by individuals. But in fact, this is only one argument that can be made or, at least, it can never be enough of an explanation. While the signs chosen for this chapter appear to speak to directly to 'surface' prevention behavior connected to HIV, in order for them to be understood and used, a number of other preconditions are required. To be clear, I am labeling 'surface' behavior as that which is proximate to the transmission of HIV. That is, imperatives to engage in safe sex, to avoid contaminated needles and so on can be understood as targeting surface behaviors. Such targeting is clearly not without merit or effect. However, as a great deal of research has shown, understanding and uptake of, as well as behavior modification because of, such messages are dependent on the personal resources available to potential addressees (see, e.g. Airhihenbuwa & Obregon, 2000). Among the factors that limit the deployment of such messages are gender, poverty, threats of violence, mistrust of addresser and lack of prophylactic resources (either material ones, such as condoms, or more general ones, such as access to medical treatment) (Amirkhanian *et al.*, 2004; Babalola, 2004; Blystad, 2004; Kapungwe, 2003; Kinsman *et al.*, 1999; Longfield *et al.*, 2004; Marston, 2004; Melkote *et al.*, 2000; Muyinda *et al.*, 2003; van Dam, 1989; Williams & Jones, 2004). In the following, I first turn to the presuppositions, entailments and lexical choices in the sign. I then turn to the important issues of education and trust, before touching on the significance of the use of English.

First sign

The primary point of health care delivery in Andaman is situated in Port Blair. The GB Pant hospital is the best equipped hospital on the island and is attended by all on the island for specialist care. It is situated adjacent to the cellular jail ruins, that is, a prison that appears to be structured according to Bentham's vision of the panopticon. While it is no longer

```
┌─────────────────────────┐
│      USE CONDOM          │
│                          │
│      AVOID HIV           │
└─────────────────────────┘
```

Figure 12.1 GB Pant hospital sign

used and is now a heritage site, it housed prisoners up until the 1930s. I will return to the siting of the hospital in my conclusion. The GB Pant hospital is also the site of the Andaman State AIDS Control Organization (ANACS). Each state in India has such an organization, which comes under the ultimate umbrella of NACO. ANACS is responsible for both the HIV prevention signs considered here.

Approaching the hospital, a neon sign is visible. 'Keep Andaman Polio Free' it urges. While the area has been officially polio free since 1999, the sign remains and immunization continues (publicized alongside the shipping news in the daily local paper). Slightly further on, visible from anywhere in the front of the hospital, is the following Figure 12.1.

Like the sign for polio, it is in neon letters, the font a simple sans serif, with no further embellishment. Both signs are blue neon against a white background. At the outset, it should be noted that neon signs are not prevalent on the island. Indeed, even street lighting is confined to areas with houses or businesses. I will return at the end of this section to the significance of the use of neon and of English; however, both can be read as appealing to discourses of progress, science and technology and hence objective reliability.

Presupposition, entailment and lexical choices

Perhaps the most basic aspect of this sign, but worth exploring nevertheless, is what is presupposed by the imperative and thus what we can read as being assumed knowledge on the part of the addressee. What a condom is and what 'using' it means are sophisticated pieces of knowledge (Elkins *et al.*, 1998). That addressees know what condoms are (if not how to use them) is also suggested by their obvious presence in paan shops and general petty shops (thus visible even to women). Thus one can assume that addressees also know where to purchase condoms. Another point to note, connected to condoms, is that the use of the lexeme itself suggests a socio-cultural entailment whereby condoms are trusted. Informant interviews in Bangalore provide anecdotal evidence that some people believe that condoms are central in the spread of HIV (see Bennell *et al.*, 2002). That is, there is a conspiracy theory that sees the West producing and distributing condoms that contain HIV and thus spread the virus.

If we accept that this sign is symptomatic of local knowledge, there is no place for such conspiracy theories. Such contrary meta-messages are labeled 'semiotic snares' by Adam who defines them as follows: 'A semiotic snare is a message where a well-understood but unspoken subtext undermines the overall thrust of the message' (Adam, 2006: 173). The absence of these snares is clear from the easy availability of condoms, and also from the way in which they are spoken about. A particularly nice exchange with an NGO working with the elusive Andaman sex workers went as follows:

Interviewer: So some CSW [commercial sex workers] were using [condoms]?

NGO: Yes – well, they are not using they are giving to their boyfriends [laughter] (lines 110–111).

I suggest that this demonstrates a sound understanding of the use of condoms purely from a content point of view, because of the disambiguation of the agent of 'using', but also because of the use of humor in relation to what is often a sensitive topic. In terms of snares, the informant's utterance could not have been produced without guile unless the condom conspiracy theory has no local adherence.

The imperative 'Use Condom, Avoid HIV' also presupposes the existence of HIV and thus assumes that addressees know what this is. Again, this is far from universal knowledge in India or indeed elsewhere in the world. This is an important point and will be explored in some comparative detail. First, the choice of 'avoid' in the sign is worth exploring. I suggest that 'avoid' signals that HIV is conceived of as a concrete entity that will be encountered on the journey of life (to stay with cognitive metaphors of this kind) (Lakoff & Johnson, 1980). That is, the usual collocation is that one is told to 'stop' or, more usually, 'prevent' HIV. The former suggests finality, a stopping of some thing (noun), while the latter conveys the forestalling of some event (verb). The collocation actually used, 'avoid', suggests a persistent obstacle to be avoided, and as such is an excellent message as it conveys object and action in one utterance.[1]

Knowledge and cultural models

The kind of knowledge that resides in structuring metaphors and that is gathered in other ways requires separate treatment. However, new information is more salient when it fits in with existing cognitive structures and metaphors. The absence of information about HIV and its transmission may be linked to exposure or to cultural models (Farmer, 1994). What is clear is that levels of knowledge about HIV are often low. Chatterjee reports

that 33% of married women in Mumbai (Bombay) are 'at risk of not knowing about AIDS' (Chatterjee, 1999: 139), even though incidence and prevalence continue to be high in this area. While estimates range from 1% (for
ante-natal patients) to 10% (for STD patients) (www.nacoonline.org/facts_
statewise.htm), among CSW the levels were thought to be over 50% in 2000
(Salunke et al., 1998). Importantly, in Chatterjee's study, the lack of awareness about HIV was not related to media exposure, but rather to years of
schooling (Chatterjee, 1999: 139). Tamil Nadu, widely considered to have
had a successful awareness raising campaign, also lacks complete coverage
in terms of knowledge of HIV/AIDS. Kattumuri reports that 'knowledge
of HIV/AIDS transmission was inadequate even among patients in
hospitals' (Kattumuri, 2003: 558), with patients viewing their HIV as a
'temporary illness' (2003: 554). As for another Indian study, again 'education was the most important predictor' of knowledge about HIV (Chaterjee,
2003: 558; see also Shrotri et al., 2003). I suggest that situating education as
a 'predictor' of HIV knowledge is a case of correlation rather than causation. However, in Andaman at least, HIV and sex education is given from
primary school; in 2004, 94% of this target population had been reached.[2]
Naturally, in such cases, an argument of causation could be made.
Nevertheless, the question of whether education represents cause or corre-
late is important. While education is a good starting place, it is not the only
intervention required. While it is a predictor, 'education' covers (and
perhaps obscures) a wide range of variables.

For an intervention to be successful, in the formal educational system
or otherwise, there has to be a robust communicative and interactive
frame. We can infer something about this from the materiality of the neon
sign. That is, the permanence, and relative expense, of neon suggests that
the addressers are reasonably confident of any shared knowledge. This
confidence is well founded, if only from the low levels of HIV. Neon can
also be read as alluding to technology and progress, and thus in turn to
objective and authoritative modes of medical science. The use of English
can be interpreted in these ways too. Further, as the sign is on a hospital,
the neon also suggests the medical technology available at this institution.
The materiality of the sign can therefore be read as reassuring, in terms of
the quality of knowledge communicated and the technological resources
available.

The relative expense may also account for the form of the message
syntactically: it is framed as an elliptical conditional, that is, the full version
is 'If you use a condom, you will avoid HIV'. When framed in the 'full'
version, the form bears a resemblance to the speech acts of warning or
threats. I do not want to argue that the message is a threat; however, in

some contexts, or rather communicative climates, it is possible to see how prevention messages could be read as something like a threat.[3] I see this as tied directly to the issue of access to and trust of medical services, which will be mentioned below. While different in their effects, there are common features shared by threats and related speech acts such as promises and warnings. I suggest that the sign's imperative can be read as a multivalent speech act in that the addresser/addressee relationship will determine how it is received (see Shon, 2005). Obviously it is intended as information (thus satisfying elements associated with warning and advising speech acts), but given the benefit to the speaker and the hearer, it falls somewhere in between (for features of the speech acts used here, see Fraser, 1998; Storey, 1995).

Relationships of trust

The issue of the addressee's relationship to the addresser is perhaps most crucial in the context of health warnings. The issue of trust here is central (see Sarangi, 2006). In Andaman, the position of government hospitals is unusual in that people are happy to attend them. As one informant put it,

> well I don't, I can't tell about people in mainland, or government in mainland – can't do that – but as far as Andaman is concerned we don't have any complaints regarding health and these things. (171–182)

The contrast made with the mainland is telling. I read the reluctance to talk about the mainland as indicating some awareness that Andaman is different in not having 'any complaints'. Certainly, fieldwork in south India suggests that trust in government health services, particularly in relation to HIV, is not always so high.

The trust in government health services in Andaman was widely attested. While it may not be enough to rely on those working in government institutions for testimony as to trust, such responses were not only commonplace but consistent among the NGOs and members of the public encountered during fieldwork. During fieldwork, many medical professionals and school teachers made a point of taking me aside and praising Dr Thulsi and outlining the specific ways in which he assists. While I have met a great number of dedicated and expert professionals in India, such unsolicited praise was unprecedented for a government official. More generally, government representatives and their institutions were seen as safe and accessible sources of information, care and advice.

Trust is often gained, at least in part, by using an appropriate language variety and register. Thus, much effort is spent in finding local terms and discourses for health campaigns. The difficulties encountered in these projects are well known and need not be discussed here. However, as the language choice of English is often understood as working against both the establishment of trust and the reception of messages, the use of English here is worth exploring.

Significantly, English is the official language in Andaman. Moreover, high levels of literacy in Andaman (77% as compared to the national 59.5%) suggest that there will also be at least some familiarity with written English. While strictly speaking English is the language of the colonizer, there is no single regional language as inhabitants of Andaman come from all Indian states. Thus, while Hindi is also used, English is more prevalent both officially and informally and rated positively (http://andamandt. nic.in; Agnihotri, 2007: 196). With respect to the national context, Agnihotri reports that at the very least 'Urban Indians generally have highly positive attitudes towards English' (2007: 195). However, he notes that 'English retains its colonial color and continues to be associated with the elite . . .' (2007: 196). At the same time, 'Indian English is a variety in its own right' (2007: 195).[4]

In order to come to terms with the 'color' of English in Andaman, we need to consider the domains of English and the presence of other Western cultural and commercial products. This is also because of the idea that the use of English in health prevention may, at best, undermine the efficacy of the message or, at worst, lead to complete rejection of the message. Certainly research suggests that local languages should be used in HIV education (see Bhaskaran & Rao, 2003; Cornwall, 2002; Hira *et al.*, 2005; McGlynn & Martin, 2009). In the Andaman signs, the use of English appears to signal the incorporation of Western medicalized models of HIV. It is exactly this incorporation that is often problematic, because these medical discourses bring with them cultural and epistemological baggage that may work against prevention messages. Because of this, and especially because of the prominence of some areas of India (Banaglore in particular) in globalization narratives, it is worth charting the flow of English language currents into Andaman. I suggest that such contamination is more likely to take place where there are negative attitudes towards material and cultural flows from the West.

Unlike most urban (and indeed semi-urban) areas of the mainland, the presence of Western food, drink and entertainment products appears to be low. To take the ubiquitous example of Coca-Cola, this was not encountered at all. No doubt it was present, as were other Western products, most notably Western brand cigarettes and the ubiquitous Nescafé; however, the level of advertising of these was such that its relative absence was recorded several times in field notes. That is to say, one of the central (and perhaps one of the few) global flows to touch Andaman is a medicalized Western discourse. Given that this will not be 'contaminated' by other less desirable flows, English apparently does not experience the challenges that it may experience elsewhere. This doubtless is related to levels of education and, in the context of health care at least, the overriding trust in government services. Indeed, such trust reclaims medical discourses in a manner analogous to re-localization or re-embedding (Giddens, 1990).

While it is important to note what is in the sign, as in the case of advertising of Western products, absences are also telling. Unusual for the Indian context, as we shall see more in the discussion of the second sign, is the absence of anything signaling relationships. Both signs, in part at least safe sex messages, provide no context about what kind of sex is involved, that is, whether it is between married people, MSM or CSW. Indeed, its presence in a public space also suggests that intended addressees are both male and female, of various ages and relationship status.

Second sign

The second sign was situated in a rural hospital/clinic located across the water from Port Blair. Although on the same island, the most efficient way of getting there was by boat. Here, the message is presented without any context of personal relationships (which is often seen as undesirable in an Indian context; Bhaskaran & Rao, 2003: 13). The 1,2,3 message is also in stark contrast to a more common (especially in USAID funded projects) ABC approach (abstinence, be faithful, condomize). The complete lack of moral message, the removal of bodies and the provision of decontextualized, autonomous, information are all noteworthy. The words in parenthesis indicate a picture. The general alignment of text has been retained (Figure 12.2).

This sign is structured in a number of ways that contribute to understanding and action. The three main causes of HIV are provided in terms of relative risk in this region (which has low levels of IDU). More importantly, each risk is elaborated and remedial action is given (Shuy, 1990). Addressees do not have to infer the danger or an avoidance strategy. It is also worth noting the detail provided in (1), that is, that unprotected sex *with an infected partner* is the risk to be avoided. While this is perhaps obvious, the preoccupation with promiscuity can tend to suggest that simply having multiple partners is in itself a risk.

This sign is clearly a warning in Fraser's and Shuy's terms (Fraser, 1998; Shuy, 1993: 98). The warning genre is a well-established one in the Port

Preventing AIDS is as simple as counting		
1. [condom]	2. [blood bag]	3. [needle]
Unprotected sex with an infected partner.	Transfusion of infected blood and blood products.	Use of contaminated needles and syringes.
Stay away from multiple sex or use condoms.	Insist on HIV free blood.	Use sterilized or disposable needles and syringes.

Figure 12.2 Clinic prevention sign

Blair region. Apart from the common postings to wear a helmet on motorcycles, there were also large billboards urging people to stay away from drugs. This was illustrated with pictures of alcoholic drinks, cigarettes and a large skull and crossbones (Figure 12.3).

This message was fortified with the practice of dry days twice a month. That is, there is prohibition on alcohol sales (alcohol belonging to the drug category) on the 7th and 31st of each month, the main pay days in the region. This was a local law, respected and appreciated, and largely intended for the well-being of women and families. The presence of other signs in the warning mode tells us at the very least that HIV prevention

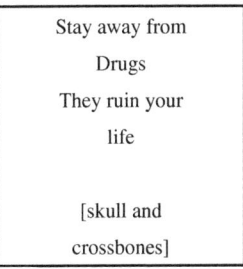

Figure 12.3 Roadside sign

messages conform to an already recognized genre. Adam points out that 'to be effective ... the [HIV] prevention message calls on an autobiograph-ical narrative that life is worth living, and that something done now makes sense because the future will be a desirable place in which to arrive' (Adam, 2006: 172). Further, 'Risk, responsibility, and subjectivity all reside inside cultural frameworks that evolve over time and shift with the communication networks that carry them' (Adam, 2006: 176). Thus, the presence of the drug warning suggests that culturally (at least locally) this positive view of the future (a frame of sorts) is established (see Beine, 2003; Farmer, 1994). The ecology is sound.

Conclusion

In Andaman, one finds little evidence of the root causes of HIV. Education and literacy are at good levels, and there is scant evidence of gender discrimination, exploitation or extreme poverty. Evidence on the ground matches up with evidence retrieved from linguistic analysis of the prevention signs. The presuppositions and entailments, the socio-pragmatic knowledge, and the cultural models needed to make sense of the signs point towards what is required for a meaningful uptake of preven-tion messages. Analysis of the signs reveals that the following are required for proper understanding: detailed knowledge about condom purchase and use, knowledge of HIV itself as something to be consistently avoided, a relationship of trust between health providers and the community, and a cultural framework that allows warnings to be interpreted as information rather than threats. The signs, being framed and presented as they are, also index the presence of these things. It is a recursive relationship: the rela-tionship between index and object. To argue that the prevention signs index success in relation to HIV prevention, that they are symptoms of success, is perhaps to suggest that the addresser and addressee share a language. This is no small thing. Further, the trust relationship that has been built up over the years is a resource that should not be underestimated.

Pointing out the importance of shared language, models and values is not perhaps new. The argument that a number of fundamental and far-reaching knowledge and practices have to be in place for prevention efforts to succeed is framed by Barnett and Whiteside in terms of socio-economic causes. They comment,

> [t]he problem is that even if people have the knowledge, they might not have the incentive or the power to change their behavior. If preven-tion is to move beyond knowledge to action, we must look at the

socio-economic causes of the epidemic and intervene there too. (Barnett & Whiteside, 2002: 42)

Socio-economic profiles are obviously causal factors in the spread and persistence of HIV. Changing these conditions, however, often involves a call for revolutionary action. We can only hope for utopia. Analyzing specific prevention messages in order to identify particular socio-economic changes is more targeted and specific and, because of that, more achievable. The reading conducted here also suggests the importance of a holistic, joined up approach. In an interview with the founder of Freedom Foundation, Ashok Rao, in Bangalore, he observed,

> you can't start something if you do not know how to finish it up somewhere down the line and I see that happening in a very large context whether it's in India or other developing countries where this prevention is something in isolation and then very grudgingly you say Ok care and support and you know but there's no proper linkages. (lines 93–96)

While Rao singles out developing nations, the argument is no less relevant for the developed world. Indeed, former colonial powers would do well to remember their past.

Upon seeing pictures of the jail I was determined to visit it to see a 'real panopticon', even one like Port Blair's cellular jail, which was in partial ruin. As Bentham ([1787], 1995) tells us, and Foucault develops in a more abstract way ([1975], 1977), the panopticon functions as a way of explaining societies of control. It seems to me that we can also interpret the concept of the panopticon in a positive sense. Rather than the punitive surveillance of the other, it is possible to recuperate it as promoting a positive regard for and awareness of self and others, a shared language and communication, and action based on trust. Rather than the panopticon being oppressive, it may be possible to use it as a concept to develop a positive social contract. While the cellular jail was in ruins, it was still possible to reconstruct its basic form. The architecture of the absolutely symmetrical original was clear from what remained. In the same way, the symmetrical relationship necessary between addressee and addresser of the signs (the conditions necessary to prevent HIV) are retrievable through linguistic analysis of the signs. If the signs, as symptoms of success, allow us to access in a detailed and schematic way the ecological conditions necessary, this may provide the architecture with which to build other positive panopticons. The author of the signs, ANACS, is sited in the GB Pant hospital. The hospital's location, in the shadow of the concrete panopticon's ruins, invites us to undertake exactly such a subversive reading.

Notes

1. WebAsCorpus.org reveals that 'avoid' and 'avoiding' have the lowest number of collocations with HIV (58,700), while 'stop' and 'stopping' occur about three times as much (156,000) and 'prevent' and 'preventing' occur nearly 20 times more frequently than 'avoid' and its variants (1,148,000).
2. From an interview with Dr Thulsi, line 317.
3. However, for a recent discussion of the utility of fear-based campaigns, see Green and Witte (2006), O'Grady (2006) and Kirby (2006).
4. In this vein, it is also worth considering whether any redemptive effects have occurred in the wake of Indian post-colonial literature, a great deal of which is written in English.

References

Adam, B.D. (2006) Infectious behavior: Imputing subjectivity to HIV transmission. *Social Theory and Health* 4, 168–179.
Agnihotri, R.K. (2007) Identity and multilinguality: The case of India. In A.B.M. Tsui and J.W. Tollefson (eds) *Language Policy, Culture, and Identity in Asian Contexts* (pp. 185–204). London: Lawrence Erlbaum.
Airhihenbuwa, C.O. and Obregon, R. (2000) A critical assessment of theories/models used in health communication for HIV/AIDS. *Journal of Health Communication* 5 (suppl), 5–15.
Altman, D. (2006) Taboos and denial in government responses. *International Affairs* 82 (2), 257–268.
Amirkhanian, Y.A., Antonova, R., Csepe, P., Gyukits, G., Kabakchieva, E., Kelly, J.A., Mihaylov, A. and Seal, D.W. (2004) Gender roles and HIV sexual risk vulnerability of Roma (Gypsies) men and women in Bulgaria and Hungary: An ethnographic study. *AIDS Care* 16 (2), 231–245.
Babalola, S. (2004) Perceived peer behavior and the timing of sexual debut in Rwanda: A survival analysis of youth data. *Journal of Youth and Adolescence* 33 (4), 353–363.
Barnett, T. and Whiteside, A. (2002) *AIDS in the Twenty-first Century: Disease and Globalization*. Basingstoke: Palgrave.
Beine, D.K. (2003) *Ensnared by AIDS: Cultural contexts of HIV/AIDS in Nepal.* Kathmandu, Nepal: Mandala Book Point.
Bennell, P., Hyde, K. and Swainson, N. (2002) The impact of the HIV/AIDS epidemic on the education sector in Sub-Saharan Africa: A synthesis of the findings and recommendations of three country studies, February 2002. Centre for International Education, University of Sussex Institute of Education. On WWW at http://www.sussex.ac.uk/education/documents/aidssynpublished.pdf. Accessed 7.9.2007.
Bentham, J. ([1787], 1995) *Panopticon.* In M. Bozovic (ed.) *The Panopticon Writings* (pp. 29–95). London: Verso.

Bhaskaran, N. and Rao, S. (2003) *Report of the TOT on Stepping Stones: A training Package on HIV/AIDS, Communication and Relationship Skills*. Bangalore: ICHAP and ActionAid India.

Blystad, A. (2004) On HIV, sex and respect: Local–global discourse encounters among the Datoga of Tanzania. *African Sociological Review/Revue Africaine de Sociologie* 8 (1), 47–66.

Chaterjee, P. (2003) Spreading the word about HIV/AIDS in India. *Lancet* 361, 1526–1527.

Cornwall, A. (2002) Body mapping: Bridging the gap between biomedical messages, popular knowledge and lived experience. In A. Cornwall and A. Wellbourn (eds) *Realizing Rights: Transforming Approaches to Sexual and Reproductive Well Being*. London: Zed books.

Dyer, G., Marcelo, R. and White, D. (2004) Poverty and denial: India is 'the ticking time-bomb of the Aids pandemic' ... while for Africa the worst is still not over. *Financial Times* 9 July, p. 15.

Elkins, D.B., Dole, L.R., Maticka-Tyndale, E. and Stam, K.R. (1998) Relaying the message of safer sex: Condom races for community-based skills training. *Health Education Research* 13 (3), 357–370.

Farmer, P. (1994) AIDS-talk and the constitution of cultural models. *Social Science and Medicine* 38 (6), 801–809.

Foucault, M. ([1975], 1977) *Discipline and Punish: The Birth of the Prison* (A. Sheridan, trans.). London: Allen Lane.

Fraser, B. (1998) Threatening revisited. *Forensic Linguistics* 5 (2), 159–173.

Giddens, A. (1990) *The Consequences of Modernity*. Cambridge: Polity Press.

Go, V.F., Sethulakshmi, J., Bentley, M.E., Sivaram, S., Srikrishnan, A.K., Solomon, S. and Celentano, D.D. (2003) When HIV-prevention messages and gender norms clash: The impact of domestic violence on women's HIV risk in slums of Chennai, India. *AIDS and Behavior* 7 (3), 263–272.

Green, E.C. and Witte, K. (2006) Can fear arousal in public health campaigns contribute to the decline of HIV prevalence? *Journal of Health Communication* 11, 245–259.

Hira, S., Khalil, S.N. and Rabia, M.W.R.M. (2005) Knowledge and attitudes towards HIV/STD among Indian adolescents. *International Journal of Adolescence and Youth* 12 (1/2), 149–168.

Kailash (1997) Human ecological stress and demographic decline: A case of Negritos of Andamans. *Indian Journal of Social Work* 58 (3), 382–402.

Kapungwe, A.K. (2003) Traditional cultural practices of imparting sex education and the fight against HIV/AIDS: The case of initiation ceremonies for girls in Zambia. *African Sociological Review/Revue Africaine de Sociologie* 7 (1), 35–52.

Kinsman, J., Harrison, S., Kengeya-Kayondo, J., Kanyesigye, E., Musoke, S. and Whitworth, J. (1999) Implications of a comprehensive AIDS education programme for schools in Masaka District, Uganda. *AIDS Care* 11 (5), 591–601.

Kirby, D. (2006) Can fear arousal in public health campaigns contribute to the decline of HIV prevalence? Commentary. *Journal of Health Communication* 11, 261–266.

Lakoff, G. and Johnson, M. (1980) *Metaphors We Live By*. Chicago: University of Chicago Press.

Laurance, W. (2007) Cursing condoms. *New Scientist* 1 September, p. 23.

Longfield, K., Glick, A., Waithaka, M. and Berman, J. (2004) Relationships between older men and younger women: Implications for STIs/HIV in Kenya. *Studies in Family Planning* 35 (2), 125–134.

Marston, C. (2004) Gendered communication among young people in Mexico: Implications for sexual health interventions. *Social Science & Medicine* 59 (3), 445–456.

McGlynn, C. and Martin, P.W. (2009) 'No Vernacular': Tensions in language choice in a sexual health lesson in The Gambia. *International Journal of Bilingual Education and Bilingualism* 12 (2), 123–136.

Melkote, S.R., Muppidi, S.R. and Goswami, D. (2000) Social and economic factors in an integrated behavioral and societal approach to communications in HIV/AIDS. *Journal of Health Communication* 5 (suppl), 17–27.

Mooney, A. and Sarangi, S. (2005) An ecological framing of HIV preventive intervention: A case study of non-government organizational work in the developing world. *Health* 9 (3), 275–296.

Muyinda, H., Nakuya, J., Pool, R. and Whitworth, J. (2003) Harnessing the Senga institution of adolescent sex education for the control of HIV and STDs in rural Uganda. *AIDS Care* 15 (2), 59–167.

O'Grady, M. (2006) Just inducing fear of HIV/AIDS is not just: Commentary. *Journal of Health Communication* 11, 261.

Peirce, C.S. (1977) *Semiotic and Significs: The Correspondence between Charles S. Peirce and Victoria Lady Welby*. In C.S. Hardwick and J. Cook (eds) Bloomington: Indiana University Press.

Peirce, C.S. (1998) A syllabus of certain topics of logic. In Peirce Edition Project (ed.) *The Essential Peirce. Selected Philosophical Writings* (Vol. 2, pp. 1893–1913). Bloomington and Indianapolis: Indiana University Press.

Salunke, S.R., Shaukat, M., Hira, S.K. and Jagtap, M.R. (1998) HIV/AIDS in India: a country responds to a challenge. *AIDS* 12 (Suppl B), S27–S31.

Sarangi, S. (2006) The micropolitics of disclosure, stigma and (dis)trust surrounding HIV/AIDS in India. In I. Markova (ed.) *Trust: Dynamic and Cultural Perspectives*. Greenwich: Information Age Publishing.

Shon, P.C.H. (2005) 'I'd grab the S-O-B by his hair and yank him out the window': The fraternal order of warnings and threats in police–citizen encounters. *Discourse and Society* 16 (6) 829–845.

Shrotri, A., Shankar, A.V., Sutar, S., Joshi, A., Suryawanshi, N., Pisal, H., Bharucha, K.E., Phadke, M.A., Bollinger, R.C. and Sastry, J. (2003) Awareness of HIV/AIDS and household environment of pregnant women in Pune, India. *International Journal of STD and AIDS* 14, 835–839.

Shuy, R. (1993) Threatening. In *Language Crimes: The Use and Abuse of Language Evidence in the Courtroom* (pp. 97–117). Cambridge, MA: Blackwell.

Shuy, R. (1990) Warning labels: Language, law and comprehensibility. *American Speech* 65 (4), 291–303.

Storey, K. (1995) The language of threats. *Forensic Linguistics* 2 (1), 74–80.

Van Dam, C.J. (1989) AIDS: Is health education the answer? *Health Policy and Planning* 4 (2), 141–147.

Williams, H.A. and Jones, C.O.H. (2004) A critical review of behavioral issues related to malaria control in Sub-Saharan Africa: What contributions have social scientists made? *Social Science & Medicine* 59 (3), 501–523.

Author Index

271

Subject Index

For Product Safety Concerns and Information please contact our EU Authorised Representative:

Easy Access System Europe

Mustamäe tee 50

10621 Tallinn

Estonia

gpsr.requests@easproject.com

www.ingramcontent.com/pod-product-compliance
Ingram Content Group UK Ltd.
Pitfield, Milton Keynes, MK11 3LW, UK
UKHW021843280426
5452IPUK00003B/35

*9 7 8 1 8 4 7 6 9 2 1 9 1 *